# BM

**Lam Library**
**in Otolaryngology**

## Landmark Papers in ... series

Titles in the series

*Landmark Papers in Otolaryngology*
Edited by John S. Phillips and Sally Erskine

*Landmark papers in Pain*
Edited by Paul Farquhar-Smith, Pierre Beaulieu, and Sian Jagger

*Landmark Papers in Neurology*
Edited by Martin R. Turner and Matthew C. Kiernan

*Landmark Papers in Rheumatology*
Edited by Richard A. Watts and David G. I. Scott

*Landmark Papers in Neurosurgery, Second Edition*
Edited by Reuben D. Johnson and Alexander L. Green

*Landmark Papers in Anaesthesia*
Edited by Nigel R. Webster and Helen F. Galley

*Landmark Papers in Nephrology*
Edited by John Feehally, Christopher McIntyre, and J. Stewart Cameron

*Landmark Papers in Allergy*
Edited by Aziz Sheikh, Thomas Platts-Mills, and Allison Worth, with Stephen Holgate

*Landmark Papers in General Surgery*
Edited by Graham MacKay, Richard Molloy, and Patrick O'Dwyer

*Landmark Papers in Cardiovascular Medicine*
Edited by Aung Myat and Tony Gershlick

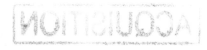

# Landmark Papers in Otolaryngology

## Seminal papers with expert commentaries

Edited by

## Mr John Phillips
Consultant ENT Surgeon
Norfolk and Norwich University Hospitals NHS Foundation Trust, UK

## Miss Sally Erskine
Specialist Registrar in ENT Surgery
Norfolk and Norwich University Hospitals NHS Foundation Trust, UK

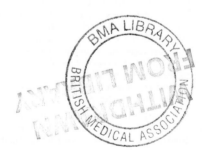

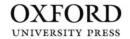

OXFORD
UNIVERSITY PRESS

# OXFORD

UNIVERSITY PRESS

Great Clarendon Street, Oxford, OX2 6DP,
United Kingdom

Oxford University Press is a department of the University of Oxford.
It furthers the University's objective of excellence in research, scholarship,
and education by publishing worldwide. Oxford is a registered trade mark of
Oxford University Press in the UK and in certain other countries

Published in the United States of America by Oxford University Press
198 Madison Avenue, New York, NY 10016, United States of America

British Library Cataloguing in Publication Data

Data available

Library of Congress Control Number: 2018937422

ISBN 978–0–19–883428–1

Printed and bound by
CPI Group (UK) Ltd, Croydon, CR0 4YY

This book is dedicated to my parents Paula and Martyn,
my wife Allyson, and my children Lydia and Benson.
J.S.P.

This book is dedicated to my parents Enid and Keith,
and my nieces and nephews,
Athena, Jess, Beth, Thomas, Harry and Joe.
S.E.E.

# Foreword

Professor Peter A. Rea

It is the supreme art of the teacher to awaken joy in creative expression and knowledge (Albert Einstein).[1]

John Phillips demonstrates mastery of his mission to stimulate interest and enrich understanding. He has attracted many of the finest current practitioners from the fields of otology, neuro-otology, rhinology, benign and malignant head and neck surgery, sleep medicine, paediatric ENT, haematology, maxillofacial surgery, anaesthesia and medico-legal practice. The enthusiasm and expertise of the international panel he has assembled is clear to see.

Reading through the selected papers I was drawn initially to the older papers we use in our practice often but have either not read for many years, or never quite got around to reading. Joe Toner's 1990 paper on surgical treatment of cholesteatoma, *Bolam* v. *Friern* [1957], which shaped our medico-legal defence for so many years, and John Epley's 1992 paper on treatment for BPPV are examples. Sistrunk's 1920 publication on surgical treatment of thyroglossal cysts allowed reflection on how little some things have changed over a century.

As I read on I became aware of many more recent papers I really ought to have read, or needed to be reminded of, to inform and consolidate current practice. And how practice really has changed enormously recently. Immunotherapy for allergic rhinitis, new work on differentiating benign from malignant thyroid nodules, the developmental consequences of general anaesthesia in infancy, and testing Eustachian tube function to name a few.

Then there were the Cochrane reviews that we do all need to know if we are to fully inform patients of their treatment options, as we are now required to do. Reviews on surgery for tympanic membrane retraction pockets, systemic vs. topical treatments for discharging ears, and surgical vs. medical treatment for chronic rhinosinusitis with nasal polyps are 'must read' examples discussed.

---

[1] Reprinted from The Ultimate Quotable Einstein, ed. Alice Calaprice ©2010, with permission from Princeton University Press. Permission conveyed through Copyright Clearance Center, Inc.

This wonderful book will therefore have broad appeal. All those involved in the care of patients with disorders of the ears, nose, or throat should have a copy. For the experienced to reminisce, to enjoy, and to be updated. For those starting out on their journey in the specialty to learn where current opinion arose from, and to see how recently such 'opinion' developed. And for those in training, to know the papers their examiners and teachers will love to quote.

Consultant ENT Surgeon
University Hospitals of Leicester
Honorary Professor of Balance Medicine
De Montfort University

# Preface

A commonly repeated question among clinicians practicing in the twenty-first century is 'what is the evidence?' This question is posed to trainees during their training and during their post-graduate exams, it is a question that practicing clinicians ask themselves, and it is a question that we are asked during our day-to-day interactions with patients and their relatives. For clinicians who are active in research and management, a good working knowledge of the up-to-date evidence is essential when designing clinical trials, and essential when interacting with commissioning groups respectively.

Unfortunately, the raw material that forms the basis of clinical evidence is not always reproduced in a manner true to its original publication. Landmark papers form the basis of guidelines and contemporary clinical practice, but often little is known about the underlying details and context of what is reported within these essential works. Landmark papers are often only highlighted as a sentence or two in a textbook. It is our principal intention that this book will address this shortcoming, presenting the latest evidence from contemporary research, alongside historical evidence that has stood the test of time. Landmark papers may not completely represent where we are today, but it is important to understand landmark papers in the context of why we currently practice otolaryngology the way we do.

For the last 5 years, the Department of Otolaryngology at the Norfolk and Norwich University Hospital has run a monthly journal club. This has always been an informal affair held in a local public house, and as such has always attracted good attendance from trainees of all levels, senior surgeons, and colleagues for allied specialties. In addition to discussing the latest publications that outline advances in our specialty, we have always discussed a classic publication from the past. It is these classic papers that have always inspired the most interesting discussions as they have been the papers that have informed practice and policy among both clinicians and those involved in the provision of health services. Moreover, this has provided an opportunity to truly appreciate the original methods and outcomes reported, without the potential misrepresentation that can occur as papers are referred to in subsequent works.

This book presents a distilled summary of the classic, ground-breaking, and significant publications in the field of otolaryngology that are of essential relevance to our specialty today. The authors of this book have been carefully selected to represent an international group of experts in their subspecialist areas, to provide a fair description of landmark publications, together with a balanced critique of their conclusions, bringing them into the context of modern day practice. It is hoped that understanding the origins of how and why we practice modern otolaryngology will inspire further evolutions that will contribute to attaining the highest quality of evidence to support the choices that we make for our patients.

John S. Phillips

# Contents

## Part II **Neurotology**

## Part III **Rhinology**

## Part IV  **Malignant head and neck disease**

## Part V  **Benign head and neck disease, laryngology, and sleep medicine**

## Part VII **Plastic and maxillofacial surgery**

## Part VIII **Miscellaneous**

# List of contributors

**Jahangir Ahmed**
Department of Otolaryngology,
Great Ormond Street Hospital for
  Children NHS Foundation Trust,
London, UK

**Christopher Aldren**
Department of Otolaryngology,
Frimley Health NHS Foundation Trust,
Slough, UK

**Andy Bath**
Department of Otolaryngology,
Norfolk and Norwich University Hospitals
  NHS Foundation Trust,
Norwich, UK

**Rajiv Bhalla**
Department of Otolaryngology,
Manchester University NHS
  Foundation Trust,
Manchester, UK

**Stephanie Cooper**
Department of Speech & Language
  Therapy,
Norfolk and Norwich University Hospitals
  NHS Foundation Trust,
Norwich, UK

**Robert Dobie**
Department of Otolaryngology,
University of California,
California, USA

**Judy Dubno**
Department of Otolaryngology,
Medical University of South Carolina,
South Carolina, USA

**James England**
Department of Otolaryngology,
Hull and East Yorkshire Hospitals
  NHS Trust,
Hull, UK

**Sally Erskine**
Department of Otolaryngology,
Norfolk and Norwich University Hospitals
  NHS Foundation Trust,
Norwich, UK

**Rebecca Field**
Department of Otolaryngology,
Christchurch Hospital,
Christchurch, New Zealand

**Hannah Fox**
Department of Otolaryngology,
The Newcastle upon Tyne Hospitals NHS
  Foundation Trust,
Newcastle upon Tyne, UK

**Jonathan Hatch**
Department of Otolaryngology,
Medical University of South Carolina,
South Carolina, USA

**Richard Haywood**
Department of Plastic Surgery,
Norfolk and Norwich University Hospitals
  NHS Foundation Trust,
Norwich, UK

**Phil Hodgson**
Department of Anaesthesia,
Norfolk and Norwich University Hospitals
  NHS Foundation Trust,
Norwich, UK

**Claire Hopkins**
Department of Otolaryngology,
Guy's and St Thomas' NHS
    Foundation Trust,
London, UK

**Casie Keaton**
Thrive Hearing and Tinnitus Solutions,
Tennessee, USA

**Veronica Kennedy**
Department of Audiovestibular Medicine,
Bolton NHS Foundation Trust,
Bolton, UK

**Walter Kutz**
Department of Otolaryngology,
University of Texas Southwestern Medical
    Center,
Texas, USA

**Paul Lambert**
Department of Otolaryngology,
Medical University of South Carolina,
South Carolina, USA

**Paul Little**
Department of Primary Care and
    Population Sciences,
University of Southampton,
Southampton, UK

**Hamish Lyall**
Department of Haematology,
Norfolk and Norwich University Hospitals
    NHS Foundation Trust,
Norwich, UK

**Liam Masterson**
Department of Otolaryngology,
Cambridge University Hospitals NHS
    Foundation Trust,
Cambridge, UK

**Don McFerran**
Department of Otolaryngology,
Colchester Hospital University NHS
    Foundation Trust,
Colchester, UK

**Gavin Morrison**
Department of Otolaryngology,
Guy's and St Thomas' NHS
    Foundation Trust,
London, UK

**Louisa Murdin**
Department of Audiovestibular Medicine,
Guy's and St Thomas' NHS
    Foundation Trust,
London, UK

**Georgios Oikonomou**
Department of Otolaryngology,
St George's University Hospitals NHS
    Foundation Trust,
London, UK

**Vinidh Paleri**
Department of Otolaryngology,
The Newcastle upon Tyne Hospitals NHS
    Foundation Trust,
Newcastle upon Tyne, UK

**John Phillips**
Department of Otolaryngology,
Norfolk and Norwich University Hospitals
    NHS Foundation Trust,
Norwich, UK

**Luke Reid**
Department of Otolaryngology, James
    Cook University, Queensland, Australia

**Tom Roques**
Department of Oncology,
Norfolk and Norwich University Hospitals
    NHS Foundation Trust,
Norwich, UK

**Hesham Saleh**
Department of Otolaryngology,
Imperial College Healthcare NHS Trust,
London, UK

**Mike Saunders**
Department of Otolaryngology,
University Hospitals Bristol NHS
  Foundation Trust,
Bristol, UK

**David Selvadurai**
Department of Otolaryngology,
St George's University Hospitals NHS
  Foundation Trust,
London, UK

**Andrew Sidebottom**
Department of Oral and Maxillofacial
  Surgery,
Nottingham University Hospitals
  NHS Trust,
Nottingham, UK

**Vedat Topsakal**
Department of Otolaryngology,
Antwerp University Hospital,
Antwerp, Belgium

**Vincent Van Rompaey**
Department of Otolaryngology,
Antwerp University Hospital,
Antwerp, Belgium

**Olivier Vanderveken**
Department of Otolaryngology,
Antwerp University Hospital,
Antwerp, Belgium

**Peter Webber**
Department of Otolaryngology,
Norfolk and Norwich University Hospitals
  NHS Foundation Trust,
Norwich, UK

**Olivia Whiteside**
Department of Otolaryngology,
Frimley Health NHS Foundation Trust,
Slough, UK

# Introduction

There is no substitute for understanding what you are doing.

*Loren P. Meissner*

The biggest challenge facing the editors and authors of this book was to determine which papers were worthy of inclusion. A robust definition of what constitutes a 'landmark paper' is difficult as such a definition is wholly subjective. Each year many thousands of articles are published in the surgical literature, so adopting some form of strict process to identify landmark papers in otolaryngology was essential. There is little doubt that the choice of papers within this book will stimulate debate in itself. With such a large choice of key publications available, we appreciate that we cannot include everything that we would wish to, and, as such, we have had to be selective.

## How does one select a 'landmark paper'?

At the outset, the editors decided to apply some 'rules' to determine whether a key publication should feature in this book. A long list of potential papers was constructed by considering several factors, initially involving an appraisal of the paper's scientific citation index and a consideration of its perceived impact on current day practice. A consistent and prominent citation of a paper within contemporary major textbooks and guidelines was considered among other key factors for inclusion, as well as papers that were considered to have invoked a paradigm shift in our thinking, or resolved an aspect of uncertainty in otolaryngology.

Certain areas of otolaryngology are far better represented in the world literature than others, attracting a greater number of publications and high citation indices. As such, great care was taken to provide a balanced and broad representation of all subspecialist areas. Current modern-day practice of otolaryngology involves overlap with other surgical specialties, such as plastic surgery and maxillofacial surgery, so a section of this book has been dedicated to these two areas. The practice of otolaryngology also involves a careful consideration of how to care for the surgical patient from a general medical and legal perspective. To address this, the final section of this book includes relevant landmark papers related to haematological and anaesthetic aspects of otolaryngology, together with relevant landmark publications related to medical law.

## Contributing authors

The contributing authors of this book were not only responsible for writing individual chapters, but also for providing a consensus opinion regarding the suitability of papers for inclusion. Contributing authors were carefully chosen for their reputable understanding of the current literature and their respected expertise in their subspecialist fields.

## Format

Each chapter provides a concise account of the context, methodology, and outcomes of the landmark paper in question. Most of the chapters follow a fixed format, although there is some intentional variation for certain types of publication. Where possible, the level of evidence will be reported according to the Oxford centre for evidence-based medicine; this scheme is outlined in the below.

| | |
|---|---|
| Level 1a | Systematic reviews (with homogeneity) of randomized controlled trials |
| Level 1b | Individual randomized controlled trials (with narrow confidence interval) |
| Level 1c | All or none randomized controlled trials |
| Level 2a | Systematic reviews (with homogeneity) of cohort studies |
| Level 2b | Individual cohort study or low quality randomized controlled trials (e.g. <80% follow-up) |
| Level 2c | 'Outcomes' research; ecological studies |
| Level 3a | Systematic review (with homogeneity) of case-control studies |
| Level 3b | Individual case-control study |
| Level 4 | Case series (and poor quality cohort and case-control studies) |
| Level 5 | Expert opinion without explicit critical appraisal, or based on physiology, bench research or 'first principles' |

Data sourced from OCEBM Levels of Evidence Working Group. 'The Oxford 2011 Levels of Evidence'. Oxford Centre for Evidence-Based Medicine. http://www.cebm.net/index.aspx?o=5653

OCEBM Table of Evidence Working Group: Jeremy Howick, Iain Chalmers (James Lind Library), Paul Glasziou, Trish Greenhalgh, Carl Heneghan, Alessandro Liberati, Ivan Moschetti, Bob Phillips, Hazel Thornton, Olive Goddard, and Mary Hodgkinson.

A summary of the main conclusions is provided, followed by a contemporary critique of how the landmark paper in question has informed current practice. It will not be surprising to many readers that the 'best' available evidence for many areas of medicine may not be of a particularly high standard. To place this into perspective, a balanced consideration of the relative merits and flaws of the landmark paper are discussed in the context of how the publication has been either superseded by more recent research, or how better evidence may be discovered in the future.

# Part I

# Otology and audiology

## Chapter 1

# Stapes surgery

Christopher Aldren

## Details of studies

Otosclerosis is the commonest cause of acquired deafness in young adults. Surgery has been performed to correct conductive hearing loss from the late nineteenth century; however, it was the development of the stapedectomy operation in 1956 by Dr John Shea that has transformed the hearing prospects for these patients. In this study the author, who invented the procedure, looks at his results from his 40 years' experience.

## Study references

### Main study

Shea JJ. Forty years of Stapes surgery. *Am J Otol* 1998;19:52–5.

### Related reference

Smyth GD, Hassard TH. Eighteen years experience in stapedectomy. The case for the small fenestra operation. *Ann Otol Rhinol Laryngol* 1978;87(Suppl. 49):3–36.

## Study design

Retrospective case series

| | |
|---|---|
| Level of evidence | 4 |
| Randomization | None |
| Number of patients | 5,444 |
| Inclusion criteria | Approximately 100 patients per year were selected randomly from each of the 40 years out of the total number of 14,449 cases performed by the author. Patient ages ranged from 6 to 89 with an average of 52 years; 64% were female |
| Exclusion criteria | None stated |
| Follow-up | Up to 30+ years |

## Outcome measures

Using an average of 500, 1,000, and 2,000 Hz success was defined as closure of the air bone gap to <10 dB (using preoperative bone conduction) and no decline in speech discrimination of >10%.

## Results

For primary stapedectomy success was achieved in 95.1% of patients at 1 year and 89.9% after 6–10 years, reducing to 62.5% after >30 years. For revision stapedectomy success was achieved in 71.1% of patients at 1 year, reducing to 59.4% after 6–36 years. Sensory hearing loss occurred in 1.8% of primary operations and 4% of revision cases. Total sensory hearing loss occurred in 0.6%. Dr Shea suggests that the excess sensory hearing loss over time when compared with controls is due to cochlear invasion by the otosclerotic process.

## Conclusions

Stapedectomy has been a successful operation that has stood the test of time with excellent initial results which slowly deteriorate over time but remain good at over 30 years.

## Critique

This study is of interest as it is the personal experience of the inventor of stapedectomy, Dr John Shea. His operation was a great success from the outset and has changed the prospects for a whole generation of deafened patients. Dr Shea describes his changes in operative technique from initial total stapedectomy, to removing the posterior half of the footplate, and then to using a laser to make a small fenestra in the centre of the footplate. His soft tissue seal of choice for the oval window was the vein graft with the adventitia placed downwards. He noticed that a gelfoam oval window seal gave less favourable results. The study is descriptive with no statistical analysis and we are therefore no wiser as to why the author changed his technique over time.

Smyth and Hassard in their 1978 paper give much more detail of their results using a variety of techniques. They noted a significant reduction in postoperative sensorineural hearing loss when switching from a stapedectomy to a 0.4 mm small fenestra stapedotomy technique. They concluded that small fenestra stapedotomy should be the technique of choice. Other authors have also concluded that small fenestra stapedotomy offers advantages over stapedectomy with Plath finding better higher frequency hearing and more stable results.

Shea declared results are good but use only three frequencies and also use preoperative bone conduction. Improvements in bone conduction with surgery therefore give a flattering postoperative air bone gap. Modern studies usually use four frequencies and postoperative bone conduction when reporting results.

Over the years since this publication, surgical refinements have improved results and decreased side effects, but the basic operation of stapedectomy as described here by its inventor remains highly successful and has benefitted many hundreds of thousands of patients worldwide.

## Additional reference

Plath P, Lenart R, Matschke RG, Kruppa E. Long-term results of stapedectomy and stapedotomy. *HNO* 1992;40:52–5.

# Chapter 2

# Cholesteatoma surgery

Christopher Aldren

## Details of studies

The optimum management of cholesteatoma patients continues to cause vigorous debate. In this study, the senior author details his experience in three consecutive case cohorts of cholesteatoma patients operated on using three different techniques over an 8-year period. The techniques were for the first cohort a two-stage combined approach tympanoplasty (CAT), then the second cohort was an open mastoidectomy with bone pate obliteration (MOT) in two stages, and the final cohort was a one-stage modified radical mastoidectomy (MRM). The author found little difference in results and so favoured the one-stage MRM.

## Study reference

### Main study

Toner JG, Smyth GDL. Surgical treatment of cholesteatoma: a comparison of three techniques *Am J Otol* 1990;**11**:247–9.

## Study design

### Case series

| | |
|---|---|
| Level of evidence | 4 |
| Randomization | None |
| Number of patients | 258 |
| Inclusion criteria | Patients operated upon for cholesteatoma by the senior author. There were three consecutive cohorts. The first group of 92 patients had combined approach tympanoplasty in two stages from 1975 to 1978. The second group, also of 92 patients, had mastoid tympanoplasty with Obliteration in two stages from 1978 to 1980. The third group of 74 patients had MRM between 1980 and 1983 |
| Exclusion criteria | None stated |
| Follow-up | Mean follow up of >7 years |

## Outcome measures

- Number of moist cavities
- Cavity volume to meatal cross-sectional area ratio for the MOT and MRM groups
- Average improvement in air conduction using of 500, 1,000, and 2,000 Hz at 1 year and at final review

## Results

Impressively dry ears were achieved in over 95% of ears in each of the three groups with no significant difference between them. Cavity volumes were smaller in the MOT group than the MRM group. Hearing improvement was greater in the CAT group at 1 year but although still better at final review the gap had decreased.

## Conclusions

The authors conclude that the proposed advantages of CAT and MOT over MRM are not maintained over time and do not justify the second staged operation. They conclude that the one-stage MRM is the optimum long-term treatment for cholesteatoma.

## Critique

This study is of interest as the senior author was noted to be an excellent surgeon who was honest and meticulous in reporting his results. Although the groups were consecutive with differing follow-ups, the lack of perceived advantage of the two-stage operations caused the authors to recommend a canal wall down MRM approach. The debate between canal wall up and down continues to rage. A recent meta-analysis by Tomlin et al. still recommends a canal wall down approach. However, a number of new techniques have emerged to improve results in intact canal wall mastoid surgery for cholesteatoma. Diffusion-weighted magnetic resonance imaging allows residual cholesteatoma to be detected without operation and so allows CAT surgery to be performed as a single-stage procedure with second stage surgery only for residual or recurrent disease. Residual cholesteatoma rates in CAT surgery have been reduced by the use of the laser and otoendoscopes. Recurrent cholesteatoma rates have been reduced by the use of primary bony obliteration of the mastoid cavity. The rights and wrongs have still not been properly determined and the debate will continue to fuel airplanes to international otology conferences for years to come.

## Additional references

James AL, Cushing S, Papsin BC. Residual cholesteatoma after endoscope-guided surgery in children. *Otol Neurotol* 2016;**37**:196–201.

Jindal M, Riskalla A, Jiang D, Connor S, O'Connor AF. A systematic review of diffusion-weighted magnetic resonance imaging in the assessment of postoperative cholesteatoma. *Otol Neurotol* 2011;**32**:1243–9.

Hamilton JW. Efficacy of the KTP laser in the treatment of middle ear cholesteatoma. *Otol Neurotol* 2005;**26**:135–9.

Tomlin J, Chang D, McCutcheon B, Harris J. Surgical technique and recurrence in cholesteatoma: a meta-analysis. *Audiol Neurootol* 2013;**18**:135–42.

van Dinther JJ, Vercruysse JP, Camp S, De Foer B, Casselman J, Somers T, et al. The bony obliteration tympanoplasty in pediatric cholesteatoma: long-term safety and hygienic results. *Otol Neurotol* 2015;**236**:1504–9.

Chapter 3

# Ossiculoplasty

Christopher Aldren

## Details of study

While short-term results of ossiculoplasty are often pleasing longer term results are often poor and frequently not reported. In this retrospective case series the senior author (V.C.) presents his long-term results for ossicular reconstruction using Plastipore and Proplast prostheses compared with those using sculptured ossicles.

## Study references

### Main study

Colletti V, Fiorino FG, Sittoni, V. Minisculptured ossicle grafts versus implants: long-term results. *Am J of Otol* 1987;**19**:52–5.

### Related reference

Palva T, Ramsay H. Myringoplasty and tympanoplasty—results related to training and experience. *Clin Otolaryngol Allied Sci* 1995;**20**:329–35.

## Study design

Retrospective case series

| | |
|---|---|
| Level of evidence | 4 |
| Randomization | None |
| Number of patients | 832 ossicular reconstructions in 655 patients |
| Inclusion criteria | All the ossicular reconstructions performed by the senior author over an 11-year period from January 1975 |
| Patient data | Patient ages ranged from 4 to 72 with a mean of 34 years; 51% of patients were female. There were far fewer ossiculoplasties performed with prostheses (52) than sculptured ossicles (529) in the partial reconstruction group. The reverse was true for the total reconstruction group with more prostheses (151) used than sculptured ossicles (90) |
| Exclusion criteria | None stated |
| Follow-up | Up to 5 years |

## Outcome measures

Using an average of 500, 1,000, and 2,000 Hz postoperative air bone gaps were defined using postoperative air conduction minus preoperative bone conduction. Postoperative air bone gaps were compared with preoperative gaps and the difference was recorded as the therapeutic efficiency. Results were compared for partial reconstructions between partial ossicular replacement prostheses (PORPS) and sculptured ossicles. These results were compared at 6 months and 1, 3, and 5 years. Similarly, results were compared between total ossicular reconstructions using total ossicular replacement prostheses (TORPS) and sculptured ossicles.

## Results

At 6 months and a year there was no significant difference in the hearing results between the PORPS and sculptured ossicles for partial ossicular reconstruction with closure of air bone gaps to <21 dB at 77.5% and 80.3% respectively. However, a significant decrease in therapeutic efficiency was noted over time and by 5 years the closure of air bone gaps to <21 dB had fallen to 31.8% for PORPS and 50.3% for sculptured ossicles. The significant superiority of the sculptured ossicles was put down to the high extrusion rate of the PORPS.

With the total ossicular reconstructions a similar pattern was seen with no significant difference between the groups at 1 year but a significant decrease in results by 5 years with the sculptured ossicles again outperforming the TORPS. At 5 years, only 23.8% of the TORPS had an air bone gap of <20 dB. The mean improvement in air bone gap for TORPS at 5 years was a barely useful 3.5 dB. With the sculptured ossicles this was significantly better at 9.6 dB.

Results were better for partial ossicular reconstruction than total ossicular reconstruction. Rates of extrusion of prostheses were reduced by interposing cartilage between the prostheses and the tympanic membrane. This was especially noticeable at one year with a reduction from 20% to 3.5%. However, even with cartilage interposition, extrusion of prostheses had reached 15.2% at 5 years. Long-term follow-up rates were poor with only 200 out of 581 partial reconstructions and 93 out of 241 total reconstructions available at 5 years.

## Conclusions

Results from ossicular replacement deteriorate significantly and progressively over time. Plastipore and Proplast are not good materials for ossicular reconstruction because of the high rates of extrusion. Cartilage interposition reduces rates of extrusion of prostheses. Autograft- or homograft-sculptured ossicles do not extrude and give better long-term hearing than Plastipore and Proplast prostheses.

A related study by Palva considered results from tympanoplasty comparing the results of Professor Palva with his trainees and other faculty members. This study demonstrated significantly better results when the surgery was performed by himself.

# Critique

This study shows that Plastipore and Proplast prostheses tend to extrude over time at a rate which makes them non-suitable for use as middle ear implants. As a result of this and other studies they have been largely replaced by materials of better biocompatibility such as hydroxyapatite and titanium. It also shows that all ossiculoplasty results get worse over time. The authors suggest, probably correctly, that the state of the Eustachian tube and the presence of residual or recurrent disease are the main factors underlying this deterioration.

The patients in this study were not randomized with the cohort of PORPS and TORPS occurring early in the study. The move to sculptured ossicles occurred later in the study owing to the observation of extrusion of the implants. Extrusion was not seen for sculptured ossicles but occurred in a significant proportion of the prostheses. This suggests that the material for reconstruction is important in determining extrusion. Subsequent studies with prostheses of titanium and hydroxyapatite have shown them to have reduced levels of extrusion, typically between 0% and 4% (O'Connell et al. 2016). While most surgeons interpose cartilage between titanium prostheses and the drum, not all feel this is necessary (Pringle et al. 2014).

Most studies and a recent meta-analysis fail to show any difference in results between different types of prostheses or indeed between prostheses and autografts (Zhang et al. 2011; Yung and Smith 2010). This may be due to lack of power where pathology has high intrinsic variability. However some studies have shown these new prostheses to give better hearing results than sculptured ossicles (Zazouk et al. 2015).

## Additional references

O'Connell BP, Rizk HG, Hutchinson T, Nguyen, SA, Lambert, PR. Long-term outcomes of titanium ossiculoplasty in chronic otitis media. *Otolaryngol Head Neck Surg* 2016;**154**:1084–92.

Pringle MB, Sunkaraneni VS, Tann N. Is cartilage interposition required for ossiculoplasty with titanium prostheses? *Otol Neurotol* 2014;**35**:482–8.

Yung M, Smith P. Titanium versus nontitanium ossicular prostheses-a randomized controlled study of the medium-term outcome. *Otol Neurotol* 2010;**31**:752–8.

Zakzouk A, Bonmardion N, Bouchetemble P, Lerosey Y, Marie J-P. Titanium prosthesis or autologous incus for total ossicular reconstruction in the absence of the stapes suprastructure and presence of mobile footplate. *Eur Arch Otorhinolaryngol* 2015;**272**:2653–7.

Zhang LC, Zhang TY, Dai PD, Luo JF. Titanium versus non-titanium prostheses in ossiculoplasty: a meta-analysis. *Acta Otolaryngol* 2011;**131**:708–15.

# Chapter 4

# Retraction pockets

David Selvadurai and Georgios Oikonomou

## Details of study

Retraction pockets of the tympanic membrane are a common clinical condition managed by otolaryngologists. They are seen when either a section or the entire tympanic membrane collapses into the middle ear, away from its natural position. Several factors are thought to be involved in the retraction formation, but chronic negative middle ear pressure is accepted as the major cause. Retractions can be completely asymptomatic; nevertheless, the most common related symptom is conductive hearing loss. They can be stable or unstable, the latter strongly related to cholesteatoma; therefore, diagnosis and correct management are critical. Diagnosis is made by clinical evaluation and several staging systems have been introduced to assess the evolution of the retraction pocket. The most commonly used ones are the Tos classification for pars flaccida retractions and the Sade classification for pars tensa retractions. Although both systems suffer from poor reproducibility they are useful for follow-up, research, and teaching purposes.

There is a wide variation between clinicians regarding the management of retraction pockets as per the indications, timing and the surgical and non-surgical options considered. The conservative 'watch and wait' policy, often coupled with medical therapies to improve Eustachian tube function, is commonly considered to be the first-line strategy as early retractions may be asymptomatic and resolve spontaneously. Surgical options include ventilation tube insertion (grommet or T-tube) alone or in combination with some form of reconstruction of the tympanic membrane (tympanoplasty with fascia or cartilage graft). Adenoidectomy for adenoid hypertrophy is also thought to improve Eustachian tube function.

The choice of treatment is not based on any consensus and Nankivell et al. (2017) have undertaken this review in an attempt to provide guidance to address this clinical uncertainty. This was the first systematic review addressing this issue making clear the lack of good evidence in the management of retraction pockets.

## Study reference

### Main study

**Nankivell PC, Pothier DD.** Surgery for tympanic membrane retraction pockets. *Cochrane Database Syst Rev* 2010;7:CD007943.

## Study design

Randomized controlled trials in which tympanic membrane retractions have been managed by any method of surgical intervention.

## Outcome measures

### Primary outcomes

- Clinical monitoring of the retraction, looking for resolution, cessation of progression, no effect or even continued progression of the disease
- Adverse events

### Secondary outcomes

Whether the intervention has any effect on those things noticeable to the patient:

- Improvement in hearing thresholds
- Reduction in ear discharge
- Improvement in otalgia
- Improvement in quality of life scores

## Results

Two studies were included ($n = 76$ patients of all ages were included):

- Barbara M. Lateral attic reconstruction technique: preventive surgery for epitympanic retraction pockets. *Otology & Neurotology* 2008;29(4):522–5.
- Elsheikh MN, Elsherief HS, Elsherief SG. Cartilage tympanoplasty for management of tympanic membrane atelectasis: is ventilatory tube necessary? *Otology & Neurotology* 2006;27(6):859–64.

No good evidence for the role of any individual surgical intervention for the management of retraction of the tympanic membrane was found. The two randomized controlled trials included in this review failed to show any statistical benefit of surgical intervention versus a 'watch and wait' policy. Comparison between cartilage tympanoplasty alone and cartilage tympanoplasty plus ventilation tube showed no statistically significant difference. No adverse events were recorded at all in one of the studies, while the other one reported only one incidence of tympanic membrane infection.

There was no difference demonstrated in the secondary outcomes assessed, reduction in ear discharge, improvement in otalgia, and improvement in quality of life scores, when assessed at all by the studies included. Hearing thresholds were reviewed only in one of the studies and no significant difference was found.

## Critique

Nankivell et al. reviewed only two relatively small and poor quality randomized controlled trials. The authors acknowledge numerous difficulties with the studies reviewed. Patients of all age groups were included and both studies were found to have a potentially significant risk of bias. In the Barbara study, a single investigator undertook the randomization, intervention, and all follow-up assessments with no evidence of blinding. Monitoring of tympanic membrane retraction pockets was performed subjectively by the investigator alone and the only objective measurements were taken with audiological assessments but no actual data were presented in the publication. The Elshiekh study mentions no randomization and blinding method. Furthermore, when it comes to the outcomes of the surgical intervention it is assessed by the authors by a single statement that all tympanic membranes returned to 'near normal'. The risk of progression to a worse stage or cholesteatoma was only calculated in the Barbara study and was not found to be statistically significant. The secondary outcomes were not assessed at all by either of the studies apart from the hearing thresholds which were reviewed only by the Elshiekh study where no statistically significant difference were found among the two surgical groups.

The Nankivell study has been the first systematic review that has tried to address the controversial issue of the management of retraction pockets. Despite reviewing only two relatively small and poor quality RCT studies, they brought to surface the poor evidence in the literature regarding retraction pockets. All the studies identified by the search were of poor design (as mostly were retrospective case series). A later study by Neumann encountered the same problems including only the same studies Nankivell et al. included, indicating the lack of robust randomized clinical studies. Nankivell et al. made a very clear comment regarding the reliability of the retraction pocket staging system. None of the various staging systems in widespread use have been validated, making interpretation of any studies performed using these systems difficult. All the studies reviewed (included or not) were affected in terms of risk of bias by the lack of common reporting method. The currently described staging systems of tympanic membrane retraction pockets had very low influence on the management of the retraction pockets. The systematic review by Alzahrani et al. (2014) 4 years later reported the same conclusion.

Nankivell et al. were the first to highlight the need for robust randomized clinical trials that include a control arm of no surgical intervention. They also outlined the fundamental need for a reliable staging method of the retraction pockets of the tympanic membrane that can be used for monitoring, which will influence the management and will also allow comparison between different studies. Currently, the staging of tympanic membrane retraction pockets is not widely used in clinical decision making. Keratin accumulation, the air bone gap level and otorrhea are more often used to guide treatment. Nonetheless there is still no consensus amongst otologists as to the optimal strategy for management of tympanic membrane retractions and no major systematic review or guidelines have been published since the Nankivell et al. study.

## Additional references

Alzahrani M, Saliba I. Tympanic membrane retraction pocket staging: is it worthwhile? *Eur Arch Otorhinolaryngol* 2014;271:1361–8.

Neumann C, Yung M. Management of retraction pockets of pars tensa and pars flaccida: a systematic review of literature. *Int Adv Otol* 2012;8:260–365.

# Chapter 5

# Tympanic membrane perforations

David Selvadurai and Georgios Oikonomou

## Details of study

Chronic suppurative otitis media (CSOM) is one of several types of otitis media characterized as a chronic infection of the middle ear with a perforated tympanic membrane and discharge. The causes and risk factors associated with CSOM are complex and poorly understood. Hearing impairment and morbidity from recurrent ear discharge are the most frequent effects of CSOM. However, untreated or undertreated CSOM may result in permanent hearing loss, speech and language delays or permanent learning disabilities in children, and intracranial complications as well as otological complications (subperiosteal abscess, facial nerve paralysis, cholesteatoma, labyrinthitis, or acute mastoiditis).

Treatment options for uncomplicated CSOM include aural toilet, systemic antibiotics (e.g. oral antibiotic preparations, or intravenous antibiotics); and topical treatment with either antiseptics or antibiotics, with or without steroids. Complications demand appropriate surgical and medical management. There has been uncertainty over whether topical or systemic antibiotic therapy is most effective. This has centred on the ability of topical agents to penetrate the middle ear and mastoid regions, and of course the sensitivity of the causative organisms. A second concern has been regarding potential ototoxicity from aminoglycoside drops. These concerns have led to the continued use of systemic antibiotics in many cases.

MacFayden et al. (2006) have tried to address this issue by comparing the results of systemic versus topical treatments (excluding steroids) for chronically discharging ears with an underlying eardrum perforation (CSOM) in participants of all ages. This was the first systematic review addressing this problem and has influenced routine practice.

## Study reference

### Main study

Macfadyen CA, Acuin JM, Gamble CL. Systemic antibiotics versus topical treatments for chronically discharging ears with underlying eardrum perforations. *Cochrane Database Syst Rev* 2006;1:CD005608.

## Study design

Individual randomized controlled trials and cluster randomized controlled trials that compared any systemic treatment excluding steroids to any topical (aural) treatment excluding steroids in patients with CSOM.

## Outcome measures

### Primary outcomes

◆ Resolution of CSOM at 2–4 weeks, and after 4 weeks, according to the investigators' criteria

### Secondary outcomes

◆ Healing of perforation at 2–4 weeks, and after 4 weeks
◆ Time to resolution of CSOM as defined by the investigators
◆ Improvement in hearing threshold, as measured by audiometry at 2–4 weeks, and after 4 weeks
◆ Time to reappearance of discharge and perforation after its previous resolution
◆ Adverse events that

  a are fatal, life-threatening, require inpatient hospitalization or prolongation of existing hospitalization, or result in persistent or significant disability/incapacity, such as permanent hearing loss, tinnitus, or vertigo

  b result in withdrawal or discontinuation of treatment

  c any other adverse events, such as ear pain, ear canal reactions and transient dizziness

## Results

Nine studies were included ($n$ = 833, age range 6–83 years):

◆ Browning et al. 1983 (published and unpublished data) Controlled trial of medical treatment of active chronic otitis media. *British Medical Journal Clinical Research Edition* 1983;287(6398):1024. Correspondence 1997, 2005.

◆ de Miguel et al. 1999. A microbial therapy in chronic suppurative otitis media. [Spanish] [Terapeutica antimicrobiana en otitis media cronica supurada]. *Acta Otorrinolaringologica Espanola* 1999;50(1):15–19.

◆ Esposito et al. 1990. Topical and oral treatment of chronic otitis media with ciprofloxacin. *Archives of Otolaryngology—Head and Neck Surgery* 1990;116(5):557–9. Esposito et al. 1992. Topical ciprofloxacin versus intramuscular gentamicin for chronic otitis media. *Archives of Otolaryngology—Head and Neck Surgery* 1992;118(8):842–4.

◆ Mira et al. 1993. Ceftizoxime as local therapy in the treatment of recurrences of chronic suppurative otitis media. *Journal of Drug Development Supplement* 1993;6(Suppl 2): 39–44.

◆ Mira et al. 1992. Clinical evaluation of ceftizoxime (EposerinR) as local therapy in the treatment of recurrences of chronic suppurative otitis media *Rivista-Italiana-di-Otorinolaringologia-Audiologia-e-Foniatria* 1992;12(4):219–25.

◆ Papastavros et al. 1989. Preoperative therapeutic considerations in chronic suppurative otitis media. *Laryngoscope* 1989;99:655–9.

- Povedano et al. 1995. Efficacy of topical ciprofloxacin in the treatment of chronic otorrhea [Eficacia del ciprofloxacino topico en el tratamiento de la otorrea cronica]. *Acta Otorrinolaryngologica Española* 1995;46(1):15–18.
- Supiyaphun et al. 2000. Comparison of ofloxacin otic solution with oral amoxicillin plus chloramphenicol ear drop in treatment of chronic suppurative otitis media with acute exacerbation. *Journal of the Medical Association of Thailand* 2000;83(1): 61–8.
- Yuen et al 1994. Ofloxacin eardrop treatment for active chronic suppurative otitis media: prospective randomized study. *American Journal of Otology* 1994;15(5):670–3.

Short courses of topical quinolone antibiotics were found to be more effective than systemic antibiotics alone for the short-term resolution of otorrhea from uncomplicated CSOM. The effects of topical non-quinolone antibiotics (without steroids) or antiseptics were unclear when compared with systemic treatment. There was no benefit to adding systemic treatment to topical antibiotics demonstrated. Moreover, no long-term outcomes regarding complications, healing of the perforation, or hearing improvement were reported. Finally, there was only weak evidence of ototoxicity.

## Critique

MacFayden et al. reviewed nine relatively small and poor-quality RCTs. The authors recognized numerous difficulties with the studies found. Many of these studies included a wide range of participants. Patients of all age groups were included and four studies included participants less than 16 years old (minimum ages 6 years). The diagnostic criteria of CSOM also varied as studies included participants with otitis externa, with draining mastoid cavities, participants post mastoidectomy, participants post tympanoplasty, participants with post-surgical otorrhea, positive fistula sign, and with cholesteatoma. There was a high risk of bias recognized in the studies. Six studies did not report on the use of blinding. Three studies contained incomplete outcome data. Trials were also inconsistent in approaches for handling participants with bilateral disease. MacFayden et al. reported results for the number of participants rather than ears to avoid having an underestimated standard error and therefore receiving an inappropriate increased weight in a meta-analysis. They suggested that this would be addressed in a later update of the review. The significant heterogeneity of the review was considered problematic by Salanti, who evaluated and downgraded the confidence of the review to low. The follow-up period in all trials included here was short (2–4 weeks). No trials assessed longer term effects of treatment, or reported time to resolution or reappearance of discharge and perforation, or results for healing of the tympanic membrane. All trials or comparisons including topical or systemic steroids were excluded and the authors suggested that steroid trials would have to be addressed in a later review.

Three questions were evaluated using this study, but the heterogeneity of the papers limited the study to only using three papers to address each query. Hence, only two trials compared topical antiseptics with systemic antibiotics and there was no statistically significant difference between groups. One trial compared topical non-quinolone antibiotics to systemic non-quinolones. There was a non-significant trend in favour of the latter. Comparison between topical quinolones and systemic non-quinolones included two trials. The results favoured a significant effect for topical quinolones and this was the first important outcome of the study. Again, no long-term data were reported and no substantial comparison was made in terms of healing of perforation and improvement in hearing thresholds. Comparison between topical and systemic quinolones included three trials and the pooled RR (95% CI) was 3.8% in favour of topical ciprofloxacin (0.2 or 0.5%). Again, no long-term data and no results on improvement in hearing thresholds were reported. Adding topical quinolone treatment to systemic quinolone antibiotic treatment is found to have higher cure rates. Nevertheless, no long-term results were reported and only two trials were included in the study. Adding a topical non-quinolone to systemic non-quinolone antibiotics was considered in only one study that did not provide full results. A statistically significant difference was found, in favour of topical antibiotic when systemic and topical non-quinolone antibiotics were compared to topical quinolones; however, follow-up was for 2 weeks only. No benefit was found when adding systemic antibiotic treatment to topical quinolone treatment. Two studies (160 participants in total) assessed this for a period no longer than 2 weeks. Despite the short follow-up this was an important finding in terms of the adding cost and risks when using combined treatment.

With respect to ototoxicity, the findings of all studies included were insufficient. It was however noted that significantly more topical side effects (such as tinnitus, fungal growth, or pain) were reported when using non-quinolone topical treatment compared to ofloxacin. Again, follow up was limited to one to two weeks. Despite the limitations outlined, this review represented the best evidence available for CSOM treatment at that time. The MacFayden review has 54 citations, the latest three were in 2016, indicating that the outcome of this review is still considered. The superiority of topical treatment compared to systemic treatment has been clearly demonstrated in this review. Furthermore, current trends for the treatment for CSOM are supported by this review, these being selection of an appropriate antibiotic drop, regular aggressive aural toilet, control of granulation tissue, and reserving systemic therapy only for cases of failure of initial topical treatment.

### Additional reference

Salanti G, Del Giovane C, Chaimani A, Caldwell DM, Higgins JP. Evaluating the quality of evidence from a network meta-analysis. *PLoS One* 2014;9:e99682.

# Chapter 6

# Eustachian tube function

Olivia Whiteside

## Details of study

Eustachian tube dysfunction is common but poorly understood. It causes a number of symptoms such as aural fullness and popping and is an important aetiological factor in the development of middle ear pathology. There is currently no 'gold standard' for the diagnosis of Eustachian tube dysfunction.

The Eustachian tube has three functions: gas transfer and pressure equalization between the middle ear and nasopharynx; mucous clearance from the middle ear; and prevention of sound, pathogens, and secretions from the nasopharynx. The tube normally lies closed, opening momentarily with actions such as swallowing.

The pressure is maintained via two mechanisms, middle ear mucosal gas exchange and Eustachian tube opening to equilibrate pressure with the nasopharynx. Though the relative contribution of each is unknown, evidence suggests that in a healthy middle ear the pressure slowly reduces and is restored by Eustachian tube opening. Clearance is my muscular peristalsis and the mucociliary escalator. Despite decades of work, there is no single, reliable test of Eustachian tube function.

Proposed tests of Eustachian tube function can measure passive tubal opening, such as by high pressure, or active tubal opening usually elicited by the patient swallowing or making a 'k' sound. There are fewer tests of patulous Eustachian tube. Manometric tests are most widely used and are designed to define the ventilatory and pressure equalization abilities of the Eustachian tube. Some depend on the drum being intact.

Tests in this review included pneumatic otoscopy; witnessed Valsalva; witnessed Toynbee; tympanometry; tympanogram Valsalva and Toynbee; tympanogram sniffing; nine-step test; inflation–deflation test; forced response test; patulous tube test; sonotubometry; tubomanometry; ETDQ7 (a patient-reported outcome measure) and combinations of tests; slow motion video endoscopy; functional imaging; clearance function tests; optotensometry; electromyography.

## Study references

### Main study

Smith M, Tysome J. Tests of Eustachian tube function: a review. *Clin Otolaryngol* 2015;40:300–11.

## Related references

Schilder A, Bhutta M, Butler C, Holy C, Levine L, Kvaerner K, et al. Eustachian tube dysfunction: consensus statement on definition, types, clinical presentation and diagnosis. *Clin Otolaryngol* 2015;40;407–11.

## Study design

Narrative systematic review to identify tests of Eustachian tube function currently available and report on their accuracy. The variation in demographics, disease presentation/severity and technological approaches limited the study to a narrative systematic review.

## Outcome measures

The sensitivity and specificity of Eustachian tube function tests
Tests included were required to measure physiological function of Eustachian tube or contribute to the diagnosis of Eustachian tube dysfunction.

## Results

Numerous tests of Eustachian tube function are available.

◆ All have significant limitations
◆ Limited accuracy data of varying quality have been published

## Conclusion

There is no 'gold standard' for the diagnosis of Eustachian tube dysfunction. Diagnostic accuracy may be improved by combining the results of different objective tests with patient-reported outcome measures. Further development of Eustachian tube function tests is needed in order to allow a standard testing regime such that research outcomes of trials into Eustachian tube dysfunction can be compared.

## Critique

This is a comprehensive review of the techniques available and demonstrates that there is no single reliable diagnostic tool for Eustachian tube dysfunction. It highlights the limited amount of good data available on Eustachian tube test accuracy due to the difficulties in validating outcome measures.

A consensus statement on the definition, types, clinical presentation, and diagnosis of Eustachian tube dysfunction in adults was subsequently produced, primarily to address the lack of consensus on the diagnostic criteria for Eustachian tube dysfunction. The panel agreed that to diagnose Eustachian tube dysfunction, the patient must present with symptoms of aural fullness or popping or discomfort/pain. Additional symptoms included clogged or underwater sensation, crackling, ringing, autophony, habitual sniffing, and muffled hearing. Acute Eustachian tube dysfunction is defined as being transient with symptoms and signs for under three months, longer than this being chronic Eustachian tube dysfunction. They concluded there are probably three subtypes of Eustachian tube dysfunction:

1 Dilatory Eustachian tube dysfunction (which may be due to functional obstruction, muscular failure: dynamic dysfunction or anatomical obstruction)

2 Baro-challenge-induced Eustachian tube dysfunction

3 Patulous Eustachian tube dysfunction

The panel agreed there is no standard set of patient-reported symptoms scores, functional tests or scoring systems to diagnose Eustachian tube dysfunction. The ETDQ7 is currently the only patient-reported outcome tool to have undergone initial validation.

The consensus panel concluded that patient-reported symptoms, otoscopy, tympanometry and pure tone audiometry should be the outcome measures included in future clinical trials.

Chapter 7

# Imaging cholesteatoma

Olivia Whiteside

## Details of study

Second-look surgery following a canal wall up procedure for cholesteatoma remains the gold standard for the diagnosis or residual and recurrent disease. With the advent of diffusion-weighted magnetic resonance imaging (DWI), surgeons are increasingly performing single stage surgery, primary reconstruction, and surgery with the possibility of burying disease such as mastoid obliteration.

Though high-resolution computed tomography (CT) scanning has a high negative predictive value in excluding cholesteatoma in the complete absence of any tympanomastoid opacification, this is rarely the case postoperatively. Most commonly there will be at least partial opacification and here both CT and conventional magnetic resonance imaging (MRI) scanning have significant limitations in distinguishing cholesteatoma from other soft tissues or fluid.

Diffusion-weighted MRI of cholesteatoma demonstrates a hyperintense signal, due to the restricted microdiffusion of water molecules in keratin and a 'T2 shine-through effect' where there is a prolonged relaxation time after a magnetic impulse passes through keratin. Two modalities of DWI have been used: echo planar imaging (EPI) is a single-shot spin echo pulse sequence, the main drawback being its susceptibility to artefact. This is of particular importance in the temporal bone where there are multiple interfaces between air, bone and soft tissue where artefact can arise. Non-EPI involves multi-shot fast spin echo or single-shot turbo spin echo which are less susceptible to interface artefact.

Jindal et al. (2011) sought to determine whether diffusion-weighted MRI could reliably detect residual or recurrent cholesteatoma after mastoid surgery. A recent further systematic review and meta-analysis by Muzaffar et al. (2017) has expanded on and supported their results.

## Study references

### Main study

Jindal M, Riskalla A, Jiang D, Conor S, Fitzgerald O'Conor A. A systematic review of diffusion-weighted magnetic resonance imaging in the assessment of postoperative cholesteatoma. *Otol Neurotol* 2011;**32**:1243–9.

### Related reference

Muzaffar J, Metcalfe C, Colley S, Coulson C. Diffusion-weighted magnetic resonance imaging for residual and recurrent cholesteatoma: a systematic review and meta-analysis. *Clin Otolaryngol* 2017;42:536–43.

## Study design

Systematic review in accordance with the PRISMA statement

| Inclusion criteria | All adult and paediatric patients |
| --- | --- |
| Number of patients | 405 |
| Intervention | DW MRI scan (EPI) and non-EPI |
| Study design | Cohort studies, randomized control trials (none found) |
| Exclusion criteria | Case reports, review articles, DWI studies in primary cholesteatoma |

## Outcome measures

Sensitivity, specificity, positive, and negative predictive values of DWI and the incidence and size of residual or recurrent choleseatoma, confirmed by revision/second look tympano-mastoid surgery.

## Results

Non-EPI scanning techniques were superior to EPI with 91% sensitivity, 96% specificity, 97% positive predictive value, and 85% negative predictive value. Non-EPI techniques were significantly superior to EPI (p<0.04).

Several studies observed that EPI would fail to identify disease of 2 to 5 mm. One 3-mm lesion was missed on non-EPI imaging in a child with motion artefact and other studies did not state the size of the lesion missed.

Incidence of residual or recurrent disease ranged from 7% to 78%.

## Conclusions

Non-EPI sequences such as half-Fourier acquisition single-shot turbo spin echo (HASTE) are more reliable in the identification of residual and recurrent cholesteatoma than EPI methods as they have fewer artefacts and better spatial resolution, allowing diagnosis of smaller lesions.

The authors recommend non-EPI techniques alongside careful otologist-based follow-up of patients with negative scans, repeating the scan after 12–18 months. Further studies were recommended to determine the place of DW imaging as an alternative to surgery.

## Critique

This was a large systematic review of a new diagnostic tool to assess the accuracy of DWI in identifying residual or recurrent cholesteatoma after canal wall up surgery. The study has significant implications for clinical practice in that the use of non-EPI DW MRI scanning could be considered as an alternative to second stage surgery.

Studies were generally felt to be of good quality but there was enormous variability across the studies in multiple factors such as the age/tuning of the scanner, slice thickness, lack of clarity as over the blinding of radiologists to surgical findings and failure to distinguish between residual and recurrent disease; this is important as often residual disease foci are smaller than recurrent disease. The time from surgery to scanning was variable and not always clearly stated. Time to the second surgery and between scanning and surgery was very variable, meaning a small cholesteatoma could be missed on a scan and have enlarged significantly by the time of surgery.

The 7–78% residual/recurrent disease rate of the Jindal study has been further analysed by Muzaffar et al., who reported a residual disease rate of 30% and a pooled residual/recurrence rate of 58%.

Muzaffar et al. also found that non-EPI performed significantly better and therefore, suggested it should be the investigation of choice. They concluded that in centres with sufficient expertise, this technique would represent a valid alternative to second-look surgery.

### Additional reference

Kosling S, Bootz F. CT and MR imaging after middle ear surgery. *Eur J Radiol* 2001;**40**:113–18.

Chapter 8

# Malignant otitis externa

David Selvadurai and Georgios Oikonomou

## Details of studies

This once rare condition is becoming more common as diabetes prevalence rises. Commonly called necrotizing otitis externa, it overlaps with true skull base osteomyelitis. It is recognized by its clinical presentation. Typically this involves a severely painful external ear canal infection in a diabetic patient. Typically examination shows a stenosed ear canal with granulation at the junction of the bony and cartilaginous canal. It may progress to cartilage destruction in the canal, temporo-mandibular joint and concha. Ultimately osteomyelitis of the skull base and cranial nerve neuropathies may occur. Intracranial complications including vascular thrombosis may also lead to mortality.

This early study outlines a large case series and provides a thorough discussion of the pathogenesis of the disease. Helpfully it outlines a potential treatment plan involving antibiotics and surgery. The surgery described varies from simple debridement to extended mastoidectomy. Today these recommendations must be taken in the context of more effective antibiotic treatments currently available and comparison with the more recent study by Hariga is recommended.

## Study references

### Main study

Chandler JR. Malignant external otitis. *Laryngoscope* 1968;**78**:1257–94.

### Related reference

Hariga I, Mardassi A, Belhaj Younes F, Ben Amor M, Zribi S, Ben Gamra O, et al. Necrotizing otitis externa: 19 cases' report. *Eur Arch Otorhinolaryngol* 2010:**267**:1193–8.

## Study design

Retrospective case note review of experience between 1959 and 1967.

| | |
|---|---|
| Level of evidence | 4 |
| Number of patients | 13 |
| Inclusion criteria | Unclear. Cases that presented with classical symptoms that were felt to meet the diagnosis were included. At least two cases from a previous study were excluded. It is not clear why these cases were not considered. Both diabetic and non-diabetic patients were considered |

| Exclusion criteria | The author excluded cases which were not under his overall care and for whom final outcome was not available. Individual case history descriptions are followed by a description of the overall outcomes. There is a discussion of surgical approaches and pathology. Finally deduced recommendations are made |
|---|---|
| Follow-up | Variable |

## Outcome measures

There was no defined outcome measure but certain features were regularly commented on. Clearly mortality was described in detail and attributed to either the condition directly or concurrent disease. Mention was made of ongoing discharge, or pain. Complete 'cure' appeared to be the absence of symptoms of discharge or pain without ongoing treatment.

## Results

| Number of patients | 13 |
|---|---|
| Average age | 73 years (range 35–87) |
| Diabetics (including IGT) | 92% |
| Cured | 7/13 |
| Died | 6/13 (four from myocardial infarction, one CVA, two osteomyelitis) |
| Microbiology | All infected with *Pseudomonas aeruginosa* |
| Treatment | All received systemic antibiotics, local toilet and varying degrees of surgical debridement |
| Other observations | Six patients were reported to have facial nerve palsy (46%) and three were bilaterally affected. Two patients died directly from the condition, one during surgery and one of intracranial disease. Two diabetic patients were more accurately described in the text as having impaired glucose tolerance |

## Conclusions

The author of this paper concludes that this is a serious condition with potentially fatal consequences. He recommends surgical debridement as the mainstay of treatment in conjunction with topical antibiotic dressings. Early and radical surgical intervention is recommended and to some extent failure to control infection is attributed to under resection of infected tissue. Little importance was given to systemic antibiotics, although all patients received some combination of either oral, intramuscular, or intravenous antibiotics.

## Critique

This is a landmark study for a number of reasons, though the passage of time has certainly affected the relevance of the treatment algorithm suggested. The term 'malignant external otitis' was coined by Chandler in this paper, and has remained in use even today. At the time of this description the need to convey the presentation of a destructive pathology with the potential to have fatal outcome was paramount, but the malignant reference has remained a source of confusion in this non-neoplastic condition.

The study itself falls short of modern research methodology. As a retrospective case study it provides only level 4 evidence. The narrative is detailed but clear inclusion and exclusion criteria are absent. There is no definition of successful outcome and the methodology of the retrospective analysis is unclear. More recent studies have demonstrated that modern management with high dose and prolonged antibiotics is both effective and avoids the disfigurement and prolonged recovery associated with the surgical approach advocated in 1968. Furthermore the advent of advanced imaging using computed tomography, magnetic resonance imaging, and radio-isotope scanning has significantly altered modern management.

Nonetheless in an era of ever-increasing antibiotic resistance the number of satisfactory outcomes obtained using a combination of surgery and limited medical therapy is noteworthy. It is also probable that the events leading to the demise of six patients would be more successfully managed today, and in many cases avoided by prophylaxis and optimal medical care. It may be that future therapy for this troublesome condition can draw on some of these old lessons in selected cases.

Chapter 9

# Tuning fork tests

Olivia Whiteside

## Details of study

Tuning forks are frequently used worldwide as an adjunct in the diagnosis of hearing impairment. Stankiewicz and Mowry evaluated the value of the Rinne, the Weber, and the Bing occlusion tests.

The Bing occlusion test: this is positive if sound is heard louder following occlusion of the ear canal. A positive result occurs in normal or sensorineural hearing loss (SNHL). It is negative in conductive hearing loss (CHL).

The Weber test: the tuning fork is heard midline with normal hearing. In unilateral SNHL, the sound is heard in the unimpaired ear. In unilateral CHL, sound is heard in the impaired ear.

The Rinne test: This is positive in normal hearing and SNHL provided air conduction is greater than bone conduction. It is negative in CHL if bone conduction is greater than air conduction.

## Study references

### Main study

Stankiewicz, JA, Mowry, HJ. Clinical accuracy of tuning fork tests. *Laryngoscope* 1979;**89**:1956–63.

### Related references

Browning G, Swan I, Chew K. Clinical role of informal tests of hearing. *J Laryngol Otol* 1989;**103**:7–11.
Sheehy J, Gardner G, Hambley W. Tuning fork tests in modern otology. *Arch Otolaryngol* 1971;**94**:132.

## Study design

A prospective double-blind study of 268 ears selected 'at random' from patients presenting to the clinic complaining of hearing loss, tinnitus, and/or vertigo.

Metal alloy forks of 256, 512, and 1,024 Hz used as described by Sheehy. Timed method used for Rinne test.

The clinical examination room was used for testing (tuning fork exceeded background noise by at least 14 dB) and testing was unmasked in order to reflect common practice.

## Outcome measures

### Accuracy of tuning fork tests

Validity/reliability and variability of a particular frequency of tuning fork. Tuning fork test results compared with amount of hearing loss, otologic examination, audiogram, and impedance studies.

## Results

With Bing occlusion testing, 72–89% of those with a CHL had a negative result and 39–91% of the normal population or those with SNHL had a negative result.

With Rinne testing, 97–100% of patients with normal hearing or SNHL had a positive test. At 256 Hz, 96% of ears with a negative result had an air–bone gap greater than 20 dB. The greater the conductive loss, the more likely a negative Rinne.

With Weber testing, 70% of normal hearing individuals heard the tone in the midline at 256 Hz. Eighty-six per cent of the bilateral SNHL group heard the tone in the midline at 256 Hz. In unilateral conductive hearing loss only 45% (256 and 1,024 Hz) to 54% (512 Hz) lateralized as traditionally expected. In unilateral SNHL 42% (256 Hz), 58% (512 Hz), and 67% (1,024 Hz) lateralized the sound appropriately.

Weber testing yielded incorrect responses in 33% patients, worsening with increasing frequency of tuning fork. Retesting showed great variability.

Physical examination was found to be extremely accurate in detecting conductive abnormalities. Used with tympanometry, audiology, and reflex testing, results were more accurate and consistent with one another than tuning fork testing.

## Conclusion

1 Tuning fork tests should not be used in the absence of other diagnostic modalities due to lack of reliability

2 Clinical use of the Bing occlusion test is not recommended due to the high rate of false positive and false negative responses

3 The Weber test is only useful in evaluating patients with bilateral hearing loss or normal hearing. In unilateral hearing loss (conductive or sensorineural), the Weber test lateralizes to the appropriate ear similarly to chance.

4 Rinne testing is valid and reliable in normal hearing ears and sensorineural hearing loss. In conductive hearing loss, the Rinne test is of no value, particularly where the air–bone gap is under 25 dB

5 The 256 Hz was the most accurate tuning fork.

## Critique

Though the methodology of this study is questionable, it does reflect how tuning forks are used in clinical practice. The overall conclusion that tuning fork tests should not be used in the absence of other diagnostic modalities such as physical examination, tympanometry, audiology, and reflex testing, has been demonstrated in numerous other studies and is echoed by current clinical practice. This study found that use of the Bing occlusion test is highly questionable, and this is reflected by its lack of use in modern day practice. The same conclusion has been found in a number of other studies.

Browning has performed further tuning fork studies and his view supports the findings of this study in that they are much less useful than is traditionally thought. He found that the Rinne test using a 256 Hz tuning fork correctly identified 95% people with a 30 dB or greater CHL with a specificity of over 90%. He concluded that audiometry, performed correctly and with appropriate masking, was the only acceptable method for differentiating between a conductive and sensorineural impairment.

Browning argues that using tuning forks to back up audiometric findings assumes that they are valid and reliable. He points out that air–bone gaps of around 20 dB are also not reliably detected by audiometry because of the difficulty in precise measurement of bone conduction thresholds, such as due to contact between the skull and bone vibrator, skull geometry, the consistency of skin, effectiveness of masking of the other ear, and unpredictability of patient response causing up to a 10 dB variation in thresholds.

Clinicians persist in using tuning forks for two main purposes. Firstly, tuning forks are used for checking that a patient does not have a dead ear following surgery by lateralizing Weber testing to the operated ear, or hearing the fork next to the ear with masking of the other ear. The scratch test has been found to be a more accurate alternative to this (scratching the head bandage in the midline and asking the patient where the sound is heard or loudest) but assumes a head bandage is present. Secondly, tuning forks are used to corroborate the audiological findings. If the audiogram suggests an air–bone gap over 30 dB that is not corroborated by tuning fork testing, particularly with Rinne testing at 256 Hz, it would seem reasonable to repeat the audiogram.

## Additional references

Browning G. Is there still a role for tuning-fork tests? *Br J Audiol* 1987;21:161–3.

Crowley H, Kaufman R. The Rinne tuning fork test. *Arch Otolaryngol* 1966;87:406.

Iacovidou A, Giblett N, Doshi J, Jindal M. How reliable is the "scratch test" versus the Weber test after tympanomastoid surgery? *Otol Neurotol* 2014;35:762–3.

# Chapter 10

# Audiological aspects of presbyacusis

Casie Keaton

## Details of study

Gates et al. (1990) set out to provide context for the inherent biological and environmental risk factors that contribute to decreased auditory function with age. At the time of the study, the decline of auditory system function with advanced age was well documented. While it was accepted that there is an intrinsic degenerative process over time within the auditory system, there was little consensus as to the degree that biologic and environmental factors contribute to presbycusis. The authors investigated the possible effects of age, gender, past otologic history, and reported exposure to noise within a subset of the Framingham Heart Study patients. The Framingham Heart Study (Kannel 1980) contributed greatly to the understanding of the pathogenesis of cardiovascular disorders and attending risk factors. With the same aim, regarding hearing ability in the elderly, the authors conducted testing on a large cohort of heart study patients in their 60th through 90th decade of life. Repeat auditory measures were completed 6 years later as part of the original Framingham biennial examination cycle.

## Study references

### Main study

Gates GA, Cooper JC, Kannel WB, Miller NJ. Hearing in elderly: the Framingham cohort, 1983-1985. 1. Basic audiometric test results. *Ear Hear* 1990;**11**;247–56.

### Related references

Bielefeld EC, Tanaka C, Chen G, Henderson D. Age-related hearing loss: is it a preventable condition? *Hear Res* 2010;**264**:98–107.

Gates GA, Mills, JH. Presbycusis. *Lancet* 2005;**366**:1111–20.

Kannel, WB, Dawber TR, McGee DL. Perspectives of systolic hypertension: the Framingham Study *Circulation* 1980;**61**:1179–82.

Wong ACY, Ryan AF. Mechanisms of sensorineural cell damage, death and survival in the cochlea. *Front Aging Neurosci* 2015;**7**:58.

## Study design

◆ An observational cohort as part of a cross-sectional study with cardiovascular risk patients

- Intention to assess auditory decline in the elderly

- Broaden the understanding of the pathogenesis of presbycusis

| | |
|---|---|
| Level of evidence | 1b |
| Randomization | None |
| Number of patients | 1662 |
| Inclusion criteria | Ambulatory members of the original Framingham cohort |
| Part A | Administered to all 1,662 subjects |
| Exclusion criteria | Non-ambulatory subjects who were unable to receive testing within the clinical setting |
| Part B | 1,026 of 1,662 without evidence of middle ear disease, prior ear surgery, or asymmetrical hearing thresholds |
| Follow-up | 6 years |

- Part A: brief auditory questionnaire, otoscopy, immittance measures, pure tone thresholds, word recognition presented at a conventional level in the better ear

- Part B: word recognition testing under earphones for the pure tone audiometry (PTA) at 40 dB SL 70 dB HL, and 90 dB HL to determine the relationship of word recognition ability to presentation level

- Data collected with respect to age and gender effects within PTA, impedance measures, and word recognition testing

## Outcome measures

### Primary endpoint

- Prevalence estimates of presbyacusis
- Impedance measures
- Quantified speech understanding ability

### Secondary endpoints

- Hearing handicap
- Tinnitus prevalence
- Results of central auditory tests, longitudinal changes in hearing, and correlations of hearing with cardiovascular status were reported in a later paper.

# Results

| | Gender | Age |
|---|---|---|
| **Hearing thresholds** | | |
| Mean PTA | Poorer in males | Increased |
| Rate of PTA decline | None | Increased |
| High-frequency thresholds | Poorer in males | Increased |
| **Acoustic impedance** | | |
| ME pressure | None | None |
| Acoustic compliance | None | Decreased |
| Contra AR at 1 kHz | Higher in females | Slightly |
| Ipsi AR at 1 kHz | None | None |
| **Articulation index** | | |
| Mean score | Higher in females | Declined |
| Rate of decline | No difference | Increased |
| Word recognition scores | | |
| 50 dB HL presentation level | Higher in females | Declined |
| Max presentation level | Higher in females | Declined |

*Poorer scores in men attributed to higher prevalence of high-frequency HL.

## Conclusion

For most measures of hearing ability, women were found to have better functional outcomes than their male counterparts. This outcome is felt to be attributed to a higher prevalence of noise exposure in men and subsequent associated high-frequency hearing loss. This also accounts for the results of articulation index calculations and word recognition testing. Immittance testing did not yield any important findings in terms of application to clinical practice. There were no interaural differences found on any measure.

## Critique

With increased access to quality medical care, there are estimates that the fastest growing sector of the population are those 65 years of age and older, and that hearing loss is the third most prevalent condition among this group. As life expectancy rises, there is a need to not only effectively care for the elderly, but to provide an understanding of how their choices earlier in life can lead to better overall health as they age.

This was a large cohort study that sought to tease apart specific factors that can contribute to reduced auditory function as we age. The evidence that followed this paper provided important correlations regarding biologic and environmental risk factors and their negative impact on hearing ability. Of interest, 61 of the 979 subjects (6.2%) that reported no hearing loss had a PTA >26 dB HL, meeting the Lloyd and Kaplan (1978) criterion for hearing impairment. This finding may speak to the effect of lifestyle on perceived hearing handicap. The authors were also able to conclude that despite the demonstrated potential benefit of amplification in the study there was a markedly low adoption rate among the cohort, with only 5.4% reporting hearing aid use of those 540 subjects meeting the criteria for benefit. Nearly 30 years later, the literature purports the adoption rate to be as high as 20%, but more investigation is needed to determine how best to close this gap. One suggestion in the literature is to change the hearing rehabilitation model from consumer driven, to a chronic disease model. The evidence strongly supports that hearing well is not just important in maintaining our social and emotional connections, but also cognitive ability. Improved hearing has been shown to ward off cognitive decline and other cognitive diseases.

Rather than accept that presbycusis is something that occurs to the same degree in everyone, the authors set out to shine a light on individual differences that can result in varying degrees of hearing impairment. The results presented were important in refocusing the discussion of presbycusis from one of singular rehabilitation, to a conversation of prevention.

## Additional references

Humes LE, Dubno JR, Gordon-Salant S, Lister JJ, Cacace AT, Cruickshanks KJ, et al.. Central presbycusis: a review and evaluation of the evidence. *J Am Acad Audiol* 2012;23:635–66.

Mamo SK, Nieman CL, Lin FR. Prevalence of untreated hearing loss by income among older adults in the United States. *J Health Care Poor Underserved* 2016;27:1812–8.

Parham K, McKinnon BJ, Eibling D, Gates GA. Challenges and opportunities in presbycusis. *Otolaryngol Head Neck Surg* 2011;144:491–5.

Ruan Q, Ma C, Zhang R, Yu Z. Current status of auditory aging and anti-aging research. *Geriatr Gerontol Int* 2014;14:40–53.

Yamasoba T, Lin FR, Someya S, Kashio A, Sakamoto T, Kondo K. Current concepts in age-related hearing loss: epidemiology and mechanistic pathways. *Hear Res* 2013;303:30–8.

# Chapter 11

# Impedance audiometry

Casie Keaton

## Details of study

This paper served to establish impedance audiometry as an invaluable diagnostic tool, especially in the assessment of young children. Impedance data were collected for analysis from over 400 patients, over the course of 1 year, within a diverse hospital population. Impedance measures were found to have broad clinical implications, which provided great diagnostic advantage when applied to the differential diagnosis of hearing disorders. The findings of this investigation were of great consequence in delineating the methods we use to assess patients then, and today.

## Study references

### Main study

Jerger J. Clinical experience with impedance audiometry. *Arch Otolaryngol* 1970;**92**:311–24.

### Related studies

Nilges TC, Northern JL, Burke KS. Zwislocki acoustic bridge. Clinical correlations. *Arch Otolaryngol* 1969;**89**:727–44.

Zwuskicki JJ, Feldman AS. Acoustic impedance of pathological ears. *ASHA Monogr* 1970;**15**:1–42.

## Study design

- Descriptive study to evaluate efficacy of impedance testing as a routine clinical procedure
- Evaluation of diagnostic value in a typical audiologic case load
- Impedance audiometry carried out by means of an electrostatic impedance bridge (Madsen, type ZO-70) and a pure tone audiometer (Beltone, type 10D)
- Tympanometry, acoustic impedance, and acoustic reflexes performed bilaterally

| | |
|---|---|
| Level of evidence | 1b |
| Number of patients | 400+, measures obtained on 96% of subjects |
| Age | 10 months to 81 years |
| Inclusion criteria | All types and degrees of hearing ability |
| Exclusion from analysis | <2 years of age, suspected or confirmed retrocochlear disorder, functional hearing problems, mixed hearing loss, ossicular discontinuity |
| Analysis sample | 316 patients, 554 ears |
| Data collection period | 1 year |

## Outcome measures

+ Analysis of distributions as a function of age and type of hearing loss
+ Case reports illustrating diagnostic value of measures

## Results

### Tympanometry

+ Results were classified into type A, B, or C pressure-compliance functions
+ Results were as expected with respect to age and type of hearing loss, except in those 2–5 years in age. This cohort presented an increase in incidence of B and C graph patterns in those with normal hearing and sensorineural hearing loss. This suggested the presence of undetected middle ear problems without audiometric evidence of a conductive component

### Acoustic impedance

+ Presented considerable overlap between normal and disordered middle ears. Found to have limited diagnostic value on its own

### Acoustic reflex

+ Analysis was conducted on normal hearing subjects only. Data were pooled since there was no frequency effect found
+ Average acoustic reflex threshold to pure tones occurred at a sensation level of 85 dB in an average normal ear
+ The sensation level was found to be reduced by the presence of loudness recruitment as a function of increasing hearing loss
+ When reflexes were observed at a particular frequency, the hearing threshold at that frequency was no greater than 80 dB HL
+ Absence of reflex may be due to conductive loss, cochlear loss greater than 80 dB, 8th nerve loss at virtually any level, or a facial nerve lesion
+ Acoustic reflexes were absent in those with otosclerosis.
+ Most useful component of impedance audiometry when results are considered singularly

## Conclusion

Impedance audiometry has significant clinical utility, which provides clinicians with a tool for differential diagnosis. Impedance measures have the most impact when considered as a test battery, and have limited value singularly. Impedance measures are helpful in supporting behavioural test results, especially in those difficult to test populations. The authors were able to provide significant evidence for a wide range of diagnostic implications, across age and hearing ability.

## Critique

The innovation of impedance audiometry was first thought to only be useful in the differentiation between ossicular discontinuity and stapes fixation. Surgeons contended that impedance had more academic value, as both conditions indicate surgical intervention. This paper launched a wider clinical benefit of impedance, demonstrating its value as part of the comprehensive audiologic test battery. Modern audiological assessment procedures owe much to the evidence provided in this landmark paper.

At the time this paper was published, impedance instrumentation was in its infancy. The time necessary to complete the impedance test battery was a limitation, particularly when trying to assess young children. Procedures were not automated as they are today with the advent of modern computers. Obtaining a proper seal with the ear canal could be somewhat problematic in all populations. New instrumentation is on the horizon with exciting research to solve these limitations and provide a more robust test for middle ear inefficiency, quickly and noninvasively. These tests (wide band acoustic immitance) are aimed at being used in conjunction with otoacoustic emission measurements in neonates. By providing more specific information as to the status of the auditory system, we can shorten and improve our early identification paths.

## Additional reference

Nakajima HH, Rosowski JJ, Shahnaz N, Voss SE. Assessment of ear disorders using power reflectance. *Ear Hearing* 2013;34: 48–53.

Sanford CA, Brockett JE. Characteristics of wideband immittance in patients with middle-ear dysfunction. *J Am Acad Audiol* 2014;25:425–40.

Chapter 12

# Otoacoustic emissions

Casie Keaton

## Details of studies

The discovery of evoked otoacoustic emissions by Kemp in 1978, greatly contributed to our modern understanding of cochlear mechanics and the dynamic role of outer hair cell function in the efferent auditory system. These findings were a continuation of work by Gold in the 1940s, which was significant in changing the way we thought about frequency coding and pitch perception within the cochlea. Bekesy's earlier work detailing the place and travelling wave theory was the accepted model at the time. His model explained the passive elements of the travelling wave, but could not account for the narrow mechanical tuning measured in the undamaged, living cochlea. This active tuning and specificity suggested there were active elements at work in the cochlea that could account for this phenomenon. Gold's research proposed that within the cochlea there is an active supply of electrical energy which acts to reduce mechanical energy loss, termed the mechanical resonator theory. These findings helped to explain the specific frequency coding and pitch perception in healthy ears. Further work by Brownell in 1983 provided evidence confirming the motility of outer hair cells, which is thought to be the source for the active electrical energy promoting the otoacoustic emission (OAE) response. Dr Kemp's work in OAEs led to an efficient and reliable way to detect early cochlear impairment, which plays a vital role in clinical assessment today.

## Study references

### Main study

Kemp, DT, Ryan S, Bray, P. A guide to the effective use of otoacoustic emissions. *Ear Hear* 1990; 11:93–8.

### Related studies

Brownell WE. Outer hair cell electromotility and otoacoustic emissions. *Ear Hear* 1990;11:82–92.

Kemp, DT. Otoacoustic emissions, travelling waves and cochlear mechanisms. *Hear Res* 1986;22:95–104.

This seminal paper was the first to report on the important applications of OAE response, providing clinicians with a practical standard for measurement interpretation. Requirements for optimal instrument design are outlined, specific to achieving reliable test performance in clinical and screening applications. Evaluation procedures for probe fit and response quality are also detailed. The authors use clinical data obtained with the test instrument that emerged from this study to illustrate the practical possibilities and problems in applying OAEs to screening and diagnostic measurement. The evidence presented in the related studies provide foundation and support for which the report is based.

## Key outcomes

◆ Seminal guideline for OAE clinical application, test instrument design, and measurement interpretation

◆ Design of TEOAE system (TLO88) that would meet specific test conduction requirements, but could be applied to the design of future instrumentation

◆ Techniques offered to achieve optimum probe placement and measurement quality outside of laboratory test conditions

◆ Signal processing methods developed to reject non-cochlear acoustic response, minimize artefact

◆ OAEs are highly stable, which allows for monitoring of minute changes of cochlear function as a result of noise, ototoxic drugs, pathology, or efferent excitation

## Foundation for clinical application

Kemp's work demonstrated that sound could be recovered from the cochlea using an ear canal microphone probe with either tone or click stimuli. OAEs represent a leakage of energy from the functional forward travelling wave due to some mechanical perturbation. The primary value of otoacoustic emissions is that their presence indicates that the preneural cochlear receptor mechanism (and middle ear mechanism) can respond to sound in a normal way. In general, only normal, or near normal ears produce acoustic emissions at all.

◆ Normal hearing threshold is only achieved with the aid of some cochlear mechanism which magnifies the vibrational stimulus internally. When this mechanism diminishes, otoacoustic emissions diminish and threshold is raised

◆ Evoked OAEs provide a unique perspective of the interaction of mechanical sound vibration and the physiological activity in the cochlea

◆ Emissions are frequency specific and frequency selective; it is possible to gain information about different parts of the cochlea simultaneously

◆ OAEs do not translate to threshold data, and cannot replace audiometric data

◆ Spontaneous emissions (SOAEs) are present in 40–60% of healthy ears, are not necessary for normal hearing, and therefore have limited clinical utility

◆ Evoked emissions, distortion product (DPOAEs), or transient evoked (TEOAEs) are easily observed in the healthy ear and have been deemed to have the most clinical utility in a variety of test conditions

## Conclusions

With the findings of this research, Kemp patented the OAE measurement technique for the purpose of early detection of auditory dysfunction, particularly in children. He formed his own company Otodynamics in 1988 to manufacture TE and DP OAE systems for screening and research use. The ILO88 TEOAE played a vital role in demonstrating the viability of universal hearing screening of neonates. Early identification of hearing loss in newborns has led to more streamlined intervention. No other clinical test can specifically assess cochlear biomechanics or combine the operational speed, non-invasivity, objectivity, sensitivity, frequency selectivity, and noise immunity of otoacoustic emissions testing. With its advent, we now possess a powerful tool in early detection of sensory hearing impairment. OAEs have become an indispensable aspect of the clinical test battery.

## Critique

While the link between OAEs and outer hair cell function is clinically useful, there is still no strong correlation between OAEs and auditory thresholds. For this reason, OAEs are limiting in providing a specific test of hearing acuity. There is also significant limitation in identification of retrocochlear disorders, such as auditory neuropathy. However, there is exciting research on the horizon investigating stimulus frequency otoacoustic emissions (SFOAE) that show a stronger correlation to behavioural thresholds. This research is still emerging and does not yet have the clinical utility of threshold prediction.

There is great evidence that OAEs provide an effective tool for the monitoring of ototoxic agents, specifically in the treatment of cancer patients. While this application has been well established, it would be encouraging to see a higher adoption rate within oncology. This would afford patients with more informed choices when considering the consequences of therapy.

### Additional references

Ellison JC, Keefe DH. Audiometric predictions using stimulus-frequency otoacoustic emissions and middle ear measurements. *Ear Hear* 2005;**26**:487–503.

Hall, JW. *Handbook of Otoacoustic Emissions.* 2000; San Diego, CA: Singular Thomson Learning.

Heitmann J, Waldmann B, Plinkert PK. Limitations in the use of distortion product otoacoustic emissions in objective audiometry as the result of fine structure. *Eur Arch Otorhinolaryngol* 1996;**253**:167–71.

Konrad-Martin D, Poling GL, Dreisback LE, Reavis KM, McMillan GP, Lapsley Miller JA, Marshall L. Serial monitoring of otoacoustic emissions in clinical trials. *Otol Neurotol* 2016;**37**:286–94.

# Part II

# **Neurotology**

# Chapter 13

# A facial nerve grading system

Walter Kutz

## Details of study

The House–Brackmann Facial Nerve Grading Scale (HBGS) scale was initially described in 1983 and adopted by the Facial Nerve Disorders Committee of the American Academy of Otolaryngology—Head and Neck Surgery in 1984. In 1983, House analysed eight current facial nerve grading systems and created a new facial nerve grading system based on the strengths of the current systems. House concluded a gross scale is the best system since it is simple, practical, and is as reliable as more complex systems that are more time intensive to complete. In addition, secondary deficits such as synkinesis and contracture are addressed in the HBGS. In 1984, the HBGS was modified by the Facial Nerve Disorders Committee and recommended as the standard facial nerve grading scale. The modified HBGS included the measurements of the eyebrow and commissure of the mouth at 0.25 mm intervals with a maximum score of 4 to help more objectively categorize patients. Although objective measurements are recommended in the HBGS, most observers do not perform measurements and subjectively estimate dysfunction. Another change from the initial version is that secondary deficits (synkinesis, etc.) can be seen in mild dysfunction.

Because of inherent limitations with the HBGS, the Facial Nerve Disorders Committee published Facial Nerve Grading Scale 2.0 (FNGS2) in 1999 (Vrabec et al. 2009). The committee felt the original HBGS had the following deficits: (1) does not discriminate between different regions of the face, (2) secondary deficits such as synkinesis are not adequately addressed, (3) too high interobserver variability, (4) inadequately discriminates between clinically different recoveries, and (5) inadequate for recovery of surgically repaired nerves. The committee revised the grading system based on the original HBGS. The FNGS2 changed measurements to a four-point scale to include the brow, eye, nasolabial fold, and oral commissure. In addition, secondary deficits were measured globally using a 0–3 point scale. The scores were calculated and the grade of facial deficit was determined based on the total score.

Despite revising the HBGS with FNGS2, the original HBGS is still most widely used. The original HBGS is easier to perform and requires less time and has been shown to be as reliable as the FNGS2 (Henstrom et al. 2011; Lee et al. 2013). In 2014, Lenzi et al. published that the modified HBGS was the most widely cited otolaryngology publication.

## Study references

### Main studies

House JW. Facial nerve grading systems. *Laryngoscope* 1983;**93**:1056–69.

House JW, Brackmann DE. Facial nerve grading system. *Otolaryngol Head Neck Surg* 1985;**93**:146–7.

### Related references

Lenzi R, Fortunato S, Muscatello L. Top-cited articles of the last 30 years (1985-2014) in otolaryngology—head and neck surgery. *J Laryngol Otol* 2016;**130**:121–7.

Vrabec JT, Backous DD, Djalilian HR, Gidley PW, Leonetti JP, Marzo SJ, et al; Facial Nerve Disorders Committee. Facial Nerve Grading System 2.0. *Otolaryngol Head Neck Surg* 2009;**140**:445–50.

## Study design

Consensus statement.

## Outcome measures

### Primary endpoint

Degree of facial movement.

### Secondary endpoints

Secondary defects (synkinesis, contracture, hemifacial spasm).

## Results

The modified HBGS of 1985 measures facial movement of the eyebrow and oral commissure using 0.25 mm increments up to 1 cm with a total possible score of 8. This score is used to determine the grade of facial dysfunction. Secondary deficits such as synkinesis and contracture results in grade II (slight), grade III (moderate), or grade IV (disfiguring). Grades V and VI do not mention secondary deficits.

| Grade | Description | Description |
|---|---|---|
| I | Normal | Normal facial function in all areas |
| II | Mild dysfunction | Gross: slight weakness noticeable on close inspection; may have very slight synkinesis<br>At rest: normal symmetry and tone<br>Motion<br>Forehead: moderate to good function<br>Eye: complete closure with effort<br>Moth: slight asymmetry |
| III | Moderate dysfunction | Gross: obvious but not disfiguring difference between two sides; noticeable but not severe synkinesis, contracture, and/or hemifacial spasm<br>At rest: normal symmetry and tone<br>Motion<br>Forehead: slight to moderate movement<br>Eye: complete closure with effort<br>Mouth: slightly weak with maximum effort |

| Grade | Description | Description |
|-------|-------------|-------------|
| IV | Moderately severe dysfunction | Gross: obvious weakness and/or disfiguring asymmetry<br>At rest: normal symmetry and tone<br>Motion<br>Forehead: none<br>Eye: incomplete closure<br>Mouth: asymmetric with maximum effort |
| V | Severe dysfunction | Gross: only barely perceptible motion<br>At rest: asymmetry<br>Motion<br>Forehead: none<br>Eye: incomplete eye closure<br>Mouth: slight movement |
| VI | Total paralysis | No movement |

Data sourced from House JW, Brackmann DE. Facial nerve grading system. *Otolaryngol Head Neck Surg* 1985;93(2):146–7.

## Conclusion

Despite some limitations, the House–Brackmann facial nerve grading system has continued to be the primary facial nerve grading system used and is the most commonly cited paper in the otolaryngology literature. The grading system has the advantage of being simple and quick to perform with relatively high interobserver reliability. The challenge with the HBGS is reliably differentiating grade III and grade IV paresis.

## Critique

Despite the publication of a multitude of facial nerve grading systems, no grading system been found to adequately address all challenges found in any grading system. In an attempt to improve the HBGS, the American Academy of Otolaryngology—Head and Neck Surgery Facial Nerve Disorders Committee updated the original House–Brackmann grading scale in 1999. The authors identified deficits in the initial scale, which included an inability to distinguish between clinically different recovery, the fact that secondary deficits were not adequately addressed, a high interobserver variability, inaccuracy in the setting of differential facial movement, and inadequacy for the surgical repair of the facial nerve. Despite the possibility of a more objective grading system using the FNGS2, subsequent studies showed the HBGS was near equal in interobserver reliability and was easier to administer. The greatest challenge in the HBGS is to differentiate moderate (grade III) and moderately severe (grade IV) grades. A patient without forehead movement but with eye closure could be considered a grade III paresis; although, some may choose a grade IV paresis since forehead movement is absent.

## Additional references

Lee HY, Park MS, Byun JY, Chung JH, Na SY, Yeo SG. Agreement between the Facial Nerve Grading System 2.0 and the House-Brackmann Grading System in patients with Bell palsy. *Clin Exp Otorhinolaryngol* 2013;6:135–9.

Henstrom DK, Skilbeck CJ, Weinberg J, Knox C, Cheney ML, Hadlock TA. Good correlation between original and modified House Brackmann facial grading systems. *Laryngoscope* 2011;121:47–50.

Chapter 14

# Medical management of Bell's palsy

John Phillips

## Details of studies

Unilateral idiopathic facial nerve palsy (Bell's palsy) affects between 11 and 40 persons per 100,000 each year. This can be associated with significant facial disfigurement, psychological problems, and facial pain. Although the true aetiology is not fully understood, there has been some work performed to suggest that herpes infection is implicated at onset. Controversy remains regarding the use of steroids and antiviral medications for Bell's palsy. To address this, Sullivan et al. performed a large double-blind, placebo-controlled, randomized trial to address our poor understanding of treatment outcomes for patients when treated during the acute phase of this condition.

## Study references

### Main study

Sullivan FM, Swan IR, Donnan PT, Morrison JM, Smith BH, McKinstry B, et al. Early treatment with prednisolone or acyclovir in Bell's palsy. *N Engl J Med* 2007;357:1598–607.

### Related references

Allen D, Dunn L. Aciclovir or valaciclovir for Bell's palsy (idiopathic facial paralysis). *Cochrane Database Syst Rev* 2004;3:CD001869.

Salinas RA, Alvarez G, Ferreira J. Corticosteroids for Bell's palsy (idiopathic facial paralysis). *Cochrane Database Syst Rev* 2004;4:CD001942.

## Study design

- A prospective multicentre, double-blind, placebo-controlled, randomized trial
- Intention to treat design
- Prednisolone was provided at a dose of 25 mg twice daily
- Acyclovir was provided at a dose of 400 mg five times daily

| | |
|---|---|
| Level of evidence | 1b |
| Randomization | Prednisolone versus acyclovir versus both agents versus placebo for 10 days |
| Number of patients | 551 |
| Inclusion criteria | Adults (16 years of age or older) |

| | | |
|---|---|---|
| | Unilateral facial-nerve weakness of no identifiable cause | |
| | Presentation within 72 hours after onset of symptoms | |
| Exclusion criteria | Pregnancy or breast-feeding | |
| | Uncontrolled diabetes or peptic ulcer | |
| | Suppurative otitis media, herpes zoster, or multiple sclerosis | |
| | Systemic infection, or sarcoidosis | |
| Follow-up | 3 months and 9 months | |

## Outcome measures

### Primary endpoint

- House–Brackmann grading system to assess facial-nerve function

### Secondary endpoints

- Health Utilities Index Mark 3 to assess health-related quality of life
- Derriford Appearance Scale 59 to assess facial appearance
- Brief pain inventory to assess pain

## Results

| | Prednisolone | | No prednisolone | |
|---|---|---|---|---|
| | **Odds ratio (95% CI)** | **p** | **Odds ratio (95% CI)** | **p** |
| Acyclovir | 1.76 (0.74–4.16) | 0.20 | 0.58 (0.28 (0.29–1.16) | 0.12 |
| No acyclovir | 3.23 (1.13–9.22) | 0.03 | 1.00 | |

## Conclusion

When provided during the acute phase of a Bell's palsy, prednisolone significantly improved the chance of complete recovery of facial nerve function at 3 and 9 months. When acyclovir was provided during the same circumstances, either alone, or in combination with prednisolone, there was no evidence of any benefit.

## Critique

This was a large multicentre trial that covered the entire population of Scotland. It was conducted to a high standard with low levels of bias, and as such these results have significant implications for clinical practice. The use of the House–Brackmann scale has been criticized for a variety of reasons, but for this study it was well suited because of its ability to reliably assign patients to a recovery status. Since the publication of this study, there has been some work to suggest that the use of corticosteroids may not be beneficial for Bell's palsies of all degrees of severity. In addition to this, although this study did not demonstrate any benefit from the administration of acyclovir, other authors have demonstrated benefit when using an alternative antiviral medication. The updated Cochrane review that considers all antiviral treatments for Bell's palsy concludes that there was some benefit from administering antivirals in combination with corticosteroids as compared with administering corticosteroids alone for the treatment of Bell's palsy in certain circumstances, but this was based on low-quality evidence. In addition to this, it was suggested that the administration of antivirals with corticosteroids reduced the long-term after-effects of Bell's palsy (excessive tear production and synkinesis) compared with corticosteroids alone.

## Additional references

Ferreira M, Firmino MJ, Marques EA, Santos PC, Duarte JA. Are corticosteroids useful in all degrees of severity and rapid recovery of Bell's palsy? *Acta Otolaryngol* 2016;**22**:1–6.

Gagyor I, Madhok VB, Daly F, Somasundara D, Sullivan M, Gammie F, Sullivan F. Antiviral treatment for Bell's palsy (idiopathic facial paralysis). *Cochrane Database Syst Rev* 2015;**11**:CD001869.

Hato N, Yamada H, Kohno H, Matsumoto S, Honda N, Gyo K, et al. Valacyclovir and prednisolone treatment for Bell's palsy: a multicenter, randomized, placebo-controlled study. *Otol Neurotol* 2007;**28**:408–13.

# Chapter 15

# Surgical management of Bell's palsy

Walter Kutz

## Details of study

Idiopathic facial nerve paralysis, or Bell's palsy, is likely to be the result of reactivation of the herpes simplex virus. Recovery to normal facial function can be expected in the majority of patients. However, there are a subset of patients that do not fully recover and can be left with poor facial function and disfiguring secondary defects such as synkinesis or hemifacial spasm. The evidence is clear that the use of oral steroids with or without antivirals is the effective medical treatment. The role of surgical decompression is more controversial.

Gantz et al. (1999) sought to answer the following questions in their landmark paper:

1 How can patients with poor prognosis for facial function recovery be identified?

2 Can poor outcomes be improved with surgical decompression?

3 If surgery is beneficial, does the timing of surgery influence outcomes?

To answer these questions, the authors developed a multicenter, case–control trial comparing the outcomes of patients presenting with Bell's palsy who were determined to have a poor prognosis for recovery using electric testing. Using previous data by Fisch and Esslen, the authors identified patients with a poor prognosis to have electroneurography with >90% degeneration, no voluntary motor unit potentials on electromyelogram, and present within 14 days of onset of paralysis. If a patient was found to meet these criteria, they were offered a middle fossa craniotomy with decompression of the meatal foramen, labyrinthine segment, geniculate ganglion, and tympanic segment. Patients were not randomized since they could choose if they wanted to undergo surgical decompression or medical therapy alone.

## Study references

### Main studies

Gantz BJ, Rubinstein JT, Gidley P, Woodworth GG. Surgical management of Bell's palsy. *Laryngoscope* 1999;109:1177–88.

## Study design

◆ Multicentre, case–control

◆ Non-randomized

- Fourteen centres participated; although only three centres had more than one patient that underwent surgery. This paper described the experience at the University of Iowa only

- Thirty patients were identified with unfavourable recovery (electroneurography >90% degeneration, no voluntary motor unit potentials on electromyelogram, and presentation within 14 days)

- Three groups were identified: patients that chose medical management alone that consisted of prednisone 80 mg daily for 7 days followed by a 7 day taper (n = 11); patients that underwent surgical decompression within 14 days of onset of facial nerve paralysis (n = 19); patients that underwent decompression between 14 and 28 days (n = 7)

## Primary endpoint

- Final facial nerve recovery measured by the House–Brackmann Facial Nerve Grading Scale

## Secondary endpoints

- Does electroneurography predict which patients fall in a poor prognostic category?

- Facial nerve outcomes if decompressed greater than 14 days after the onset of paralysis

- Facial nerve outcomes based on time of onset of paralysis to decompression within the 14-day period

## Results

The mean ages of the three groups were as follows: (1) steroid-only group was 47 years (range 23–66 years); surgical decompression within 14 days was 32 years old (range 9–58 years); and decompression greater than 14 days was 41 years (range 20–57 years). A good outcome (House–Brackmann Grade of I or II) was achieved in 91% of patients who underwent surgical decompression within 14 days of the onset of facial paralysis compared to only 42% of patients achieving a good outcome with treatment of oral steroids alone. This difference was found to be significant (p < 0.0002). The surgical decompression patients outside the 14 days showed similar recovery to the steroid-only group with both groups combining to achieve a good recovery 33% of the time. No patient in any group had a recovery worse than a House–Brackmann grade III. Of the 54 patients that did not meet inclusion criteria because electroneurography showed <90% degeneration, 100% had a good recovery, with 89% achieving a House–Brackmann grade I. Finally, the authors reported better outcomes with earlier decompression. Surgical complications included a patient with a conductive hearing loss of 20 dB and another patient with a cerebrospinal fluid leak that required a temporary lumbar drain.

## Conclusion

Surgical decompression through a middle fossa approach should be considered in patients with Bell's palsy who have no visible motion, electroneurography showing >90% degeneration, no voluntary motor unit potentials on electromyelogram, and present within 14 days of onset of paralysis. Earlier decompression is correlated with more favourable outcomes.

## Critique

The management of facial paralysis in the setting of Bell's palsy continues to be controversial. This study is a well-designed study showing benefit of a middle fossa approach and facial nerve decompression over oral steroids alone. Despite the evidence presented here, the universal adoption of facial nerve decompression has not been established. In 2011, Smouha et al. sent a questionnaire to the members of the American Otologic Society and the American Neurotology Society asking about decompression for facial paralysis from Bell's palsy. Approximately two-thirds of the respondents said they would decompress the nerve if the electric testing was unfavourable and within 10 days of the onset of paralysis. Only 22% reported performing more than five decompressions in a 10-year period.

A potential weakness in the study is the lack of randomization since patients could chose whether or not they wanted to proceed with surgical decompression. The lack of randomization is the reason this study is not included in the Cochrane review of the surgical management of Bell's palsy. Also, the patients that elected surgical decompression were younger than patients that chose steroids alone, 32 years versus 47 years, respectively. Another limitation of this study is the use of electroneurography, which is not available at all centres. In addition, electroneurography is not useful if a patient presents with bilateral Bell's palsy since there is not a normal side to use a control. Finally, although a middle fossa decompression surgery is generally safe, there are potential serious side effects of haemorrhage, hearing loss, cerebrospinal leak, further damage to the facial nerve, and seizure.

## Additional references

McAllister K, Walker D, Donnan PT, Swan I. Surgical interventions for the early management of Bell's palsy. *Cochrane Database Syst Rev* 2013;2:CD007468.

Smouha E, Toh E, Schaitkin BM. Surgical treatment of Bell's palsy: current attitudes. *Laryngoscope* 2011;**121**:1965–70.

Chapter 16

# The anatomical location of tinnitus

Don McFerran

## Details of studies

Defined as the conscious perception of an auditory sensation in the absence of a corresponding external stimulus, tinnitus is a common symptom with point prevalence figures quoted at between 10% and 20% of the adult population. The exact pathophysiology of tinnitus is incompletely understood and medical management is currently aimed at ameliorating the impact rather than eradicating the perception. A serendipitous observation occurred in 1935 (Bárány) when a patient undergoing nasal surgery reported temporary relief from tinnitus following an intranasal injection of the ester local anaesthetic, procaine. Subsequent work showed that temporary tinnitus relief also occurs following intravenous injection of certain other local anaesthetic drugs, from both ester and amide groups. Most ensuing studies have investigated lidocaine, the most commonly used local anaesthetic agent, which temporarily reduces tinnitus in approximately 60% of subjects. A small number of subjects experience the opposite effect and report exacerbation of their tinnitus. Possible sites of action for this tinnitus reducing effect include the cochlea, cochlear nerve and/or the central auditory system. To try and confirm the presence of a central site of action, Baguley et al performed a double-blind, placebo-controlled, crossover randomized trial, administering intravenous lidocaine to patients who had undergone translabyrinthine removal of a vestibular schwannoma within the previous decade.

## Study references

### Main study

Baguley DM, Jones S, Wilkins I, Axon PR, Moffat DA. The inhibitory effect of intravenous lidocaine infusion on tinnitus after translabyrinthine removal of vestibular schwannoma: a double-blind, placebo-controlled, crossover study. *Otol Neurotol* 2005;**26**:169–76.

### Related reference

Bárány R. Die Beeinflussung des Ohrensausens durch intravenös Injizierte lokalanästhetica. *Acta Otolaryngolog* 1935;**23**:201–3.

## Study design

A prospective single-centre, double-blind, placebo-controlled, randomized crossover trial.

| | |
|---|---|
| Level of evidence | 1b |
| Randomization | Lidocaine versus placebo (normal saline) |
| Number of patients | 16 |
| Inclusion criteria | Patients who had undergone translabyrinthine removal of a unilateral, sporadic, histologically proven vestibular schwannoma within the previous 10 years |
| Exclusion criteria | Patients who had undergone removal of a vestibular schwannoma by other routes such as the suboccipital route. Non-specified medical conditions that would contraindicate lidocaine administration |

## Outcome measures

### Primary measures

Visual analogue scale (VAS) measures of tinnitus pitch, intensity and tinnitus-related distress. Measures pre-infusion and at 5 and 20 minutes post infusion.

### Secondary measure

Tinnitus Handicap Inventory (THI) questionnaire.

## Results

THI was performed at the recruitment stage and the median value was 31 (range 0–82); 12 (75%) subjects reported reduction of their tinnitus; two (12.5%) reported no change; two (12.5%) reported worsening of all parameters. The Wilcoxon signed-rank test was performed on the VAS data.

| | | p values for difference in VAS scores between lidocaine and placebo infusions | | |
|---|---|---|---|---|
| | | **Tinnitus loudness** | **Tinnitus pitch** | **Tinnitus distress** |
| Time after lidocaine infusion | 5 minutes | 0.036 | 0.026 | 0.04 |
| | 20 minutes | 0.066 | 0.173 | 0.058 |

## Conclusions

Intravenous infusion of lidocaine significantly reduced all measured tinnitus parameters. This effect was brief. The site of action of lidocaine in this trial must be in the central auditory pathways.

# Critique

This was a small trial with a highly original design that produced evidence that, within a specific cohort of patients, the tinnitus suppressing site of action of lidocaine was central. This evidence was used to suggest that drugs that have similar action within the central auditory system should be investigated for possible tinnitus inhibiting effect. The study did not claim that lidocaine cannot also have a peripheral action: other studies have pointed to both central and peripheral actions. Martin and Colman (1980) extrapolated from work with lidocaine on chronic pain to suggest a central site of action. A retrocochlear site was supported by Ruth et al. (1985), who showed that lidocaine administered intravenously produced prolongation of wave V of brainstem evoked response audiometry in healthy non-tinnitus volunteers. In a similar fashion, Lenarz et al. (1986) demonstrated prolongation of interpeak latencies of brainstem evoked response audiometry in some tinnitus patients when given lidocaine. Proponents of a peripheral source of action have used evidence from lidocaine's effect on otoacoustic emissions (Haginomori et al. 1995; Laurikainen et al. 1996) and electrocochleography (Majumdar et al., 1983) to suggest that the cochlea is implicated. Englesson et al. (1976) demonstrated that radiolabelled lidocaine is taken up in the modiolus of the cochlea.

The main mechanism of action of lidocaine is blockage of fast voltage gated sodium channels in neurons. A compound that has such fundamental action may well have effect at multiple sites within the auditory system. Furthermore the pathogenesis of tinnitus appears heterogeneous (Landgrebe et al. 2010) and different patients may have different pharmacological targets.

The main study had flaws. The number of participants was small and the randomization produced an unbalanced allocation. The trial did not prove that the site of lidocaine's action was central: the participants all had functioning peripheral auditory systems on the contralateral side to their vestibular schwannoma. The blinding of the trial may have been incomplete: some participants were aware of perioral tingling when receiving the lidocaine but not when receiving the placebo. A crossover design was used but only amalgamated pre-and post-crossover data were presented. Patients with tinnitus following vestibular schwannoma surgery may not be representative of the wider tinnitus community.

## Additional references

Englesson S, Larsson B, Lindquist NG, Lyttkens L, Stahle J. Accumulation of 14C-lidocaine in the inner ear. Preliminary clinical experience utilizing intravenous lidocaine in the treatment of severe tinnitus. *Acta Otolaryngol* 1976;**82**:297–300.

Haginomori S, Makimoto K, Araki M, Kawakami M, Takahashi H. Effect of lidocaine injection of EOAE in patients with tinnitus. *Acta Otolaryngol* 1995;**115**:488–492.

Landgrebe M, Zeman F, Koller M, Eberl Y, Mohr M, Reiter J, et al. The Tinnitus Research Initiative (TRI) database: a new approach for delineation of tinnitus subtypes and generation of predictors for treatment outcome. *BMC Med Inform Decis Mak* 2010;**10**:42.

Laurikainen EA, Johansson RK, Kileny PR. Effects of intratympanically delivered lidocaine on the auditory system in humans. *Ear Hear* 1996;17:49–54.

Lenarz T. Treatment of tinnitus with lidocaine and tocainide. *Scand Audiol Suppl* 1986;26: 49–51.

Majumdar B, Mason SM, Gibbin KP. An electrocochleographic study of the effects of lignocaine on patients with tinnitus. *Clin Otolaryngol Allied Sci* 1983;8:175–80.

Martin FW, Colman BH. Tinnitus: a double-blind crossover controlled trial to evaluate the use of lignocaine. *Clin Otolaryngol Allied Sci* 1980;5:3–11.

Ruth RA, Gal TJ, DiFazio CA, Moscicki JC. Brain-stem auditory-evoked potentials during lidocaine infusion in humans. *Arch Otolaryngol* 1985;111:799–802.

Chapter 17

# Tinnitus in normal hearing individuals

Don McFerran

## Details of study

Among the recurring questions regarding tinnitus is whether it is possible to experience tinnitus with normal peripheral auditory system function. To try and ascertain whether people with normal hearing could experience tinnitus in abnormally quiet environments Heller and Bergman (1953) placed 80 volunteers in a sound-proofed chamber, asked them to listen carefully and record any sounds they perceived. The ambient sound in the chamber was less than the available equipment could detect and was estimated at between 15 dB and 18 dB.

## Study reference

### Main study

Heller MF, Bergman M. Tinnitus aurium in normally hearing persons. *Ann Otol Rhinol Laryngol* 1953;**62**:73–83.

## Study design

Cross-sectional study.

|  | Participants with hearing loss | Participants with normal hearing |
| --- | --- | --- |
| Number of participants | 100 | 80 |
| Study location | Outpatient clinic | Soundproof chamber |
| Inclusion criteria | Armed forces veterans with audiometrically confirmed hearing loss | Adults between 18 and 60 with self-reported normal hearing, no tinnitus and good general health. Sedentary occupations |
| Exclusion criteria | None stated | History of previous aural disease |

## Outcome measures

### Participants with hearing loss

- Otological history and examination
- Pure tone audiometry
- Presence or absence of tinnitus and qualitative description of any tinnitus

## Participants Laryngol hearing

◆ Qualitative description of any perceived sound

# Results

The prevalence of participants with a hearing loss who reported hearing sounds (tinnitus) in their normal daily life is shown.

|  | Number of participants with hearing loss | Percentage of participants with hearing loss |
|---|---|---|
| Reporting hearing a sound (tinnitus) | 73 | 73 |
| Reporting hearing no sound (no tinnitus) | 27 | 27 |
| Total | 100 | 100 |

The prevalence of participants with normal hearing who reported hearing one or more sounds when placed in a soundproof chamber is shown.

|  | Number of participants with normal hearing | Percentage of participants with normal hearing |
|---|---|---|
| Reporting hearing a sound (tinnitus) | 75 | 93.75 |
| Reporting hearing no sound (no tinnitus) | 5 | 6.25 |
| Total | 80 | 100 |

There were 39 different descriptions of sounds perceived. Those that occurred at least three times in either group are tabulated.

| Sound | Number of reports in hearing loss group | Percentage of those with hearing loss reporting sound | Number of reports in normal hearing group | Percentage of those with normal hearing reporting sound |
|---|---|---|---|---|
| Bell | 3 | 3 | 0 | 0 |
| Buzz | 12 | 12 | 13 | 16.25 |
| Hiss | 3 | 3 | 3 | 3.75 |
| Hum | 10 | 10 | 16 | 20 |
| Ring | 32 | 32 | 11 | 13.75 |
| Steam | 4 | 4 | 0 | 0 |
| Roar | 5 | 5 | 2 | 2.5 |
| Whistle | 9 | 9 | 3 | 3.75 |

| Sound | Number of reports in hearing loss group | Percentage of those with hearing loss reporting sound | Number of reports in normal hearing group | Percentage of those with normal hearing reporting sound |
|---|---|---|---|---|
| Click | 3 | 3 | 0 | 0 |
| Falling water | 3 | 3 | 4 | 5 |
| Insects/crickets | 2 | 2 | 6 | 7.5 |
| Squeak | 0 | 0 | 3 | 3.75 |
| Pulse | 0 | 0 | 7 | 8.75 |
| Thumping pulsation | 0 | 0 | 4 | 5 |

## Conclusions

Heller and Bergman concluded that head noises perceived among normal hearing people placed in a sound-proof room occurred at about the same frequency as tinnitus occurs in people with hearing loss in normal ambient sound and that the quality of the perceived sounds was broadly similar. They suggested that tinnitus is constantly present in normal hearing people but is masked by the ambient sound of our environment. Their logical, if unsettling, conclusion was that tinnitus is a normal physiological phenomenon which, because it is omnipresent, cannot be eradicated. Treatment, at best, can only ever make it sub-audible.

## Critique

The main study was very much 'research of its time' and subsequently came in for criticism. In particular, the true hearing of the group that self-defined as normal was questioned. No hearing test had been performed on this group. Also, the sound level in the test chamber had been estimated rather than accurately measured.

Several subsequent studies have re-explored the theme using greater scientific rigour. Tucker et al. (2005) investigated 120 young people with audiometrically normal hearing between 250 Hz and 8 kHz, finding that tinnitus-like sounds were perceived in 64% overall. They found that gender did not affect outcome but there were some differences between Caucasians and African Americans.

Knobel and Sanchez (2008) investigated how attention affects the emergence of sound perception: participants with normal hearing between 250 Hz and 8 kHz were asked to solve a Tower of Hanoi puzzle, pay visual attention, or pay auditory attention. Auditory phantom perception was reported in 19.7%, 45.5%, and 68.2%.

Some criticism was directed at this later research, pointing out that normal pure tone audiometry between 250 Hz and 8 kHz does not guarantee an absence of cochlear pathology. It was suggested that defining normal hearing in this manner meant that the subjects might have subtle cochlear defects that were being overlooked.

Del Bo et al. (2008) undertook the most rigorous study to date using much tighter definitions of normal cochlear function and normal hearing. Fifty-three young (mean age 22 years) people with normal extended range audiograms (250 Hz to 16 kHz), normal tympanometry, normal distortion product otoacoustic emissions and normal stapedial reflexes were asked to listen while in an anechoic chamber. For the first experiment, the chamber was empty. In the second experiment a fake loudspeaker was introduced. When the loudspeaker was absent 83% reported perceiving at least one sound. When the loudspeaker was present the figure rose to 92%. The investigators concluded that tinnitus perceptions do emerge in silent environments and suggestive mechanisms play only a minor role. Although these subsequent trials did not quite reach the levels demonstrated by Heller and Bergman they all showed that when people with normal hearing are asked to listen in a silent environment the majority will experience tinnitus like activity.

## Additional references

Del Bo L, Forti S, Ambrosetti U, Costanzo S, Mauro D, Ugazio G, et al. Tinnitus aurium in persons with normal hearing: 55 years later. *Otolaryngol Head Neck Surg* 2008;**139**: 391–4.

Knobel KA, Sanchez TG. Influence of silence and attention on tinnitus perception. *Otolaryngol Head Neck Surg* 2008;**138**:18–22.

Tucker DA, Phillips SL, Ruth RA, Clayton WA, Royster E, Todd AD. The effect of silence on tinnitus perception. *Otolaryngol Head Neck Surg* 2005;**132**:20–4.

Chapter 18

# A neurophysiological model of tinnitus

Don McFerran

## Details of studies

In the UK and much of the rest of the world, the medical management of tinnitus uses either psychological modalities such as cognitive behaviour therapy and mindfulness meditation or an audiological strategy using sound therapy, education, counselling, and stress management techniques. In 1990 an American neurophysiologist, Pawel Jastreboff, published a lengthy review paper describing the existing scientific knowledge regarding tinnitus. This work subsequently became known as the neurophysiological model of tinnitus. Jastreboff collaborated with a British otologist Jonathan Hazell, and in 1993 they published an article on the clinical implications of the previous work. This laid the foundations for a systematic protocol for delivering audiological tinnitus management which subsequently became known as tinnitus retraining therapy (TRT). The first part of this article was essentially a synopsis of the 1990 work. Various theories regarding the site of generation of tinnitus in the auditory system were expounded.

| Hypothesized site of tinnitus generator | Proposed mechanism by which tinnitus could be generated |
|---|---|
| Discordant damage of outer hair cells (OHCs) and inner hair cells (IHCs) | If OHCs are lost but IHCs remain, local collapse of the tectorial membrane onto the IHCs could occur, causing depolarization of those cells |
| Crosstalk between cochlear nerve fibres | Pressure on the nerve from an adjacent blood vessel or a tumour could cause a breakdown of the insulation properties of the nerve causing electrical activity to spread between neurons |
| Ionic imbalance within the cochlea | Calcium homeostasis is fundamental to normal cochlear functioning. Altered calcium levels could affect multiple areas including the link between OHCs and the tectorial membrane, the OHCs body, or neurotransmitter release mechanisms |
| Dysfunction of cochlear neurotransmitter systems | Increased levels of neurotransmitter release either spontaneously or in response to sound could increase cochlear neural activity. Increased effectiveness of the neurotransmitter due to increased sensitivity of the post-synaptic site could also achieve this |
| Heterogeneous activation of the efferent system | Reduced inhibition by the efferent system could increase cochlear neural activity or enhance one of the other tinnitus generating mechanisms |
| Heterogeneous activation of type I and type II cochlear afferents | Type I fibres synapse with IHC; type II with OHC. If OHCs are lost, imbalanced neural activity results which could cause imbalance at higher centres in the auditory system |

Although this part of the paper focused very much on cochlear and auditory nerve pathology, Jastreboff and Hazell went on to explain that the central auditory system plays a pivotal role in the development of tinnitus. They suggested that there are three separate stages.

| Stage of tinnitus emergence | Anatomical site | Process |
| --- | --- | --- |
| Generation | Usually in the peripheral auditory system (cochlear or auditory nerve) | Production of a neural signal that can then misconstrued as a sound |
| Detection | Sub cortical brain centres | Pattern recognition processes highlight the tinnitus signal from other neuronal activity |
| Perception and evaluation | Within the auditory cortex and other areas, particularly the limbic system and the pre-frontal cortex. | The sound sensation is perceived and activation of systems of emotion creates distress. The distress causes enhanced perception which results in a vicious circle being generated |

The remainder of the study describes how the two authors manage patients with tinnitus in their respective clinics. They recognize that although the tinnitus generator signal is usually in the cochlea or auditory nerve they cannot directly treat this. They stress the importance of a multidisciplinary team with access to otologists, audiologists, neurophysiologists and clinical psychologists. They describe the diagnostic processes that they undertake, putting stress on the importance of checking for hyperacusis: they regard hyperacusis as a marker of increased gain within auditory pathways and recommend the routine measurement of loudness discomfort levels at multiple frequencies.

| Component | Delivery | Rationale |
| --- | --- | --- |
| Directive counselling | Explaining to the patient the processes that lead up to tinnitus and addressing any concerns or questions | To retrain the patient's thinking regarding tinnitus and to reclassify tinnitus as a benign and harmless phenomenon |
| Sound therapy | Wearable ear level sound generators (maskers) to deliver low-level neutral acoustic signal, typically white noise. Alternatively, if there is associated hearing loss, hearing aids may be used to increase awareness of normal environmental sound | Interferes with perception of the tinnitus generator signal. Meaningless and therefore relatively easy to habituate to. Delivered at a low level which does not significantly impede normal hearing |
| Management of associated emotional disturbance | Clinical psychologist | Anxiety control using thought blocking and relaxation techniques. Measures for dealing with associated insomnia |

## Study references

### Main study

Jastreboff PJ, Hazell JW. A neurophysiological approach to tinnitus: clinical implications. *Br J Audiol* 1993;27:7–17.

### Related reference

Jastreboff PJ. Phantom auditory perception (tinnitus): mechanisms of generation and perception. *Neurosci Res* 1990;8:221–54.

## Study design

Review and expert opinion. Level of evidence, 5.

## Critique

Jastreboff and Hazell did not present any new scientific or clinical research in either the main or related study. However, they did provide a very useful synthesis of the available knowledge regarding tinnitus. They also supplied broad treatment principles which are still in use a quarter of a century later though there was not enough detail supplied in the paper to enable clinicians to deliver the treatment they were recommending. Both authors set up training courses and for a long time this was the only method of learning how to deliver TRT. It was over a decade later that a detailed description of how to undertake TRT was made available (Jastreboff and Hazell 2004). Various subsequent papers were published expanding the underpinning theories and a useful diagram of the neurophysiological model was published in 1996, with an enhanced version appearing in 1999. In the original study, Jastreboff and Hazell mention that they had achieved good results using their management strategy but no figures were supplied to validate this claim. Many subsequent studies have purported to test TRT but often, when these studies are examined in detail, the investigators have deviated from the strict protocol of TRT. A Cochrane review looked at trials of TRT and found only one admissible study (Phillips and McFerran 2010): this study did show some benefit when using TRT.

Although there are many areas where TRT can be criticized its introduction had an enormous impact on the world of tinnitus management.

### Additional references

Jastreboff PJ. The neurophysiological model of tinnitus and hyperacusis. 1999. In: Hazell J (ed.). *Proceedings of the Sixth International Tinnitus Seminar.* Cambridge: The Tinnitus and Hyperacusis Centre; 32–38.

Jastreboff PJ, Gray WC, Gold SL Neurophysiological approach to tinnitus patients. *Am J Otol* 1996;7:236–40.

Jastreboff PJ, Hazell JWP. *Tinnitus retraining therapy. Implementing the neurophysiological model.* Cambridge UK: Cambridge University Press, 2004.

Phillips JS, McFerran D. Tinnitus retraining therapy (TRT) for tinnitus. *Cochrane Database Syst Rev* 2010;3:CD007330.

# Chapter 19

# The head thrust test

Louisa Murdin

## Details of studies

An accurate diagnostic clinical examination at the bedside has long been regarded as a key medical professional skill. Clinical signs are ideally simple to elicit and have high diagnostic sensitivity and specificity. A good clinical examination helps to avoid unnecessary, expensive and intrusive diagnostic investigations. This paper by Halmagyi and Curthoys in 1988 described such a clinical sign, which has been shown to be both simple and useful.

## Study references

### Main study

**Halmagyi GM, Curthoys IS.** A clinical sign of canal paresis. *Arch Neurol* 1988;45:737–9.

## Study design

The study was designed to test the value of the head thrust test as a sign of canal paresis. The authors used the scleral search coil (a highly accurate means of eye movement recording) to record eye movement during rapid head accelerations with visual fixation in patients with clearly defined vestibular deficits; and to compare these results with 'gold standard' caloric test outcomes.

- Level of evidence: not applicable
- Randomization: not applicable
- Number of patients: 12
- Inclusion criteria: unilateral vestibular neurectomy for vestibular schwannoma or intractable vertigo
- Exclusion criteria: none
- Follow-up: not applicable

## Outcome measures

- Primary endpoint: Search coil evidence of refixation saccades when the head was turned ipsilesionally; caloric test results

## Results

In all 12 patients clinically evident contraversive refixation saccades were elicited during ipsilesional head rotation. None of the control subjects showed this sign. The results were similar in those with surgery one week previously and those tested after 1 year. Peak head acceleration was 3,000 degrees/second.

## Conclusions

Oppositely directed saccades during rapid horizontal head movements indicate a severe horizontal semicircular canal lesion on the side to which the head is being rotated.

## Critique

This test is a simple and well-tolerated clinical assessment of the vestibulo-ocular reflex (VOR) which can be easily used at the bedside. The test was devised on the basis of a detailed understanding of the physiology of the vestibular system including Ewald's second law, which states that excitatory stimuli to the labyrinth produce a stronger response than inhibitory stimuli. Saccades, pursuit and VOR eye movement systems can all be used to maintain visual fixation. The initiation of the VOR is extremely fast; and a unilateral deficit of vestibular function means that other (slower) pathways must be used. This is visible as a 'catch-up' saccade.

To carry out the test, the patient is instructed to fixate on a suitable target (often the examiner's nasal bridge); the hands of the examiner are placed over the sides of the patient's head which is then subjected to low amplitude but high acceleration thrusts. These should be unpredictable in timing and direction for best response. Some co-operation is required as the patient must be able and willing to fixate on a visual target; the test cannot be performed in individuals with significant cervical spine disease or pain; however it can be readily achieved in most outpatient situations.

The paper from Halmagyi and Curthoys shows that that there is a high degree of sensitivity and specificity in patients with total unilateral loss of vestibular function. The paper does not report the test against the more common scenario in clinical practice of a partial unilateral loss of vestibular function; however, it is known that the test can be positive in such patients. This paper only reports on 12 patients and up to 1 year follow-up. It is now known that in the longer term, the test will often normalize due to the learned use of pre-programmed compensatory saccades.

It is also now recognized that the head thrust test can be effectively carried out in the vertical planes as well as the horizontal plane. A vertical head thrust can, with practice, be carried out in either the plane of the right anterior–left posterior canals (RALP) or the left anterior–right posterior canals (LARP). This allows a detailed anatomical characterization in conditions such as vestibular neuritis.

Automated systems have been designed to record the output of the head thrust test (video head impulse test (VHIT)) and can measure gain of the reflex as well as document the presence of saccades. The VHIT can also detect saccades that occur very early while the head is still moving (covert saccades) rather than simply those visible to the naked eye of an external observer which are only apparent once the head movement has ceased (overt saccades).

The clinical value of the head thrust test has been underlined by work on the assessment of patients with acute vertigo. Many such patients will have a unilateral vestibular disorder such as vestibular neuritis, and will show an associated positive head thrust test in the side of the pathology. A normal head thrust test indicates that the VOR is intact, indicating that the origin of the vertigo is central rather than peripheral. It has been shown that a careful clinical examination including this key sign is a more sensitive indicator of posterior circulation stroke in the early stages than magnetic resonance imaging.

The head thrust test has therefore been transformative in neuro-otology because it is a simple and well-tolerated technique for assessing vestibular function in a way that has been clearly linked to important clinical outcomes.

## Additional reference

Kattah JC, Talkad AV, Wang DZ, Hsieh Y-H, Newman-Toker DE. Hints to diagnose stroke in the acute vestibular syndrome three-step bedside oculomotor examination more sensitive than early MRI diffusion-weighted imaging. *Stroke* 2009;**40**:3504–10.

Chapter 20

# Benign paroxysmal positional vertigo

Louisa Murdin

## Details of studies

Benign paroxysmal positional vertigo (BPPV) is the commonest cause of episodic vertigo with 1-year incidence estimates ranging from 0.06% to 0.6% (Murdin 2014). Despite its name, it is not benign in terms of associated disability, being also the commonest cause of presentations with isolated vertigo to emergency departments (Cutfield 2011) and a significant contributing factor for falls in older people (Lawson 2005). Prior to the publication of this paper in 1992, treatment options included the Brandt–Daroff exercises (Brandt and Daroff 1980), the Semont liberatory manoeuvre and posterior semicircular canal plugging. Previous treatments had been designed primarily around the pathomechanism of cupulolithiasis (Schuknecht 1969). Epley (1992) postulated that symptoms could also be related to canalolithiasis and designed a repositioning manoeuvre (canalith repositioning manoeuvre (CRP)) accordingly.

## Study references

### Main study

Epley JM. The canalith repositioning procedure: for treatment of benign paroxysmal positional vertigo. *Otolaryngol Head Neck Surg* 1992;**107**:399–404.

### Related references

Brandt T, Daroff RB. Physical therapy for benign positional vertigo. *Arch Otolaryngol Head Neck Surg* 1980;**106**:484–5.

Dix MR, Hallpike CS. The pathology, symptomology and diagnosis of certain common disorders of the vestibular system. *Ann Otol Rhinol Laryngol* 1952;**87**:987–1016.

Schuknecht HF. Cupulolithiasis. *Arch Otolaryngol* 1969;**90**:765–78.

## Study design

♦ Observational case series

♦ Designed to record the effectiveness of the canal CRP

| | |
|---|---|
| Level of evidence | 4 |
| Randomization | None |
| Number of patients | 30 |

| Inclusion criteria | All patients with 'classic' posterior canal BPPV treated with CRP over an 18-month period; diagnosed by the Dix–Hallpike manoeuvre |
| --- | --- |
| Exclusion criteria | Patients who had had previous CRPs |
| Follow-up | 30 months |

## Outcome measures

| Primary endpoint | Resolution of vertigo and positional nystagmus |
| --- | --- |
| Secondary endpoints | Time to recurrence of symptoms |

## Results

Ninety per cent had vertigo and nystagmus resolved at initial follow-up, and 10% had resolution of nystagmus but ongoing non-positional vertigo. BPPV recurred in 30% patients. One patient had four recurrences and was offered surgery which was declined. The authors noted significant but temporary nausea as an unwanted effect.

## Conclusions

The CRP technique was concluded to be effective and generally well tolerated.

## Critique

A recent systematic review considered that the Epley CRP manoeuvre was a 'safe, effective treatment for posterior canal BPPV, based on the results of 11, mostly small, randomized controlled trials with relatively short follow-up' (Hilton 2014). The development of simple effective treatment procedures for BPPV, the commonest cause of vertigo has been said to be 'the most important therapeutic breakthrough in the field of neuro-otology in 25 years' (Baloh 2005).

Epley designed the CRP based on his understanding of the pathophysiology of benign paroxysmal positional vertigo of the posterior canal and published this observational study to show that it was safe and effective. The manoeuvre has been widely adopted into clinical practice, and allows treatment of what can be a highly disabling condition with a short non-invasive intervention with very low risk of any harm. The intervention is simple and can be done in almost all patients with nothing more than an examination couch required by way of equipment. Patients with spinal disorders (especially if cervical) or mobility problems are the main groups for whom the procedure can be difficult.

Epley recommended the use of mastoid vibration and for patients to stay upright for a period after the intervention. Subsequent studies have not confirmed a specific advantage of these aspects of the procedure over and above the basic CRP manoeuvre.

Complications are rare. Epley noted that the provocation of symptoms (dizziness and nausea) is a significant aspect of the procedure and advocated pre-treatment with anti-nausea agents.

One complication not mentioned in the paper is the possibility to transform posterior canal BPPV into other forms (e.g. of the anterior or horizontal canal), but this is an unusual occurrence.

Hi-tech versions of the CRP that involve mechanized chairs into which patients can be strapped to allow whole body rotation rather than head on trunk manipulation have been devised. These may have a role for those rare cases of spinal disease or poor mobility where the CRP cannot be performed in the normal clinic environment. However, given the simplicity and low expense of the CRP as originally along with its very high efficacy and acceptability it seems unlikely that expensive technologies will find a role in most settings.

## Additional references

Baloh RW. Preface. *Audiolog Med* 2005;3:2–3.

Cutfield NJ, Seemungal BM, Millington H, Bronstein AM. Diagnosis of acute vertigo in the emergency department. *Emerg Med J* 2011;**28**:538–9.

Hilton MP, Pinder DK. The Epley (canalith repositioning) manoeuvre for benign paroxysmal positional vertigo. *Cochrane Database Syst Rev* 2014:CD003162.

Lawson J, Johnson I, Bamiou DE, Newton JL. Benign paroxysmal positional vertigo: clinical characteristics of dizzy patients referred to a Falls and Syncope Unit. *QJM* 2005;**98**:357–64.

Murdin L, Schilder AGM. Epidemiology of balance symptoms and disorders in the community: a systematic review. *Otol Neurotol* 2015;**36**:387–92.

Chapter 21

# Ménière's disease

Louisa Murdin

## Details of studies

Prosper Ménière's described his eponymous disorder in 1861, noting a condition in which there was a liability to vertiginous episodes lasting several minutes, associated with aural fullness, tinnitus, and fluctuations in hearing. More than 150 years later, this condition continues to be a challenge to individual sufferers and their clinicians at every level of diagnosis and management.

The evidence base for management decisions in Ménière's disease has historically been rather weak. It could be argued that it is a condition which is especially challenging for the researcher; with its variable phenotype and natural history, absence of a single diagnostic marker, and the prominence of subjective symptoms. These features all make the execution and reporting of outcomes in clinical trials particularly problematic. The need for standardization of diagnosis and outcomes reporting in Ménière's disease is well-recognized. The papers here illustrate the progress to date in this difficult area.

## Study references

### Main study

Pearson BW, Brackmann DE. Committee on hearing and equilibrium guidelines for reporting treatment results in Ménière's disease. *Otolaryngol Head Neck Surg* 1985;**93**:579–81.

### Related references

Committee on Hearing and Equilibrium guidelines for the diagnosis and evaluation of therapy in Ménière's disease. *Otolaryngol Head Neck Surg* 1995;**113**:181–5.

Lopez-Escamez JA, Carey J, Chung WH, Goebel JA, Magnusson M, Mandalà M, Newman-Toker DE, Strupp M, Suzuki M, Trabalzini F, Bisdorff A. Diagnostic criteria for Ménière's disease. *J Vestib Res* 2015;**25**:1–7.

## Study design

The 1985 paper is an editorial piece; reporting on guidelines developed by the Committee on Hearing and Equilibrium of the American Academy of Otolaryngology and Head and Neck Surgery. The paper develops from an original publication by the AAO-HNS in 1972.

- Level of evidence: not applicable
- Randomization: not applicable

- Number of patients: not applicable
- Inclusion criteria: not applicable
- Exclusion criteria: not applicable
- Follow-up: not applicable
- Primary endpoint: not applicable

## Results

The diagnostic criteria proposed depended on a combination of clinical descriptors of the attacks and also pure tone audiometric features. The committee proposed a method of quantifying the attacks and also the hearing loss of Ménière's disease for standardization purposes to allow comparability between different clinical trials; and also a grading system for disability. The system relies on the number of definitive episodes per month; and the pure tone audiometric threshold at 0.5, 1, 2, and 3 kHz.

## Conclusions

The proposed diagnostic and treatment reporting criteria are affirmed. However the authors rightly recognize that these criteria and reporting standards will inevitably evolve as understanding of the condition further develops.

## Critique

The 1985 AAO-HNS paper was a landmark in Ménière's disease because of its influence on the evidence-based culture in neuro-otology. It consolidated the view that progress in evidence-based medicine could only be made with standardization of diagnosis and reporting, and was a key point in the path towards such standardization.

In 1972, the AAO-HNS had defined diagnostic criteria for Ménière's disease as

1  Fluctuating, progressive, sensorineural deafness.
2  Episodic, characteristic definitive spells of vertigo lasting 20 minutes to 24 hours with no unconsciousness; vestibular nystagmus always present.
3  Tinnitus (ringing in the ears, from mild to severe); often the tinnitus is accompanied by ear pain and a feeling of fullness in the affected ear. Usually the tinnitus is more severe before a spell of vertigo and lessens after the vertigo attack

The opening position of the 1985 paper is the comment on the need for a restrictive diagnosis including only those cases with the full complement of classic symptoms.

The paper discusses issues around the choice of audiometric criteria; in particular the decision to use 3 kHz but not to use 0.25 kHz. The authors argue that this is a more useful strategy for monitoring effectiveness of treatment in the longer term, and note the importance of higher frequencies in normal hearing. The authors acknowledge the impact of tinnitus, unsteadiness and aural pressure but says that because of a lack of objectivity 'they can play no part in the objective evaluation of treatment'.

The AAO-HNS guidelines were reviewed and further updated in 1995. The audiometric criteria were further developed, focusing on asymmetry and low frequency predominance. The audiometric criteria are used to define the stage of the Ménière's disease. The dizziness disability scale is expanded in terms of detail and categories. The 1995 paper also makes a distinction between 'definite', 'certain', 'probable', and 'possible' Ménière's disease. This is a significant change from the earlier 1985 paper which sought to identify only a restricted group. The Committee states that these latter groups 'might constitute important groups to study ... it would be desirable to have a treatment that would prevent progression to successive stages and further loss of hearing.'

The AAO-HNS guidelines were a definitive influence on research into Ménière's disease. Most published trials have attempted to use them to report outcomes. However; there are reports that many papers do not use them correctly. Uptake is improving: a recent paper recorded an increase in the proportion of published studies fulfilling the AAO-HNS criteria for diagnosis (86.5–97%) and treatment outcome (49–55.4%) when comparing two consecutive decades of literature. Nonetheless the observation that only 55% use the treatment outcome still seems rather low.

The guidelines were an influence on the international document from the Barany Society and other national and international groups. This document refers only to 'definite' and 'probable' Ménière's disease; describes audiometric criteria in more detail; and provides more detail about the differential diagnosis and clinical characteristics.

There are a number of criticisms that can be made of all of these diagnostic criteria. For example, the AAO-HNS criteria are an example of diagnosis by committee, meaning that a group of self-selected experts have produced a list of the criteria that they consider to be valuable, without any apparent reference to external validation beyond acceptance by the international community in neuro-otology. There is also the 'catch-all' use of 'not better accounted for by another disorder', which would not be necessary if the authors were truly confident about the nature of the entity they were dealing with. This last and easily overlooked line of the diagnostic criteria serves to remind us how much more there is still to understand about this diagnosis.

## Additional references

Equilibrium CoHa. Committee on Hearing and Equilibrium. Report of Subcommittee on Equilibrium and its Measurement. Ménière's disease: criteria for diagnosis and evaluation of therapy for reporting. *Trans Am Acad Ophthalmol Otolaryngol* 1972;**76**:1462–4.

Lopez-Escamez JA, Carey J, Chung WH, Goebel JA, Magnusson M, Mandalà M, et al. Diagnostic criteria for Ménière's disease. *J Vest Res* 2015;**25**:1–7.

Syed MI, Ilan O, Leong AC, Pothier DD, Rutka JA. Ménière's syndrome or disease: time trends in management and quality of evidence over the last two decades. *Otol Neurotol* 2015;**36**:1309–16.

# Chapter 22

# Endolymphatic sac decompression

Walter Kutz

## Details of study

Treatment of Ménière's disease continues to be controversial because there is no one universally accepted treatment paradigm. The high placebo effect makes studying treatment options challenging. Thomsen et al. (1981) had doubts of the efficacy of the endolymphatic sac shunt surgery, and designed a prospective, randomized trial comparing endolymphatic sac shunt surgery with a regular mastoidectomy (placebo). The authors randomized patients that failed medical therapy into an active group that underwent endolymphatic sac shunt surgery with placement of Silastic that drained into the mastoid cavity and a placebo group that underwent a regular mastoidectomy. The endolymphatic sac was not decompressed in the placebo group. The presence of active disease was established by a three-month lead in period where the participants filled out a dizziness questionnaire. The definition of active disease was not described. After surgery, the subjects rated their symptoms on a 0–3 scale. Each month the subject's otologist, who was blinded to the operation type, determined the subject's present state of the disease by giving a score from 0 to 10. Pure tone audiometry was measured before and after treatment. Subjects pre- and postoperative results were categorized using to the American Academy of Ophthalmology and Otolaryngology (AAOO) classification for Ménière's disease (1972). The median values of the patients total score for the five parameters was determined and used for statistical analysis.

## Study references

### Main study

Thomsen J, Bretlau P, Tos M, Johnsen NJ. Ménière's disease: endolymphatic sac decompression compared with sham (placebo) decompression. *Ann NY Acad Sci* 1981;**374**:820–30.

### Related studies

Bretlau P, Thomsen J, Tos M, Johnsen NJ. Placebo effect in surgery for Ménière's disease: a three-year follow-up study of patients in a double blind placebo controlled study on endolymphatic sac shunt surgery. *Am J Otol* 1984;**5**:558–61.

Bretlau P, Thomsen J, Tos M, Johnsen NJ. Placebo effect in surgery for Menière's disease: nine-year follow-up. *Am J Otol* 1989;**10**:259–61.

Thomsen J, Bretlau P, Tos M, Johnsen NJ. Placebo effect in surgery for Ménière's disease. A double-blind, placebo-controlled study on endolymphatic sac shunt surgery. *Arch Otolaryngol* 1981;**107**:271–7.

## Study design

- Randomized, controlled trial
- Double-blinded
- Thirty subjects randomized equally to endolymphatic sac shunt surgery versus simple mastoidectomy (placebo)
- Subjects filled out daily questionnaire with score from 0 to 3
- Median of total scores were used for statistical analysis
- Minimum follow up was 12 months. None lost to follow-up

## Outcome measures

### Primary endpoint

- Improvement in all Ménière's symptoms

### Secondary endpoints

- Nausea and vomiting
- Dizziness or vertigo
- Tinnitus and subjective hearing impairment
- Pressure in the ear
- Global score
- Objective hearing

## Results

Both the active and placebo groups showed improvement in overall symptoms ($p < 0.1$), and no significant difference was seen between the groups. All subjects in the active group showed improvement, while four subjects in the placebo group showed decline in function. Nausea and vomiting also improved in both groups ($p < 0.1$), and no significant difference was seen between groups. Both groups showed improvement in dizziness and vertigo scores ($p < 0.01$), and the active group had a significantly improved score compared to the placebo group ($p < 0.05$). The authors describe this as 'slightly significant' and determined the difference disappears when two of the placebo subjects are removed from analysis. No difference was found between groups when looking at tinnitus and subjective hearing impairment. There was significant improvement in both groups in pressure in the ear, but no difference was found when comparing groups. The median monthly global score for both the active and placebo groups improved ($p < 0.005$); however, there was no difference between the groups. The pure-tone audiogram showed no difference in pre- and postoperative objective hearing between groups when the three-tone average (250, 500, and 1000 Hz) was analysed. There was a larger number of active patients compared to placebo subjects categorized as class A or B on the AAOO post-treatment reporting criteria, but this was not found to be significant.

## Conclusion

Thomsen et al. concluded that the endolymphatic sac shunt surgery and placebo surgery resulted in improvement in all symptoms of Ménière's disease. The authors also found no benefit of endolymphatic sac shunt surgery over a regular mastoidectomy.

## Critique

Ever since this manuscript was published, there have been critics of the methodology, data analysis, and conclusions. One glaring concern is the inclusion of five patients with bilateral disease. The authors do not describe how they determined which ear was the active ear before treatment. Also, the authors do not discuss if postoperative symptoms could be caused by the untreated ear. The study is also underpowered and creates the risk of a type II error where no difference is found between groups when a difference exists. When comparing the effect of treatment on dizziness and vertigo, the authors found a 'slightly significant' difference ($p < 0.05$) between the active and placebo groups. Most statisticians would consider $p < 0.05$ to be significant. The authors then proceed to remove two of the scores in the placebo group, which make the $p > 0.05$. The authors concluded there was no difference in the pure-tone average, but the data is not described. Finally, the authors admit this study cannot be replicated since the adoption of the Declaration of Helsinki since the declaration mandates participants in medical studies be aware of the specifics of the study making a surgical placebo study unethical.

In a comprehensive re-evaluation of the data, Welling and Nagaraja (2000) concluded the active group undergoing an endolymphatic shunt significantly improved in most categories compared with the placebo group. The authors extracted the data from the charts in the manuscript using three observers and then reanalysed the data. Welling and Nagaraja (2000) make the point that Thomsen et al. (1981) did not describe their statistical methods adequately. Vaisrub (1981) also had similar concerns regarding the statistics used and that it was unclear if preoperative, postoperative, or the difference in scores were used to compare between the active and placebo groups. Welling and Nagaraja concluded the active group showed significant improvement in all categories except subjective hearing loss over the placebo group. Pillsbury et al. (1983) also performed an alternative analysis and argued that the active group showed more improvement when using the 1972 AAOO criteria for treatment of Ménière's disease. The authors show that 87% of the active group resulted in a class A or B compared to only 47% of the placebo patients. The authors also support Vaisrub's concerns that the data was averaged within patients and not across patients, which could result in missing interactions and trends. Pillsbury et al. (1983) also showed that vertigo control was better in all months in the active group than the placebo.

### Additional references

Arenberg IK. Placebo effect for Ménière's disease sac shunt surgery disputed. *Arch Otolaryngol* 1981;107:773–4.

Pillsbury HC 3rd, Arenberg IK, Ferraro J, Ackley RS. Endolymphatic sac surgery. The Danish sham surgery study: an alternative analysis. *Otolaryngol Clin North Am* 1983;16:123–7.

Vaisrub N. Summary statement to 'Placebo effect for Ménière's disease sac shunt surgery disputed.' *Arch Otolaryngol* 1981;107:774.

Welling DB, Nagaraja HN. Endolymphatic mastoid shunt: a reevaluation of efficacy. *Otolaryngol Head Neck Surg* 2000;122:340–5.

Chapter 23

# Vestibular migraine

Louisa Murdin

## Details of studies

Migraine would currently be considered one of the commonest pathologies seen in any clinic specializing in dizziness. For decades it had been recognized that migraine and vertigo might be linked (Kayan 1984). The entity of basilar type migraine, in which vertigo is a recognized posterior circulation aura symptom occurring before a migraine headache, has long been recognized by migraine specialists. However, a number of epidemiological studies had highlighted a potentially broader connection between migraine and vertigo. It had become increasingly clear that the vertigo associated with migraine was not restricted to such a specific aura phenomenon. Furthermore, there was a clear clinical need for research to identify how to best to manage this patient group. Workers in this field were using varied terminology including migraine related dizziness/vertigo, migraine vestibulopathy and migraine associated dizziness/vertigo without any clear consensus on definitions; meaning that clinical and scientific advances in the field were limited. This paper by Neuhauser et al. (2001) was a landmark in reconciling these different perspectives.

## Study references

### Main study

Neuhauser H, Leopold M, von Brevern M, Arnold G, Lempert T. The interrelations of migraine, vertigo and migrainous vertigo. *Neurology* 2001;**56**:436–41.

### Related references

Lempert T, Olesen J, Furman J, Waterston J, Seemungal B, Carey J, et al. Vestibular migraine: diagnostic criteria. *J Vestib Res* 2012;**22**:167–72.

## Study design

Prospective observational study set in dizziness, migraine and orthopaedic clinics.

- ◆ Level of evidence: not applicable
- ◆ Randomization: not applicable
- ◆ Number of patients: 200

- Inclusion criteria: patients attending dizziness, migraine and orthopaedic clinics
- Exclusion criteria: none given
- Follow-up: not applicable

## Outcome measure

Primary endpoint: prevalence of migrainous vertigo (defined by the authors) in the different settings

Secondary endpoints: prevalence of migraine in the dizziness and orthopaedic clinics

## Results

The prevalence of migraine was higher in the dizziness clinic group (38%) than the orthopaedic clinic control group (24%, p 0.01). The prevalence of migrainous vertigo was 7% in the dizziness clinic group, and 9% in the migraine clinic group. In 15 of 33 patients with migrainous vertigo, vertigo was regularly associated with migrainous headache. In 16 patients, vertigo occurred both with and without headache, and in two patients headache and vertigo never occurred together. The duration of attacks varied from minutes to days.

## Conclusions

These results substantiate the epidemiologic association between migraine and vertigo and indicate that migrainous vertigo affects a significant proportion of patients both in dizziness and headache clinics. The study also proposed a clear definition of migrainous vertigo.

## Critique

The paper provided additional clear evidence of an epidemiological link between migraine and vertigo in a well-designed study with an appropriate control.

This paper was influential in neuro-otology primarily in terms of the clear definition of migrainous vertigo that was given: (1) recurrent vestibular symptoms (rotatory/positional vertigo, other illusory self or object motion, head motion intolerance); (2) migraine according to the criteria of the International Headache Society (IHS); (3) at least one of the following migrainous symptoms during at least two vertiginous attacks: migrainous headache, photophobia, phonophobia, visual or other auras; and (4) other causes ruled out by appropriate investigations. The definition was derived from the clinical experience of the authors rather than from any pathophysiological or theoretical basis.

It has been widely adopted into clinical practice and research. It formed the basis of the consensus document between the IHS and the Barany Society with changes including that the duration of vertigo attacks was required to be at least 5 minutes and up to 72 hours. The name was also changed to 'vestibular migraine'.

The paper also emphasizes the important clinical point that for many patients the dizziness and vertigo symptoms frequently occur in the absence of headache.

The validity and stability of the criteria have also been demonstrated over time. What has yet to be proven is the existence of any specific treatment strategies for vestibular migraine as distinct from other forms of migraine. The current Cochrane review of trials of prophylactic agents for vestibular migraine had no trials of an adequate standard for review, but at the time of writing such trials are underway.

## Additional references

Kayan A, Hood JD. Neuro-otological manifestations of migraine. *Brain* 1984;**107**:1123–42.

Lempert T, Olesen J, Furman J, Waterston J, Seemungal B, Carey J, et al. Vestibular migraine: diagnostic criteria. *J Vestib Res* 2012; **22**:167–72.

Radtke A, Neuhauser H, von Brevern M, Hottenrott T, Lempert T. Vestibular migraine—validity of clinical diagnostic criteria. *Cephalalgia* 2011;**31**:906–13.

# Chapter 24

# Semicircular canal dehiscence

Paul Lambert

## Details of study

Bony dehiscence of the superior semicircular canal was first described by Minor et al. in 1998. It had been long recognized that sound or pressure induced vestibular and eye (oscillopsia) symptoms (Tullio's phenomenon and Hennebert's sign respectively) could be caused by various pathologies including Ménière's disease, syphilis, and chronic otitis media/cholesteatoma erosion into the horizontal semicircular canal. Bony dehiscence of the superior semicircular canal is now known to be the most common condition eliciting these symptoms. Further studies have expanded the initial clinical description to a syndrome that can include autophony, exaggerated bone conduction (e.g. 'hearing' mastication or walking on a hard surface; bone conductive thresholds better than 0 dB HL), pulsatile tinnitus, and pseudo-conductive hearing loss with intact acoustic reflexes. In addition to the description by Minor et al. of the superior semicircular canal dehiscence, surgical plugging of the dehiscence via a middle cranial fossa craniotomy was proposed as a therapeutic intervention.

## References

### Main study

Minor LB, Solomon D, Zihreich, JS, Zee DS. Sound—and/or pressure-induced vertigo due to bone dehiscence of the superior semicircular canal. *Arch Otolaryngol Head Neck Surg* 1998;**124**:249–58.

### Related references

Chien WW, Carey JP, Minor LB. Canal dehiscence. *Curr Opin Neurol* 2011;**24**:25–31.

Minor LB. Clinical manifestation of superior semicircular canal dehiscence. *Laryngoscope* 2005;**115**:1717–27,

## Study design

- Level of evidence: 4
- Randomization: None
- Number of patients: eight
- Case series from a single institution collected over a 2-year period

## Outcome measures

♦ Catalogue of signs and symptoms

♦ Temporal bone CT findings

♦ Description of eye movements and response to sound and pressure using video-oculography or a scleral search coil

♦ Audiometric findings

♦ Symptom status in two patients undergoing surgery (plugging of superior semicircular canal dehiscence)

## Results

Patients with sound and/or pressure induced vertigo, disequilibrium, and/or oscillopsia underwent fine cut (1 mm) temporal bone CT scans. Eight patients were identified with a bony dehiscence of a superior semicircular canal (SSCD). The most common complaints in these patients were sound induced eye movements in six out of eight, pressure induced eye movements in five out of eight, and chronic disequilibrium in five out of eight. The most common findings were sound evoked eye movements in six of eight patients and pressure induced eye movements in six of eight patients. In seven patients the symptoms had been present from 3 months to 7 years and in a 41 year old it had been present for 'as long as he could remember.'

Seven of the eight patients had vertical-torsional eye movements in the plane of the affected superior semicircular canal in response to pressure (Valsalva manoeuvre or pressure applied to the external auditory canal) or sound (various tones from 250–3,000 Hz at 90–110 dB). Neither electronystagmography nor rotary chair testing were predictive of a SSCD. Three of the eight patients showed a 10–20 dB conductive hearing loss in the 500–1,000 Hz range.

A thorough explanation of the problem and avoidance counselling of provoking stimuli was satisfactory treatment for six of the eight patients. Two patients persisted with disabling disequilibrium and underwent plugging of the dehiscence through a middle cranial fossa craniotomy. One patient had near total resolution of disequilibrium and nystagmus with unchanged hearing. The other patient had symptom relief for 2 months, then recurrence of symptoms necessitating re-exploration. Disequilibrium and pressure induced imbalance improved after the second surgery, but pure tone thresholds and speech recognition scores began fluctuating; iatrogenic endolymphatic hydrops was postulated.

## Conclusion

The authors concluded that a bony dehiscence over the superior semicircular canal creates a third mobile window into the inner ear, allowing transmission of sound and pressure into the membranous labyrinth, stimulating the superior semicircular canal and causing a myriad of symptoms. A possible surgical approach to this condition was proposed, but the long-term efficacy and potential complications such as sensorineural hearing loss were not defined.

## Critique

Prior to this landmark article, many patients with vague symptoms of disequilibrium, ear pressure, autophony, and/or pulsatile tinnitus were misdiagnosed. As a consequence, a potpourri of medications and/or surgical procedures were employed for presumed Eustachian tube dysfunction (especially a patulous Eustachian tube), inner ear fistula, Ménière's disease, and various other vestibulopathies. An entity termed 'cochlear conductive hearing loss' was applied to patients with presumed otosclerosis who were discovered at surgery to have a mobile ossicular chain. It is now recognized that the third window phenomenon explains these cases, as it often causes a 10–30 dB conductive hearing loss, predominantly in the lower frequencies.

The authors carefully characterized eye movements induced by pressure and sound in patients with SSCD. In so doing, they nicely demonstrated the effects of excitation and inhibition within the superior semicircular canal (ampullofugal and ampullopetal deflection of the cupula). For example, forcing air into the middle ear by a Valsalva manoeuvre against a pinched nose displaces the stapes into the vestibule, causing an ampullofugal movement of the superior canal ampulla (an excitatory response). The same response can be elicited by positive pressure within the ear canal transmitted to the middle ear or by a loud sound (90–110 dB). A Valsalva manoeuvre against a closed glottis increases intracranial pressure (via increased intrathoracic pressure and decreased central venous return) and causes an ampullopetal movement of the superior canal ampulla (an inhibitory response). Vertical torsional eye movements will occur with these sound and pressure stimuli.

This report also alerted otolaryngologists and radiologists to carefully examine the bony integrity of the skull base and otic capsule in the area of the superior semicircular canal. SSCD became more frequently diagnosed, often in patients who were symptom free. Conversely, some patients with symptoms that could be attributed to a SSCD had only thinning of bone over the superior canal without obvious dehiscence. These scenarios were the impetus to explore and develop various physiologic tests, such as electrocochleography and vestibular evoked myogenic potentials, as diagnostic aids.

Multiple studies have demonstrated that a SSCD is associated with generalized thinning of the tegmen. A recent investigation by Rizk et al. in 2016 noted the mean skull base thickness in these patients to be 17% thinner than in spontaneous CSF otorrhoea controls and 31% thinner than in obese (BMI >30 kg/m$^2$) controls. Interestingly, the BMI in the SSCD group was significantly less (28.6 kg/m$^2$) than the group with spontaneous CSF otorrhoea (37.7 kg/m$^2$). These data suggest that pathologic processes, independent from obesity, are contributory to the dehiscence. Dehiscence of the bone over the superior canal has been found in 0.5% of 1,000 temporal bones. Clearly, the prevalence of a SSCD syndrome is much less than this, underscoring our incomplete understanding of the pathogenesis of this condition.

Despite the disparate symptoms a SSCD can cause, surgical correction remains an option for patients who are unable to avoid provoking factors. The middle cranial fossa approach with plugging of the defect, with or without adjunctive resurfacing of the dehiscent area, has demonstrated high success improving symptoms for the majority of patients. More recently a transmastoid approach has been employed, although the location of the dehiscence and the position of the tegmen can impose access limitations. Regardless of the approach, **complete** resolution of all vestibular and auditory symptoms is often not achieved. Appropriate preoperative counselling in this regard is important.

## Additional references

Rizk HG, Hatch JL, Stevens, SM, Lambert PR, Meyer TA,. Lateral skull base attenuation in superior semicircular dehiscence and spontaneous cerebrospinal fluid otorrhea. *Otolaryngol Head Neck Surg* 2016;155:641–8.

Sharon JD, Pross SE, Ward BK, Carey JP. Revision surgery for superior canal dehiscence syndrome. *Otol Neurotol* 2016;37:1096–103.

Chapter 25

# Histopathological aspects of presbyacusis

Paul Lambert and Judy Dubno

## Details of study

Age-related hearing loss (presbycusis) in humans is complex because many factors in addition to ageing can result in hearing loss in older adults, such as exposure to noise, oto-toxic drugs, or otologic disease. Subcategories of presbycusis resulting from ageing and/or environmental exposures are difficult to identify solely from human audiometric meas-ures. As such, assessment of the pathology of presbycusis from human temporal bones is a critical tool to advance understanding of inner ear disease in humans. The earliest work attempted to correlate histopathological abnormalities of the cochlea observed in human temporal bones with specific audiometric patterns (e.g. Schuknecht 1955,1964; Suga and Lindsay 1976). For many reasons, including long delays between audiometric measures and temporal bone donations, results were often inconsistent and contradictory (Nelson and Hinojosa 2006). Nevertheless, for many years, four categories of presbycusis were commonly accepted (alone or in combination), based on extensive studies of human tem-poral bones and audiometric findings (Schuknecht 1974; Schuknecht et al. 1974): (1) sen-sory, characterized by atrophy and degeneration of sensory hair cells and supporting cells; (2) neural, typified by loss of spiral ganglion neurons; (3) metabolic, characterized by atrophy and degeneration of the lateral wall of the cochlea, especially the stria vascularis; and (4) mechanical, where the basilar membrane is hypothesized to change its conductive or stiffness characteristics.

## Study references

### Main study

Schuknecht HF, Gacek MR. Cochlear pathology in presbycusis. *Ann Otol Rhinol Laryngol* 1993;102:1–16.

### Related references

Nelson EG, Hinojosa R. Presbycusis: a human temporal bone study of individuals with downward sloping audiometric patterns of hearing loss and review of the literature. *Laryngoscope* 2006;116: 1–12.

Schuknecht HF. Presbycusis. *Laryngoscope* 1955;65:402–19.

Schuknecht HF. Further observations on the pathology of presbycusis. *Arch Otolaryngol*
  1964;80:369–82.

Schuknecht HF. Presbyacusis. In: *Pathology of the Ear*. Cambridge, MA: Harvard University Press, 1974.

Suga F, Lindsay J. Histopathological observations of presbyacusis. *Ann Otol Rhinol Laryngol*
  1976;85:169–84.

## Study design

From a collection of 1,500 temporal bones at the Massachusetts Eye and Ear Infirmary,
21 cases were identified as being consistent with age-related hearing loss (bilateral symmetrical sensorineural hearing loss with gradual onset and no evidence of other otologic
disease). All 21 were older adults with audiometric testing ranging from 2 months to
16 years before autopsy. Temporal bones were decalcified, embedded in celloidin, and
serially sectioned (20 μm). Because the sample was too small for statistical analyses, analyses consisted of 'visual correlation' between audiometric results and cytocochleograms
and assignment of cases to one of six classifications (sensory, neural, strial, cochlear conductive, mixed, or indeterminate presbycusis).

## Outcome measures

- Patient data (age, sex, occupation, time from audiometry to autopsy, cause of death)
- Histopathologic findings (presence/absence of inner and outer hair cells, sensory le-
  sion (mm), strial tissue volume loss (%), neuronal count, neuronal loss (% of neonatal))
- Audiometric results (pure-tone thresholds, word recognition scores)
- Matched chart of audiogram and cytocochleogram
- Criteria and classification of 21 cases

## Results

The major findings relate to sensory, neural, and strial presbycusis. For sensory
presbycusis, it was noted that many cases showed an 'island' of hair cell loss in the 8–
12 mm region (~4 kHz), which was attributed to noise exposure. This hair cell lesion
often merged with what was assumed to be the sensory presbycusic region, making it difficult to differentiate age-related and noise-induced effects. Earliest losses were limited
to stereocilia, followed by a loss of supporting and sensory cells. Apical losses and inner
hair cell losses were minimal.

Neural presbycusis was described as 'the most consistent pathologic change in the aging
ear', occurring across the cochlea, with some increased loss at the base. The neuronal loss
was found to be total, including the soma, axons, and dendrites, which indicated primary
neuronal degeneration, rather than secondary degeneration due to loss of sensory cells.
The authors emphasized the lack of an association between elevated pure-tone thresholds
and a loss of cochlear neurons, estimating that the neuronal loss would have to reach 90%
to affect pure-tone thresholds. Rather than neuronal loss leading to reduced detection,

the authors hypothesized an association between neuronal loss and declines in word recognition, but also noted cases with 50% neuronal loss and near-normal word recognition.

Strial presbycusis was described as a 'common pathologic entity' with a slow progression and a flat or gradually sloping audiometric configuration, good word recognition, and normal stimulus coding (loudness and auditory processing). The atrophy was described as patchy in the middle and apical turns, but also with a complete loss of strial cells. The authors emphasized that a significant consequence of strial tissue loss is the change in endolymph and the subsequent functional changes in the cochlea related to the reduction in the endocochlear potential (EP), the positive 80-mV DC potential in the scala media. Given that the stria vascularis is responsible for endolymph formation and for generating the EP, age-related degeneration of strial tissues may also underlie the loss of energy needed for normal cochlear function.

Although many of the 21 cases were identified as one of the four classic types, several were identified as mixed presbycusis and included those with combinations of sensory, neural, and strial losses. Moreover, approximately 25% of the cases did not show pathologic changes in any cochlear structure so could not be classified, despite having audiometric results consistent with one or more classifications. The authors speculate that these cases could be attributed to impaired cellular function (such as reduced numbers of synapses or electrochemical changes in the endolymph) that cannot be detected by the light microscopic techniques used in this study.

## Conclusion

The authors concluded that the results of this study, conducted many decades after the original histopathologic studies of human temporal bones, provided further support for the four pathologic subtypes of human presbycusis. Three limitations of this approach were identified: (1) many cases show pathologic changes in more than one cochlear structure; (2) one-quarter of cases could not be classified; and (3) imperfect relationships exist between patterns of pure-tone thresholds and presbycusic classifications.

In their conclusions, following many years of research on human temporal bones, Schuknecht and Gacek made significant revisions to their classification scheme, paraphrased as follows: "(1) sensory cell losses are the least important type of loss in the aged ear; (2) neuronal losses are constant and predictable expressions of aging; and (3) atrophy of the stria vascularis is the predominant lesion of the aging cochlea." Thus, the revision and updating of the classic presbycusis classifications by Schuknecht and Gacek downplays the significance of age-related loss of sensory cells, emphasizes the importance of age-related degeneration of the stria vascularis and auditory nerve, and brings consistency between results from human temporal bones and from experiments with aging animals.

## Critique

This landmark article updates earlier classic studies of human temporal bone histopathology and audiometric findings from older adults. Because of limitations due to light microscopy, detection of cellular changes was limited to advanced pathology. Cases of missing hair cells classified as sensory presbycusis were more likely related to noise exposure (consistent with occupational noise histories) rather than aging alone, as subsequent reports have demonstrated an absence of hair cell loss in laboratory animals raised in quiet (e.g. Mills et al. 1990). With regard to neural presbycusis, the authors emphasize the lack of association with pure-tone threshold elevation and speculate that poor word recognition in older adults with normal thresholds is an indication of neuronal loss. Of course, this general topic is currently under intense study, following the work of Kujawa and Liberman (2009,2015) showing primary neural degeneration (synaptopathy) in laboratory animals after noise exposure and in the aging cochlea.

Of primary significance in this landmark article is a new emphasis on the degeneration of the stria vascularis and their description of this finding as 'a predominant lesion of the aging cochlea.' These conclusions are consistent with more recent evidence from an animal model of metabolic (strial) presbycusis (Schmiedt et al. 2002). In these cases of reduced EP and loss of voltage to the cochlear amplifier, audiometric patterns are characterized by a mild flat low-frequency loss coupled with a gradually sloping loss in the higher frequencies, which is similar to the most common audiometric configuration of older adults without significant noise exposure histories.

## Additional references

Kujawa SG, Liberman MC. Adding insult to injury: cochlear nerve degeneration after "temporary" noise-induced hearing loss. *J Neurosci* 2009;**29**:14077–85.

Kujawa SG, Liberman MC. Synaptopathy in the noise-exposed and aging cochlea: Primary neural degeneration in acquired sensorineural hearing loss. *Hear Res* 2015;**25**: 191–9.

Mills JH, Schmiedt RA, Kulish LF. Age-related changes of auditory potentials of Mongolian gerbil. *Hear Res* 1990;**46**:201–10.

Schmiedt RA, Lang H, Okamura HO, Schulte BA. Effects of furosemide applied chronically to the round window: a model of metabolic presbyacusis. *J Neurosci* 2002;**22**:9643–50.

Chapter 26

# Sudden sensorineural hearing loss

Paul Lambert and Jonathan Hatch

## Details of the study

Sudden sensorineural hearing loss (SSNHL) is currently defined as a loss of greater than 30 dB over three or more contiguous frequencies occurring within a 72-hour period. It may also be associated with tinnitus and vertigo. The aetiology of SSNHL is uncertain but theories proposed include viral infections, vascular compromise, autoimmune processes, and structural disruption within the inner ear. Most cases, however, are diagnosed as idiopathic. The treatment options are as varied as to the proposed aetiologies. In the past, several medications and procedures have been put forth. In practice currently, the most common treatment includes some form of corticosteroids, either administered orally or transtympanically. Early studies addressing this topic are the foundation for ongoing research investigations and help shape the current diagnostic and treatment recommendations.

## Study references

### Main studies

Mattox DE, Simmons FB. Natural history of sudden sensorineural hearing loss. *Ann Otol Rhinol Laryngol* 1977;**86**:463–80.

Wilson WR, Byl FM, Laird N. The efficacy of steroids in the treatment of idiopathic sudden hearing loss. A double-blind clinical study. *Arch Otolaryngol* 1980;**106**:772–6.

### Related references

Stachler RJ, Chandrasekhar SS, Archer SM, Rosenfeld RM, Schwartz SR, Barrs DM, et al. Clinical practice guideline: sudden hearing loss. *Otolaryngol Head Neck Surg* 2012;**146**:S1–35.

## Study design

Mattox et al. (1977)

- Multicentre, prospective, observational study

| | |
|---|---|
| Level of evidence | 2b |
| Number of patients | 88 |
| Inclusion criteria | Abrupt (less than 12 hours) idiopathic hearing loss |
| Exclusion criteria | Positive diagnoses (Meniere's, trauma, etc.), insufficient information, Non-abrupt |
| Treatment | Discretion of the treating physician |

## Outcome measures

- Recovery of hearing loss
- Classify types of hearing loss
- Results of treatment

## Results

- 65% of patients had spontaneous recovery without medical treatment
- Most patients that recovered hearing did so within a 2-week timeframe
- Low-frequency hearing loss was more recoverable than high frequency
  - Losses at frequencies less than 8 kHz had good or complete recovery in 78% of cases
  - Losses at frequencies at 8 kHz or greater had good or complete recovery in only 29% of cases
- Factors adversely affecting hearing recovery rates included advancing age and presence of severe vestibular symptoms
- Varied treatment modalities did not affect outcome (108 treatment epochs)
- Recovery was always better at the apex of the cochlea compared to the base

## Conclusion

Recoverable hearing rates following idiopathic sudden sensorineural hearing loss are high and treatment options may not necessarily affect outcome. A wide variety of aetiologies have been proposed but are difficult to prove.

## Study design

Wilson et al. (1980)

- Multicentre, double-blinded, placebo-controlled, randomized trial

| Level of evidence | 1b |
| --- | --- |
| Randomization | Steroids versus observation |
| Number of patients | 33 treatment arm and 86 in control arm (34 received placebo, 52 observation) |
| Inclusion criteria | 30 dB loss at three contiguous frequencies in less than 3 days<br>Seen within 10 days of onset<br>No prior treatment received |
| Exclusion criteria | Other diagnoses that were treatable causes of hearing loss<br>Contraindication to steroid use |
| Follow-up | Audiograms obtained 4 and 12 weeks afterwards |

- Corticosteroid administered and dosage range
  - Dexamethasone 0.75–4.5 mg daily to twice daily
  - Methylprednisolone 4–16 mg daily to three times daily

## Outcome measures

- Recovery of hearing defined as complete (within 10 dB of speech reception threshold or pure-tone average of pre-hearing loss), partial (greater than 50% of pre-hearing loss) or no recovery (less than 50% of pre-hearing loss)

## Results

- Overall recovery rate was 61% in the steroid group and 32% in the placebo group
- Three groups were identified
  - Mid-frequency hearing loss (40 dB or less); these patients in both treatment arms had 100% complete recovery; steroids offered no improvement
  - Profound hearing loss patients (90 dB or greater in all frequencies) had no recovery in 76% of patients; limited response to steroids
  - Moderate hearing loss (1, 2, 4 kHz range with greater than 40 dB loss but less than a 90 dB loss) were combined into a single group.
    - This group had the most improvement with steroids (78% in the treatment arm and 38% in the placebo arm)
- Younger age was found to be significant for favouring recovery. The effect of vertigo on recovery was not significant.

## Conclusion

Steroids have a significant impact on hearing recovery in young patients with moderate to severe hearing loss. Patients with severe loss or mild to moderate mid-frequency loss have limited benefit from steroid use.

## Critique

The paper by Mattox et al. presents one of the first attempts to gain objective insight in sudden sensorineural hearing loss (SSNHL). At the time of publication, 1977, several etiologic theories had been proposed. However, there was lack of uniformity of the parameters constituting SSNHL: time course, frequencies involved, and severity. Further, treatment options were highly variable. In the study, they gathered key data including the onset of symptoms, the severity of hearing loss, preceding activity potentially contributing to the hearing loss, and complete audiometric analysis. A wide net was cast in hopes of collecting new information. However, the work-up and treatment of patients was variable and left to the discretion of the provider and/or institution.

Ideally the workup and treatment would have been more standardized with well-defined criteria for inclusion. The lack of uniformity may have affected their statistical analysis.

The study by Wilson et al. is widely touted as the basis for steroid treatment of SSNHL. The main criticisms of the paper are the types, dosages and duration of steroids. Steroids used included dexamethasone and methylprednisolone which the authors state are roughly equivalent. However, the data from the separate institutions show disparity between the steroid type and hearing recovery. Also, the dosages and schedule were not controlled. The authors' main conclusion was that patients with moderate hearing loss had the best response to steroids. The data supports this conclusion but drug choice, dosage or duration of treatment cannot be determined.

Since the appearance of these two landmark articles, SSNHL has received more attention, including the recently published clinical guidelines by the American Academy of Otolaryngology—Head and Neck Surgery. The aetiology and pathophysiology of SSNHL remains elusive, despite multiple clinical and histological studies. Likely, SSNHL is not a single process but rather a common pathway for a variety of insults. The uses of steroids, both oral and intratympanic, are well-accepted treatment approaches.

## Additional references

El Sabbagh NH, Sewitch MJ, Bezdjian A, Daniel SJ. Intratympanic dexamethasone in sudden sensorineural hearing loss: a systematic review and meta-analysis. *Laryngoscope* 2017;**127**:1897–908.

Labus J, Breil J, Stützer H, Michel O. Meta-analysis for the effect of medical therapy vs. placebo on recovery of idiopathic sudden hearing loss. *Laryngoscope* 2010;**120**:1863–71.

Lawrence R, Thevasagayam R. Controversies in the management of sudden sensorineural hearing loss: an evidence-based review. *Clin Otolaryngol* 2015;**40**:176–82.

Chapter 27

# Conservative management of vestibular schwannoma

Vincent Van Rompaey

## Details of studies

The vestibular schwannoma is a benign tumour originating from the Schwann cells insulating the vestibulocochlear nerve's axons. It is the most frequent tumour in the cerebellopontine angle with an approximate incidence of 23 patients per million per year. The most frequently reported symptoms are hearing loss, tinnitus, feeling of pressure in the ear, and vertigo. Magnetic resonance imaging (MRI) of the cerebellopontine angle leads to the diagnosis of the vestibular schwannoma.

Knowledge of this lesion's natural evolution is essential in its management. Since there is a significant amount of non-growing tumours, active treatment (including radiotherapy and microsurgical resection) is often not indicated because of poorer quality of life compared to conservative management. The latter is the so-called wait-and-scan policy, in which serial MRI scans are performed to measure the tumour's growth. It has been suggested that conservative management of small vestibular schwannomas would lead to a progressive hearing loss over time, which would end up in losing the option to attempt surgery with a hearing preservation objective. To address this matter, Stangerup et al. performed a large retrospective review to study the natural progression of hearing loss in patients with diagnosed vestibular schwannoma.

## Study references

### Main study

Stangerup S-E, Caye-Thomasen P, Tos M, Thomsen J. Change in hearing during 'wait and scan' management of patients with vestibular schwannoma. *J Laryngol Otol* 2008;**122**:673–81.

### Related reference

Stangerup SE, Tos M, Thomsen J, Caye-Thomasen P. Hearing outcomes of vestibular schwannoma patients managed with 'wait and scan': predictive value of hearing level at diagnosis. *J Laryngol Otol* 2010;**124**:490–4.

## Study design

A retrospective single-centre observational study with prospective inclusion.

| | |
|---|---|
| Level of evidence | 2b |
| Randomization | N/A |
| Number of patients | 636 |
| Inclusion criteria | Diagnosed with a unilateral cerebellopontine angle tumour on MRI resembling a vestibular schwannoma. |
| | Maximum largest extrameatal diameter of 20 mm. |
| Exclusion criteria | Not reported. |
| Follow-up | The mean observation time was 3.9 years, with a range of 0.3 to 11.4 years. |

Included patients were allocated to the 'wait-and-scan' management, with the intention of performing annual MRI and clinical assessment, including audiological examination.

## Outcome measures

### Primary endpoints

+ Growth or no growth on MRI at last evaluation, defined as either development of an extrameatal extension of a previously purely intrameatal tumour, or an increase in the size of the extrameatal part in an extrameatal tumour exceeding 2 mm.
+ Pure-tone audiometry and speech discrimination at last evaluation

### Secondary endpoints

+ American Academy of Otolaryngology—Head and Neck Surgery hearing class in vestibular schwannoma ears.
+ Word recognition score hearing class

## Results

### Primary endpoints

#### Growth or no growth on MRI at last evaluation

Of the 636 patients included in this study, at least two MRI scans and two audiograms were available in 90%. The observation period was terminated by surgery in 118 patients and by radiotherapy in 118 patients. In most cases active treatment was performed because of significant tumour growth: 19.8% of intrameatal tumours and 33.2% of extrameatal tumours.

#### Pure-tone audiometry at last evaluation

The deterioration of pure tone hearing during the observation period was similar in all age groups. There was no significant difference in hearing deterioration between the intrameatal tumours, small and medium tumours, at diagnosis or at the last evaluation.

At diagnosis, the hearing in ears with tumour growth was not different from that in ears without tumour growth.

### Speech discrimination at last evaluation

At diagnosis, the mean speech discrimination score in the tumour ear was 62.4%, compared with 46.7% at the last evaluation.

## Secondary endpoints

### American Academy of Otolaryngology—Head and Neck Surgery hearing class in vestibular schwannoma ears.

At diagnosis, class A hearing (i.e. pure-tone average of 30 dB and speech discrimination score of 70% or higher) was observed in 20% of the tumour ears. Class A hearing was preserved in 48.1% of these patients at the last evaluation available.

### Word recognition score hearing class

At diagnosis, class I hearing (i.e. speech discrimination score of 70% or higher) was observed in 52.5% of the tumour ears. Class I hearing was preserved in 55% of these patients at the last evaluation available.

## Conclusion

Of all patients with normal speech discrimination score 88% maintained good hearing, while patients with a small speech discrimination loss at diagnosis lost serviceable hearing after a few years in 45%. The authors conclude that in vestibular schwannoma patients with a small tumour and normal speech discrimination, the main indication for active treatment should be established tumour growth.

## Critique

This study is one of the largest series of unilateral vestibular schwannomas managed by means of 'wait-and-scan'. It draws its strength through the centralization of all patients in Denmark diagnosed with a vestibular schwannoma in one centre and therefore covers the entire national population. Because of its sample size, its prospective inclusion of data and its minimal referral bias, these results have had significant implications for clinical practice.

The present study has reported a relatively low growth percentage of 19.8–33.2%, while more recent reports suggest growth rates of 40%. (Hunter et al. 2016) These differences might be explained in cases of intrameatal tumours by using different definitions: i.e. growth can be defined as extrameatal extension (used in the present study) or a diameter increase of 2 mm (used in the study by Hunter et al.).

In a more recent study, published by the same group of authors in 2010, data were reported on 932 patients allocated to "wait-and-scan" over a 33-year period with at least two available pure-tone and speech discrimination audiograms. (Stangerup et al. 2010) At diagnosis, hearing level of 10 dB or better at 4000 Hz was found in only 18 of the 932 vestibular schwannoma ears, while good speech discrimination was found in 159 patients (17%). Of the latter patients, 138 maintained good hearing after observation (86.8%).

The success of the wait-and-scan approach lies in identifying the right subset of patients and tumours that are most likely to grow in an indolent fashion and follow them up with strict imaging guidelines, thereby enabling the patients to escape any form of treatment. The 'wait-and-scan' policy has now been widely adopted in intracanalicular and small non-growing vestibular schwannoma cases (Kondziolka et al. 2012; Liu et al. 2015). However, a failed wait and scan after a period could lead to difficult and unfavourable situations because of the problems of active treatment (microsurgical resection or radiotherapy) on a larger tumour, advanced age, and symptom progression.

## Additional references

Hunter JB, Francis DO, O'Connell BP, Kabagambe EK, Bennett ML, Wanna GB, et al. Single institutional experience with observing 564 vestibular schwannomas: factors associated with tumor growth. *Otol Neurotol* 2016;37:1630–6.

Kondziolka D, Mousavi SH, Kano H, Flickinger JC, Lunsford LD. The newly diagnosed vestibular schwannoma: radiosurgery, resection, or observation? *Neurosurg Focus* 2012;33:E8

Liu W, Ni M, Jia W, Zhou D, Zhang Q, Jiang Y, Jia G. How to address small- and medium-sized acoustic neuromas with hearing: a systematic review and decision analysis. *World Neurosurg* 2015;84:283–91.e1.

Chapter 28

# Hearing preservation in vestibular schwannoma surgery

Vincent Van Rompaey

## Details of studies

Three management options are typically available when considering the treatment of patients with a vestibular schwannoma: wait-and-scan, radiotherapy, and microsurgical resection. The objectives of microsurgical resection of vestibular schwannoma have evolved significantly in the last 120 years from its first removal in 1895, credited to Thomas Annandale in Edinburgh. In this early era mortality was as high as 80% because of lack of understanding of the anatomy and physiologic importance of the anterior inferior cerebellar artery (AICA) and because haemostasis was limited to packing. Survival was primordial to cranial nerve deficits of the facial and vestibulocochlear nerve. In the absence of X-rays, computed tomography, or magnetic resonance imaging, clinicians had to rely on the evolution of symptoms and surgeons therefore were dealing with larger tumours with significant compression of the brainstem. Interestingly, in these early days it was quite difficult to determine the laterality of the tumour, explaining the use of a bilateral suboccipital approach to confirm the tumour side (Bruns 1897; Nguyen-Huynh et al. 2007).

Mortality rates improved significantly from 80% to 20% by 1917 and 4% by 1931 thanks to some innovations related to haemostasis introduced by Harvey Cushing, including the use of bone wax, vessel clips, and electrocautery (Cushing 1917). William House popularized the use of the binocular microscope while concurrent medical advances in anaesthesia, antibiotics and blood transfusion also improved outcome (House 1964). By 1979, Delgado et al. published the first report of facial nerve monitoring to guide facial nerve dissection (Delgado et al. 1979). While facial nerve outcome has improved significantly the last few decades, attention has turned to the anatomical preservation of the cochlear nerve and functional preservation of the cochlea. To address this matter, Gardner and Robertson performed a review of the literature on hearing preservation in unilateral vestibular schwannoma (then called acoustic neuroma) surgery.

## Study references

### Main study

**Gardner G, Robertson JH.** Hearing preservation in unilateral acoustic neuroma surgery. *Ann Otol Rhinol Laryngol* 1988;97:55–66.

### Related reference

**Maniakas A, Saliba I.** Microsurgery versus stereotactic radiation for small vestibular schwannomas: a meta-analysis of patients with more than 5 years' follow-up. *Otol Neurotol* 2012;33:1611–20.

## Study design

A review of the literature.

| | |
|---|---|
| Level of evidence | 4 |
| Randomization | N/A |
| Number of patients | 621 |
| Inclusion criteria | Studies on attempted hearing preservation in the surgical treatment of unilateral vestibular schwannoma. |
| Exclusion criteria | Languages other than English. |
| Follow-up | No comprehensive data available. One of 13 studies had 1-year follow-up |

Non-systematic review of 13 case series with total of 492 patients in whom hearing preservation was stated to have been attempted.

## Outcome measures

### Primary endpoints

To categorize hearing preservation cases by means of a newly suggested audiometric classification.

### Secondary endpoints

None.

## Results

### Primary endpoints

#### Audiometric criteria

Thirteen case series were reviewed, including 492 patients in whom hearing preservation was stated to have been attempted, 77 patients in which hearing preservation may have been attempted and 12 patients with limited data. Using the suggested audiometric criteria (Table 28.1), it was possible to classify 100 patients from 6 of the 13 studies. Twenty-seven patients had class 1 hearing, 28 in class 2, 28 in class 3, none in class 4, and 17 in class 5.

The authors report their own case series of 155 surgically treated unilateral vestibular schwannoma, of which 10 were operated with the intent of hearing preservation. Successful hearing preservation (i.e. class 1) was achieved in two patients. Of note, all patients underwent total microsurgical removal.

**Table 28.1.** Classification for hearing preservation

| Class | PTA or SRT (dB)* | Speech discrimination (%) |
|---|---|---|
| 1 | 0–30 | 70–100 |
| 2 | 31–50 | 69–50 |
| 3 | 51–90 | 49–5 |
| 4 | 91–max loss | 4–1 |
| 5 | No response | No response |

PTA, pure-tone average; SRT, speech reception threshold; dB, decibel.

*The better score was used. If PTA/SRT score and speech discrimination scores do not qualify for same class, the class appropriate for the poorer of two scores was used.

Reprinted from Gardner G, Robertson JH. Hearing preservation in unilateral acoustic neuroma surgery. *Ann Otol Rhinol Laryngol* 1988;97:55–66 with permission from Sage.

## Conclusion

Studies have been reviewed that reported 394 patients in whom hearing preservation was attempted in cases where a unilateral vestibular schwannoma was surgically removed. In 131 of these cases hearing preservation was claimed. Because many studies are case reports that do not report on the total number of cases where hearing preservation was attempted, the exact hearing preservation success rate is difficult to calculate.

Hearing preservation is a reasonable goal in unilateral vestibular schwannoma surgery, although the number of available candidates is relatively small. Intelligent selection of patients and high-quality surgical technique are keys to success.

## Critique

The Gardner and Robertson review, although troubled by the inaccurate case series they had to review, has paved the way for systematic audiometric outcome reporting after hearing preservation attempt. The 1995 American Academy of Otolaryngology—Head and Neck Surgery guidelines were based largely on the criteria suggested by Gardner and Robertson. More recently, they have been replaced by the guidelines suggested by Gurgel et al. (2012) The latter promote individual reporting of pure-tone averages and word recognition scores by means of a scattergram (Gurgel et al. 2012).

Shortcomings of the reviewed articles included the lack of valid preoperative audiometry for all patients (only available in three of 13 studies), tumour size, comprehensive facial nerve outcome reporting by means of the House–Brackmann grading system or total tumour removal achieved.

Selection of potential hearing preservation candidates is essential and this generally includes vestibular schwannoma cases up to 20 mm in size with the fundus of the internal auditory meatus free of tumour, with up to 50 dB PTA hearing loss and at least 50% of speech discrimination (Zhang et al. 2016) A recent meta-analysis studied the hearing preservation outcome in cases with at least 5 years of follow-up after stereotactic radiotherapy (n = 410) and microsurgical resection (n = 153). Hearing preservation was observed in the former group in 70.2% and 50.3% in the latter group (middle fossa and retrosigmoid approach combined) (Ansari et al. 2012; Maniakas and Saliba 2012).

## Additional references

Ansari SF, Terry C, Cohen-Gadol AA. Surgery for vestibular schwannomas: a systematic review of complications by approach. *Neurosurg Focus* 2012;33:E14.

Bruns L. *Die Geschwülste des Nervensystems*. Berlin: Karger, 1897.

Committee on Hearing and Equilibrium guidelines for the evaluation of hearing preservation in acoustic neuroma (vestibular schwannoma). American Academy of Otolaryngology-Head and Neck Surgery Foundation, INC. *Otolaryngol Head Neck Surg* 1995;113:179–80.

Cushing H. *Tumors of the Nervus Acusticus and the Syndrome of the Cerebellopontine Angle*. Philadelphia, PA.: WB Saunders; 1917.

Delgado TE, Bucheit WA, Rosenholtz HR, Chrissian S. Intraoperative monitoring of facila muscle evoked responses obtained by intracranial stimulation of the facila nerve: a more accurate technique for facila nerve dissection. *Neurosurgery* 1979;4:418–21.

Gurgel RK, Jackler RK, Dobie RA, Popelka GR. A new standardized format for reporting hearing outcome in clinical trials. *Otolaryngol Head Neck Surg* 2012;147:803–7.

House WF. Transtemporal bone microsurgical removal of acoustic neuromas. report of cases. *Arch Otolaryngol* 1964;80:617–67.

Maniakas A, Saliba, I Microsurgery versus stereotactic radiation for small vestibular schwannomas: a meta-analysis of patients with more than 5 years' follow-up. *Otol Neurotol* 2012;33:1611–20.

Nguyen-Huynh AT, Jackler RK, Pfister M, Tseng J. The aborted early history of the translabyrinthine approach: a victim of suppression or technical prematurity? *Otol Neurotol* 2007;28:269–79.

Zhang Z, Nguyen Y, De Seta D, Russo FY, Rey A, Kalamarides M, et al. Surgical treatment of sporadic vestibular schwannoma in a series of 1006 patients. *Acta Otorhinolaryngol Ital* 2016;36:408–14.

# Chapter 29

# Cochlear implant design

Vedat Topsakal

## Details of study

The cochlear implant has become the preferred method of rehabilitation for profound postlingually deaf adults. Improved multichannel speech processing strategies have enhanced the performance of implants. Debate continues about the most appropriate prosthesis design and inter-individual variability in performance. Gantz et al. (1988) study the differences of single versus multichannel implants in a multicentre design.

## Study references

### Main study

Gantz BJ, Tyler RS, Knutson JF, Woodworth G, Abbas P, McCabe BF, et al. Evaluation of five different cochlear implant designs: audiologic assessment and predictors of performance. *Laryngoscope* 1988;98:1100–6.

### Related references

Clark GM, Blamey PJ, Brown AM, Gusby PA, Dowell RC, Franz BK, et al. The University of Melbourne nucleus multi-electrode cochlear implant. *Adv Otorhinolaryngol* 1987;38:V–IX, 1–181.

Eddington DK, Dobelle WH, Brackmann DE, Mladejovsky MG, Parkin JL. Auditory prostheses research with multiple channel intracochlear stimulation in man. *Ann Otol Rhinol Laryngol* 1978;87:1–39.

Fretz RJ, Fravel RP. Design and function: a physical and electrical description of the 3M House cochlear implant system. *Ear Hear* 1985;6:14S–19S.

Hochmair-Desoyer IJ, Hochmair ES, Burian K, Fischer RE. Four years of experience with cochlear prostheses. *Med Prog Technol* 1981;8:107–19.

## Study design

| | |
|---|---|
| Level of evidence | 2 |
| Randomization | None |
| Number of patients | 54 |
| Stratification | Single (two centres) vs. multichannel implanted patients (three centres) |
| Centres | 5 |
| Inclusion criteria | postlingually deaf adults with bilateral sensorineural unable to understand speech with proper hearing aids |
| Follow Up | at least 9 months |
| Exclusion criteria | None defined or applicable for this study design |

## Outcome measures

1   Audiological battery to test sound recognition, speech recognition
2   Residual hearing: quantified by own scoring system
3   Electric stimulation in a subset of 17 multichannel patients
4   Psychophysical test

## Secondary outcome measures

Correlations with duration of deafness, age at implantation, preoperative residual hearing, and motivation of patient.

## Results

### Main results

There is a significant difference in performance in sound recognition and speech recognition between single and multichannel devices. The multichannel devices outperform the single channel devices.

| Outcome measure | Single channel | Multichannel |
| --- | --- | --- |
| Sound recognition | + (0–50 %) | + (11–95%) |
| Word recognition | 3% (only 1 case) | 90 % (35 of 39) |

### Secondary outcomes

Strong negative correlation of implant performance with duration of deafness and age at implantation and positive correlation.

## Conclusion

There is a significant effect of implant design on the level of audiological performance. The addition of place or spectral information provided by multichannel speech processing systems enables most postlingually deafened adults to recognize speech.

## Critique

The study has shortcomings in the number of study cases and a substantial variability among participants within groups. Selection criteria may have been different over the participating centres resulting in a selection bias. Demographics and etiological factors could have been studied more specifically. Although differences between multichannel devices were generally not significant there seemed to be an artificial effort to find better performance in specific centres.

# Part III

# Rhinology

Chapter 30

# Guidelines for the management of rhinosinusitis

Claire Hopkins

## Details of study

The last 20 years have seen the publication of a growing number of evidence-based guide-lines and consensus documents for chronic rhinosinusitis (CRS). Perhaps the best known of these is the European Position Paper (EPOS). This was first published in 2005, initiated by the European Academy of Allergology and Clinical Immunology, and endorsed by the European Rhinological Society. There had been such an explosion of trials and other lit-erature that it was felt necessary to update this first edition only 2 years later.

The next iteration was published in 2012, with 29 international authors, each charged with undertaking a critical review of published literature in a given topic, and to make evidence-based recommendations on this. All contributions were circulated and con-sidered prior to a 4-day consensus meeting, when final recommendations were made. The Oxford Centre of Evidence Based Medicine levels of evidence and strength of recom-mendations were used throughout the publication. A key change for the 2012 EPOS was the clear separation of CRS with and without nasal polyps (CRSwNP and CRSsNP).

## Study references

### Main reference

Fokkens WJ, Lund VJ, Mullol J, Bachert C, Alobid I, Baroody F, et al. European Position Paper on Rhinosinusitis and Nasal Polyps 2012. *Rhinol Suppl* 2012;**23**:3 pp. preceding table of contents.

### Related reference

Orlandi RR, Kingdom TT, Hwang PH, Smith TL, Alt JA, Baroody FM, et al. International consensus statement on allergy and rhinology: rhinosinusitis. *Int Forum Allergy Rhinol* 2016;**6**:S22–209.

# Results

## CRSwNP management scheme for ENT specialists

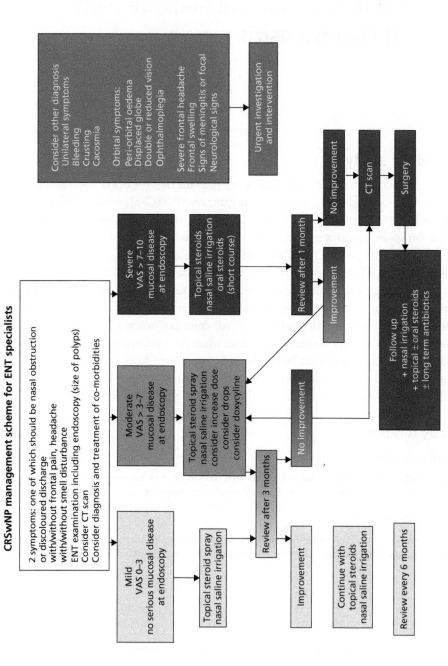

Reproduced from Fokkens WJ, Lund VJ, Mullol J et. al. European Position Paper on Rhinosinusitis and Nasal Polyps 2012. Rhinol Suppl. 2012;(23):3 p preceding table of contents, 1–298, with permission from Rhinology International.

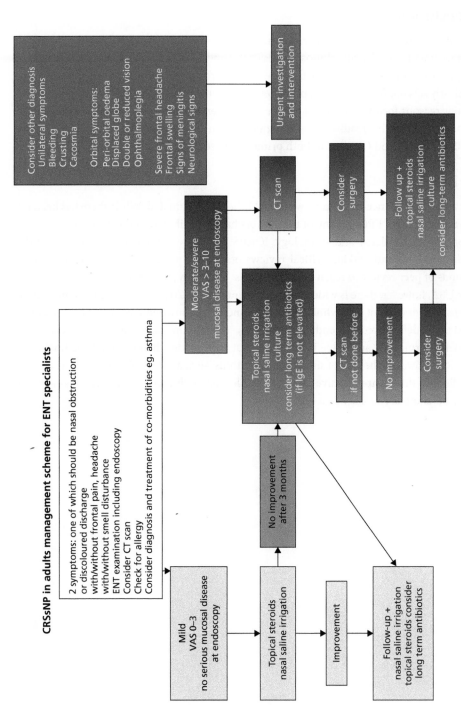

## CRSsNP in adults management scheme for ENT specialists

2 symptoms: one of which should be nasal obstruction
or discoloured discharge
with/without frontal pain, headache
with/without smell disturbance
ENT examination including endoscopy
Consider CT scan
Check for allergy
Consider diagnosis and treatment of co-morbidities eg. asthma

Consider other diagnosis
Unilateral symptoms
Bleeding
Crusting
Cacosmia

Orbital symptoms:
Peri-orbital oedema
Displaced globe
Double or reduced vision
Ophthalmoplegia

Severe frontal headache
Frontal swelling
Signs of meningitis
Neurological signs

Urgent investigation
and intervention

Mild
VAS 0–3
no serious mucosal disease
at endoscopy

Moderate/severe
VAS > 3–10
mucosal disease at endoscopy

Topical steroids
nasal saline irrigation

Topical steroids
nasal saline irrigation
culture
consider long term antibiotics
(if IgE is not elevated)

CT scan

No improvement
after 3 months

Improvement

CT scan
if not done before

No improvement

Consider
surgery

Consider
surgery

Follow-up +
nasal saline irrigation
topical steroids consider
long term antibiotics

Follow up +
topical steroids
nasal saline irrigation
culture
consider long-term antibiotics

Reproduced from Fokkens WJ, Lund VJ, Mullol J et. al. European Position Paper on Rhinosinusitis and Nasal Polyps 2012. Rhinol Suppl. 2012;(23):3 p preceding table of contents, 1–298, with permission from Rhinology International.

## Conclusion

EPOS provides a comprehensive summary on the pathophysiology, investigation, and management of both acute rhinosinusitis (ARS) and CRS, with special sections dedicated to paediatric disease, immunodeficiency, cystic fibrosis, and aspirin-exacerbated disease. It clearly sets out future research priorities. However, the strength of EPOS, and one of the major reasons for its widespread uptake are the very clear evidence-based management schemes. These give readily accessible guidance on the management of ARS, paediatric CRS, CRSwNP, and CRSsNP in both primary and secondary care.

## Critique

As with any evidence-based review, it quickly becomes outdated. While there has been no further update of EPOS, many of the authors have contributed to the 2016 International Consensus on Allergy and Rhinology. ICARS adopted a similar methodology of individual authors undertaking critical reviews of discrete topics, but relied on sequential rounds of peer review to reach final consensus. There is a predominance of authors from the USA; however, there is widespread representation. ICARS achieve greater consistency across the document as a whole, by using a more standardized format for each section, and a well defined recommendation template, summarizing aggregate grade of evidence, benefit, harm, cost, and value judgements that were made when reaching the final conclusion. However, the lack of simplified algorithms, such as those of EPOS, may make the findings of this comprehensive piece of work less accessible to those in primary care and in general otolaryngology practice.

Chapter 31

# Radiological staging of rhinosinusitis

Rajiv Bhalla

## Details of study

Staging scores are useful in the management of disease as they allow comparison between patients, and before and after treatment. Several aspects of sinus disease potentially
benefit from scoring systems including endoscopy, radiological investigations, and symptoms. Various tools have been proposed and the two which are now most commonly used
in the management and research of chronic rhinosinusitis (CRS) are the Lund–Mackay
score and the SNOT-22.

## Study references

### Main study

Lund VJ, Mackay IS. Staging in rhinosinusitis. *Rhinology* 1993;107:183–4.

### Related references

Hopkins C, Browne JP, Slack R, Lund V, Brown P. The Lund-Mackay staging system for
    chronic rhinosinusitis: how is it used and what does it predict? *Otolaryngol Head Neck Surg*
    2007;**137**:555–61.
Gaskins RE. A surgical staging system for chronic sinusitis. *Am J Rhinol* 1992;**6**:5–12.
Kennedy DW. Prognostic factors, outcomes and staging in ethmoid sinus surgery. *Laryngoscope Suppl*
    1992;**57**:1–18.

## Study design

Level 5 evidence: descriptive paper.

| | |
|---|---|
| Level of evidence | 5 |
| Randomization | None |
| Number of patients | ? |
| Inclusion criteria | A staging system evolved over 3 years in an attempt to categorize the extent of CRS in patients undergoing endoscopic sinus surgery |
| Exclusion criteria | n/a |
| Follow-up | n/a |

## Results

### Scores were proposed for

Radiological grading comprising three parts:

1  Sinus systems: (now known as 'modified Lund Mackay Score')
   - Score of 0 (absent), 1 (partial opacification) or 2 (complete opacification)
   - Given to right and left maxillary sinuses, anterior ethmoids, posterior ethmoids, sphenoids, and frontals
   - Ostiomeatal complex is scored as 0 (not obstructed) or 2 (obstructed)
   - Total 24

2  Anatomic variants
   - Scored as 0 (absent) or 1 (present)
   - frontal sinus, concha bullosa, paradoxical middle turbinate, everted uncinate process, Haller cells, Agger nasi cells

3  Surgical score
   - Scored as 0 (not performed) and 1 (performed)
   - Uncinectomy, middle meatal antrostomy, anterior ethmoidectomy, posterior ethmoidectomy, sphenoidotomy, frontal recess surgery, reduction of middle turbinate

Further scores included a pre- and postoperative symptom score with five symptoms each graded scores 0 to 10 and an endoscopic score (to include appearances of polyps, discharge, oedema, scarring or adhesions, and crusting).

## Conclusions

The authors propose use of the tool as a standardised way of describing patients with CRS.

## Critique

This is a brief but seminal paper elaborating on a staging system developed over a period of 3 years for the management of CRS. Since publication alternative symptom-based questionnaires have evolved to further consider aspects of sinus disease and management.

The modified Lund–Mackay score which comprises the 'sinus systems' radiological grading described in this paper is very simple; each group of sinuses is judged on cross sectional images to be completely clear, partly opacified or completely opacified. All clinicians are able to accurately score scans without radiological training and inter observer reliability is high. This modified Lund–Mackay score has therefore come to be the most widely used radiological scoring system for CRS in clinical and research practice.

## Additional references

Oluwole M, Russell N, Tan L, Gardiner Q, White P. A comparison of computerized tomographic staging systems in chronic sinusitis. *Clin Otolaryngol* 1996;**21**:91–95.

Metson R, Gliklich RE, Stankiewicz JA, Kennedy DW, Duncavage JA, Hoffman SR, et al. Comparison of sinus computed tomography staging systems. *Otolaryngol Head Neck Surg* 1997;**117**:372–9.

# Chapter 32

# Nasal polyposis

Rajiv Bhalla

## Details of studies

Chronic rhinosinusitis with nasal polyps is a condition of unknown aetiology but is characterized by benign swelling of the nasal mucosa, likely to be the result of chronic mucosal inflammation. This condition has various clinical manifestations from being completely asymptomatic to causing severe nasal blockage, congestion, facial pain/pressure, and anosmia. It is a common condition with prevalence rates of between 0.2% and 4%, increasing with advanced age with a higher male–female 2:1 ratio. Further, this condition represents a significant disease burden; in the USA it is responsible for 12 million doctor visits and 70 million restricted activity days annually.

At the time of writing, there was no universally accepted management protocol for chronic rhinosinusitis with nasal polyps. To address this Rimmer et al. (2014). performed a Cochrane intervention review looking at the effectiveness of surgical versus medical interventions for this condition.

## Study reference

### Main study

Rimmer J, Fokkens W, Chong LY, Hopkins C. Surgical versus medical interventions for chronic rhinosinusitis with nasal polyps (Review). *Cochrane Database Syst Rev* 2014;**11**:CD006990.

## Study design

| Type of study | Cochrane Collaboration intervention review—qualitative analysis. Meta-analysis was not able to be performed/not possible due to the heterogeneity of the studies and the selective (incomplete) outcome reporting by the studies: there was a wide variation in the surgical and medical interventions performed in the review studies |
|---|---|
| Intention to treat analysis | Not maintained/not performed |
| Level of evidence | 1a |
| Randomization | Yes |
| Number of patients | 231 participants across four studies that yielded three comparison pairs |

| | |
|---|---|
| Inclusion criteria | All randomized controlled trials where the unit of randomization was the patient, patients 16 years old or greater with bilateral nasal polyps confirmed by direct visualization |
| Exclusion criteria | 'Split nose' studies (where the patient acted as their own control), patients <16 years old, patients undergoing revision surgery, patients with a known malignancy, and unilateral polyps shown to be inverting papillomas |
| Follow-up | 12 months |
| Intervention(s) | Any surgical intervention; including simple polypectomy or more extensive endoscopic sinus surgery (ESS) vs. any medical treatment (including placebo) |

## Outcome measures

### Primary

- Disease severity, as measured by patient-reported disease specific symptoms scores
- Health-related quality of life, using disease specific health-related quality of life scores (such as the Sino-Nasal Outcome Test—22 (SNOT-22))
- Health-related quality of life, using generic quality of life scores such as SF-36

### Secondary

- Endoscopic appearance (there is no single accepted endoscopic grading system)
- Complications from surgical or medical treatment; epistaxis, infection, orbital complications, intracranial complications, intolerance to medication or other medication side effects
- Recurrence rates: if available the authors used disease free interval
- Objective physiological measures; nasal peak flow, nasal volume, nasal cross sectional area, nasal nitric oxide (nNO), ciliary function (including saccharine clearance time)
- Olfaction tests

# Results

| Intervention groups | Results (at 12 months post intervention) |
|---|---|
| ESS vs. systemic steroids (one study, n = 109) | **Primary**<br>No difference in patient reported disease specific symptoms (nasal obstruction, nasal discharge, sneezing and loss of smell)<br>Disease specific quality of life measurement not performed<br>No difference using generic health related quality of life measures<br>**Secondary**<br>Polyp size significantly improved in both groups with the ESS group significantly better<br>14.3% vs. 0% complication rate (ESS vs. medical therapy) (epistaxis 3.6%, orbital fat exposure 7.1% and CSF leak with meningitis 1.8%)<br>No objective measures performed for recurrence |
| Polypectomy versus systemic steroids (two studies, n = 87) | **Primary**<br>No difference in symptom scores<br>Disease specific quality of life measurement not performed<br>Generic quality of life measurement not performed<br>**Secondary**<br>Endoscopic appearance not reported or not performed<br>Unclear reporting of complications; 4% suffered 'serious adverse events' but judged by the investigators to be 'unlikely to have been caused by either medication or surgery'<br>No difference in recurrence rates<br>No difference in nasal peak expiratory flow/olfaction |
| ESS plus topical steroids versus antibiotics plus high dose topical steroids (one study, n = 35) | **Primary**<br>Small improvement in the surgical intervention group from baseline symptom score<br>No difference in disease specific quality of life scores<br>No difference in generic quality of life scores<br>**Secondary**<br>No difference in endoscopic appearance scores<br>Complications rates were low in both groups (epistaxis 4.4% vs. 2.2% ESS vs. medical treatment). 4.4% suffered a postoperative infection<br>No difference in objective physiological measures |

# Conclusions

The evidence presented in this review does not show that one treatment is better than the other in terms of patient reported symptom scores and quality of life measurements.

# Critique

This study was a qualitative Cochrane Collaboration Intervention Review with a laudable aim of determining whether surgical interventions were superior to medical ones in the treatment of chronic rhinosinusitis (CRS) with nasal polyposis. Despite an exhaustive literature search including searching unpublished data there were only four studies (with

231 randomized participants) available for review. This is interesting given widespread application of ESS in the treatment of CRS with nasal polyps since the 1980s. Further, several of those studies in the review described interventions that are no longer considered as standard/contemporary procedures (i.e. the removal of 'visible' polyps under local anaesthetic).

Including non-standard interventions in the evidentiary base means no firm conclusions can definitively be made about the superiority of surgical to medical interventions. However the aphorism, 'the absence of evidence is not evidence of absence' is particularly pertinent here as multiple non-randomized control trial style studies have shown surgery to have a place in the treatment of CRS with nasal polyps. In particular it is generally accepted practice that those refractory to medical therapy after 3 months benefit from surgery.

The question of determining appropriate inventions in the treatment of CRS is an important one and requires further investigation.

## Additional reference

Fokkens WJ, Lund VJ, Mullol J, Bachert C, Alobid I, Baroody F, et al. European position paper on rhinosinusitis and nasal polyps 2012. *Rhinol Suppl* 2012:50:1–12; 3 pp preceding table of contents.

Chapter 33

# Endoscopic sinus surgery

Rebecca Field

## Details of study

Prior to the introduction of well-lit, cool, near-vision optics as in the Hopkins rod endoscope, practised sinus surgery was radical and non-physiological, utilizing the operating microscope and aggressive, obliterative techniques. In the early 1970s, Messerklinger's endoscopic studies revealed disturbed mucociliary clearance and narrow areas within the osteomeatal complex (middle turbinate, uncinate process, bulla ethmoidalis). He proposed the underlying pathogenesis of sinus disease was rhinogenic in aetiology rather than a problem within the sinus chambers themselves and that inflammation or infection spread, subsequently, to the dependent (or subordinate) maxillary and frontal sinuses.

At around the same time Stammberger in Europe and Kennedy in the USA developed endoscopic surgical techniques that aimed to restore function to the sinuses by removing obstructing and diseased mucosa from the osteomeatal complex and ethmoid. This was said to improve ventilation and drainage of the dependent maxillary and frontal sinuses via their natural ostia without actually interfering with those sinuses directly, thereby addressing the underlying cause of sinus disease. The papers by Stammberger (1986) and Kennedy (1985) effectively changed forever the way in which sinus surgery was conducted, introducing the concepts of minimally invasive and targeted sinus surgery, which still prevail today.

## Study references

### Main study

**Stammberger H.** Endoscopic endonasal surgery—concepts in treating recurring rhinosinusitis. Part II. Surgical Technique. *Otolaryngol Head Neck Surg* 1986;**94**:147–56.

### Related reference

**Kennedy DW.** Functional endoscopic sinus surgery. Technique. *Arch Otolaryngol* 1985;**111**:643–9.

## Study design

- University of Graz ENT clinic, Graz, Austria
- Qualitative study
- Retrospective review of surgical technique

| Level of evidence | 4 |
|---|---|
| Randomization | None |
| Number of patients | Over 2500 alluded to |
| Inclusion criteria | Endoscopic and X-ray or computed tomography evidence of sinus disease |
| Exclusion criteria | None stated |
| Follow-up | Postoperative debridement regime described but no standardized follow-up to assess efficacy of technique |

## Outcome measures

### Primary endpoint

Completion of endoscopic sinus surgery (ESS).

### Secondary endpoints

None.

## Results

- >2,500 patients
- No serious dural or orbital complications
- No cerebrospinal fluid leaks
- Negligible blood loss reported (but not measured or recorded)
- Only isolated cases of breach of lamina papyracea resulting in subcutaneous emphysema
- Angled endoscopes useful to observe sinus ostia
- Objective of surgery to skeletonize roof of ethmoid, lamina papyracea and frontal recess
- Stressed importance of postoperative care, including debridement and antimicrobials or antifungals

## Conclusions

The use of the endoscope to perform sinus surgery significantly enhanced the quality and finesse of the intervention.

- Excessive surgery could be avoided
- Surgery could be targeted more effectively
- Surgery could be tailored to the disease and the individual more effectively
- Surgery could be performed under surface and local anaesthesia
- Postoperative debridement and medical therapies were considered important adjuncts to surgery

# Critique

This seminal paper by Stammberger (1986) and subsequent publications changed the landscape of how sinus surgery was conducted. Two extremely important changes occurred subsequently:

- the use of the endoscope, and
- targeted, less destructive sinus surgery

Although purely descriptive, alluding to over 2,500 cases and only making a vague case for the absence of complications and bleeding, the paper provided a framework for researchers to subsequently better quantify indications and complications of ESS. Over the past 30 years the surgical ethos has not altered radically but, if anything, has become even more targeted with a focus on mucosal preservation to encourage inherent mucociliary function.

## Additional references

Kennedy DW, Zinreich SJ, Rosenbaum AE, Johns ME. Functional endoscopic sinus surgery. Theory and diagnostic evaluation. *Arch Otolaryngol* 1985;**111**:576–82.

Stammberger H. Endoscopic endonasal surgery—concepts in treatment of recurring rhinosinusitis. Part I. Anatomic and pathophysiologic considerations. *Otolaryngol Head Neck Surg* 1986;**94**:143–7.

Stammberger H, Posawetz W. Functional endoscopic sinus surgery. Concept, indications and results of the Messerklinger technique. *Eur Arch Otorhinolaryngol* 1990;**247**:63–76.

Weber R, Hosemann W. Comprehensive review on endonasal endoscopic sinus surgery. *GMS Curr Top Otorhinolaryngol Head Neck Surg* 2015;**14**:1–108.

# Chapter 34

# Assessing quality of life in rhinosinusitis

Claire Hopkins

## Details of studies

The impact of chronic rhinosinusitis (CRS) on health-related quality of life (HRQOL) was first quantified by Gliklich and Metson (1995), in a landmark paper using the SF-36 to compare patients with CRS and other chronic conditions to normative data. This paper reported significant differences in several domains, and greater impact on bodily pain and social function. The relative burden of chronic sinusitis came as a surprise to the authors but helped to define the healthcare implications and societal costs of the condition. Although generic instruments such as the SF-36 facilitate comparison between different medical conditions and healthy cohorts, they may lack the sensitivity to detect small but clinically important changes in HRQOL. For this reason, a myriad of disease-specific HRQOL instruments have been developed, including items rated by patients themselves as being important when afflicted with the disease in question. One of the most widely used and translated of these is the SNOT-20 (20-item Sino-Nasal Outcome Test).

## Study references

### Main reference

Piccirillo JF, Merritt MG, Richards ML. Psychometric and clinimetric validity of the 20-item Sino-Nasal Outcome Test (SNOT-20). *Otolaryngol Head Neck Surg* 2002;**126**:41–7.

### Related references

Gliklich RE, Metson R. The health impact of chronic sinusitis in patients seeking otolaryngologic care. *Otolaryngol Head Neck Surg* 1995;**113**:104–9.

Hopkins C, Gillett S, Slack R, Lund VJ, Browne JP. Psychometric validity of the 22-item Sinonasal Outcome Test. *Clin Otolaryngol* 2009;**34**:447–54.

## Study design

Psychometric validation of the SNOT-20, a modification of the RSOM-31, in patients with CRS.

| | |
|---|---|
| Number of patients | 102 |
| Inclusion criteria | All adult patients undergoing treatment for CRS an academic hospital setting |
| Follow-up | Patients completed SNOT-20 questionnaires at 0, 6, and 12 months |

## Outcome measures

To confirm validity, internal consistency, reliability, construct validity, and content validity were assessed. Sensitivity to change was assessed using the standardized response mean.

## Results

Cronbach's α was 0.90, demonstrating good internal consistency. Test–retest reliability was established in a group of 15 patients that repeated the SNOT-20 2 weeks after baseline. Discriminant validity was shown by comparing the SNOT-20 in CRS patients with 10 healthy volunteers. Concurrent validity was established by comparing SNOT-20 scores with a global rating of HRQOL. A change of SNOT-20 of more than 0.8 was calculated to be the minimal clinically important difference.

## Conclusion

The SNOT-20 was shown to be a valid patient-reported outcome measure suitable for use in adult patients with CRS.

## Critique

The SNOT-20 was one of the first PROMs that achieved widespread uptake in both research and routine clinical practice. A literature search reveals more than 200 studies utilizing the SNOT-20, with many validated translations. Importantly, Piccirillo and his colleagues demonstrated responsiveness and also quantified what was a clinically meaningful change in SNOT-20 scores, which allowed better appreciation of the effectiveness of different treatments; too often statistically significant changes may be reported by trials, yet the actual magnitude of change is not detectable as improvement by the patient.

It is interesting that both nasal obstruction and anosmia were items that were deleted from the RSOM-31 during factor analysis and do not appear in the SNOT-20. Both American and European guidelines on the diagnosis of chronic rhinosinusitis include these symptoms within their defining criteria, and it is surprising that factor analysis identified them as redundant. Now, the SNOT-22 is the more widely used tool, it uses SNOT-20 but adds on these additional factors of nasal obstruction and anosmia (Hopkins et al. 2009).

The authors also believe their importance rating (where participants choose the five items that are the most important items affecting their health) is a key aspect of the SNOT-20. However, they found that the items identified by patients as the most important had statistically significantly higher individual item scores and could therefore be identified by the item score alone. One wonders if this additional burden on the respondent adds to the utility of the instrument.

Chapter 35

# Surgical outcomes for rhinosinusitis

Luke Reid

Chronic rhinosinusitis (CRS) is a common condition affecting up to 11% UK adults and has been shown to have a significant impact on quality of life. When medical treatment has failed, surgical intervention is often considered. As with many surgical procedures, high quality randomized controlled trials are limited and large cohort studies provide estimates of effectiveness in a 'real-world' setting. The UK comparative audit is the largest prospective study evaluating outcomes of surgery for CRS.

## Study references

### Main reference

Hopkins C, Browne J, Slack R, Lund V, Topham J, Reeves B, et al. The national comparative audit of surgery for nasal polyposis and rhinosinusitis. *Clin Otol* 2006;**31**:390–8.

### Related references

Hopkins C, Gillett S, Slack R, Lund VJ, Browne JP. Psychometric validation for the SNOT22. *Clin Otol* 2009;**34**:447–54.

Hopkins C, Slack R, Lund V, Brown P, Copley L, Browne J. 5 year results of the national audit of surgery for rhinosinusitis and nasal polyposis. *Laryngoscope* 2009;**119**:2459–65.

## Study design

Prospective, multicentre longitudinal outcome study of patients undergoing surgery for CRS, reporting 3-year follow-up (level 2 evidence).

| | |
|---|---|
| Level of evidence | 2a |
| Recruitment | Consecutive patients in 87 NHS hospitals in England and Wales were recruited at the time of endoscopic sinus surgery |
| Number of patients | 3,128 |
| Inclusion criteria | All adult patients undergoing elective surgery for CRS, including both primary and secondary cases, and CRSwNP (with nasal polyps) and CRSsNP (without nasal polyps) |
| Exclusion criteria | Patients undergoing non-CRS related surgery |
| Follow-up | Patients completed follow-up questionnaires at 3, 12, and 36 months. |

## Outcome measures

The primary outcome was change in SNOT-22, a patient reported outcome measure.

Secondary outcomes were complications of surgery reported at 3 months, and revision surgery rates were reported at each follow-up point.

## Study results

A total of 2,176 included patients had CRSwNP, the remainder had CRSsNP. Two-thirds of CRSwNP patients were male, compared with less than half the CRSsNP patients. The mean age was 49 years. Forty-eight per cent of patients had undergone previous sinus surgery. The mean Lund–Mackay score was 10.6, but this was significantly higher in the CRSwNP group (13.2) than the CRSsNP group (6.5). Thirty-nine per cent of patients had a Lund–Mackay score of ≤4. The mean preoperative SNOT-22 score was 42.0, with 19% of patients reporting mild symptoms with a preoperative score of ≤22.

Consultants performed half of the recorded procedures. Mean operative time was 40 minutes.

There was a large improvement in SNOT-22 scores from baseline (42.0 mean) to 3 months (25.5 mean). Greater improvement was seen in patients with CRSwNP (41.0 to 23.1) than with CRSsNP (44.2 to 31.2). The rate of major complications was low (0.2% orbital complications, all orbital haematomas, and 0.06% intracranial; both CSF leaks). At 36 months 11.4% patients had undergone revision surgery.

## Conclusions

This study highlights that some patients are submitted to elective surgery in the setting of mild symptoms and/or limited disease on computed tomography imaging, and that this needs further study. However, it found that sinus surgery has a low risk of major complications, and results in large reductions in mean symptom scores, with maintenance of benefit over 36 months although a proportion had required revision in this time.

## Critique

This is the largest prospective outcome study of sinus surgery to date, and is notable in that it was funded entirely by participating trusts. At the time of recruitment in 2000 49% invited trusts across the UK declined to submit data, the vast majority quoting financial restrictions as the cause of refusal. It is quite likely to be that in times of increasing austerity, this study could never be repeated with a similar funding model.

The value of this study is that it demonstrates the real-life effectiveness of sinus surgery, as it demonstrates improvement in patients treated under 298 different consultants across the UK, using a wide variety of surgical techniques. While most procedures were performed endoscopically, surgery varied significantly in terms of its extent. Despite this, there was little difference in outcome between different extents of surgery. There was a significant reduction in SNOT-22 scores, with persistent benefit at 36 months shown in this study, and at 60 months in a subsequent follow-up. Given the paucity of randomized trials, and increased pressure to only commission surgical procedures with proven efficacy, it is likely to be that this study has contributed to the continued ability to offer surgery within both state-funded and the private healthcare market.

The limitation of the study is the lack of randomization to any particular technique or control arm, and there is certainly selection bias in the choice of procedures offered in addition to other confounders. Any estimates of effectiveness must be considered with this in mind.

The study was one of the first large studies within ENT to utilize a patient reported outcome measure. The SNOT-22 was a derivative of the SNOT-20, and was developed for the purpose of the audit. The steering group felt that although the SNOT-20 had gone through rigorous psychometric validation, it lacked content validity due to the absence of the symptoms of nasal obstruction and change in sense of smell. Both symptoms are key in diagnostic criteria. The resulting SNOT-22 has since been formally revalidated, and now one of the most widely used patient reported outcome measures in CRS. As such the results of the UK audit often form the benchmark against which other studies are compared.

Chapter 36

# Allergic rhinitis and asthma

Hesham Saleh and Jahangir Ahmed

## Details of study

Allergic rhinitis and asthma are systemic inflammatory conditions and are very often comorbidities. A conservative estimate is that allergic rhinitis occurs in over 500 million people around the world and is likely to increase in most countries. They are both highly complex diseases with many aetiological factors, mechanisms of onset, and multifarious interplay between epidemiology and quality of life. There is also a strong causal association between disease of the upper airway and that of the lower airways (Hakansson et al. 2015). The literature makes frequent reference to either one-airway disease or sinobronchial syndrome. The ARIA document (Allergic Rhinitis and its Impact on Asthma) was intended to be a state-of-the-art reference for the specialist as well as for the general practitioner and other healthcare professionals to

- update their knowledge of allergic rhinitis
- highlight the impact of allergic rhinitis on asthma
- provide an evidence-based documented revision on diagnostic methods
- provide an evidence-based revision on treatments, and
- propose a stepwise approach to management (Bousquet et al. 2008).

## Study references

### Main study

Bousquet J, Khaltaev N, Cruz AA, Denburg J, Fokkens WJ, Togias A, et al. Allergic rhinitis and its impact on asthma (ARIA) 2008. *Allergy* 2008;**63** (Suppl. 86):8–160.

### Related references

Brozek JL, Bousquet J, Baena-Cagnani CE, Bonini S, Canonica GW, Casale TB, et al. Allergic rhinitis and its impact on asthma (ARIA) guidelines: 2010 revision. *J Allergy Clin Immunol* 2010;**126**:466–76.

Fokkens W, Lund, V, Mullol J, Bachert C, Cohen N, Cobo R, et al. European position paper on rhinosinusitis and nasal polyps 2007. *Rhinology Suppl* 2007;**20**:1–136.

Fokkens W, Lund V, Mullol J, Bachert C, Alobid I, Baroody F, et al. EPOS 2012: European position paper on rhinosinusitis and nasal polyps 2012. A summary for otorhinolaryngologists. *Rhinology* 2012;**50**:1–12.

## Study design

- Multicentre international collaboration of panel of experts in 1999
- Review of 2241 publications up to December 1999 related to rhinitis and asthma

| | |
|---|---|
| Level of evidence | 3a |
| Randomization | Not applicable |
| Number of patients | Not applicable |
| Inclusion criteria | All publications relating to rhinitis and asthma up to December 1999 |
| Exclusion criteria | None stated |
| Follow-up | Not applicable |

## Outcome measures

### Primary endpoint

Not applicable.

### Secondary endpoints

None.

## Results

The paper was divided into subsections with exhaustive elaboration of aetiological causes, mechanisms of inflammation, epidemiology and disease burden, diagnosis and technical adjuncts, management and prevention, links between rhinitis and asthma, impact on quality of life, appraisal of comorbidities (e.g. allergic conjunctivitis, rhinosinusitis, adenoidal hypertrophy, Eustachian tube dysfunction, otitis media with effusion, chronic cough, laryngitis, reflux), and rhinitis in children. There was also specific discussion in areas such as rhinitis in athletes.

Objectives achieved by the working group included

- a new classification for allergic rhinitis, which was subdivided into 'intermittent' (IAR) or 'persistent' (PER) disease, and
- severity of allergic rhinitis was classified as 'mild' or 'moderate/severe' depending on symptoms but also on quality of life

It was also identified that over 80% of asthmatics have rhinitis and 10–40% of patients with rhinitis have asthma. Thus, most patients with asthma have rhinitis suggesting the concept of 'one airway one disease' alluded to above. The document also discussed chronic rhinosinusitis without and with nasal polyps, in addition to rhinitis, with some crossover, therefore, with the first evolution of the EPOS guideline (Fokkens et al. 2007).

## Conclusions

This was a very useful, comprehensive resource examining in great detail the literature pertaining to allergic rhinitis and asthma.

## Critique

While being a very useful single-point resource for over 2000 publications assessing the relationship between allergic rhinitis and asthma, this document illustrates quite clearly the difficulty in pulling together subsection literature reviews from multiple authors. The working group formed in 1999; the paper was eventually published in 2008: a mammoth task. The magnitude of the effort required to pull together such a complex document is unfortunately, therefore, reflected in certain aspects of the paper. There is considerable repetition both within and between sections, perhaps a reflection of authors being given sections or subsections to review. Additionally, there is no systematic appraisal of the literature referenced, without either inclusion or exclusion criteria and with variable critique of the reviewed literature by the section authors. What the paper does do well, however, is provide a framework to direct further reading of the current literature in small, manageable amounts.

## Additional references

Hakansson K, Bachert C, Konge L, Thomsen SF, Pedersen AE, Poulsen SS, et al. Airway inflammation in chronic rhinosinusitis with nasal polyps and asthma: the united airways concept further supported. *PLoS One* 2015;**10**:1–11.

Scadding G, Walker S. Poor asthma control?—then look up the nose. The importance of co-morbid rhinitis in patients with asthma. *Prim Care Resp J* 2012;**21**:222–8.

Terzakis D, Georgalas C. Polyps, asthma, and allergy: what's new. *Curr Opin Otolaryngol Head Neck Surg* 2017;**25**:12–18.

# Chapter 37

# Allergic fungal rhinosinusitis

Hesham Saleh and Jahangir Ahmed

## Details of studies

Fungal sinusitis encompasses a spectrum of diseases that differ in clinical presentation, histopathology, and prognosis from other forms of rhinosinusitis and are consequently managed differently. Specific diagnostic criteria have been much debated in the literature. Fungal sinusitis is commonly categorized into invasive and non-invasive forms. The former are further subclassified into acute, chronic, and granulomatous invasive fungal sinusitis that are almost exclusive to immunocompromised individuals. Non-invasive categorization includes fungal colonization, fungal ball, and allergic fungal rhinosinusitis (AFRS).

AFRS is the commonest form of fungal sinusitis and has attracted significant controversy regarding its clinicopathological definition, aetiology, and management. Prior to this landmark publication by Bent and Kuhn in 1994, rhinologists worldwide were reporting on a heterogeneous group of immunocompetent patients with chronic rhinosinusitis (CRS), refractory to conventional medical treatment, with relatively rapid recurrence of symptoms following sinus surgery. These patients were atopic, had nasal polyposis, and demonstrated characteristic sinus radiology. Tenacious mucus was universally found intraoperatively. The underlying pathophysiology was assumed to be a type 1 hypersensitivity reaction to fungal antigens in parallel to allergic bronchopulmonary aspergillosis, although the most common organisms isolated from sinuses were of the *Dematiaceous* variety and not *Aspergillus* species. Up to 7% of CRS patients could retrospectively be recategorized as AFRS, with an even higher prevalence in warm humid climates such as in southern and southeastern USA. Nevertheless, there were no uniformly accepted diagnostic criteria, posing a problem for comparative investigation and the creation of uniformly acceptable management protocols. This case series sought to establish such a set of diagnostic criteria and despite its size, is still referenced in many publications about fungal sinus disease.

## Reference

### Main study

Bent JP 3rd, Kuhn FA. Diagnosis of allergic fungal sinusitis. *Otolaryngol Head Neck Surg* 1994;111:580–8.

## Study design

Level of evidence: 4

## Method

### Prospective case series

Fifteen consecutive patients with presumed allergic fungal sinusitis based on a broad set of non-inclusive criteria (see Results)

- Six females and nine males
- Mean age 27.6 (13–51) years
- Study period 15 months. No follow-up included
- Documentation of 11 characteristic items to determine common criteria (see table in Results)

## Results

Symptoms, signs, radiological and pathological features that aroused suspicion of AFRS were actively sought in these patients.

| Clinicopathological features sought | Present in x/15 |
|---|---|
| 1. Type 1 hypersensitivity (on history/elevated total serum immunoglobulin (Ig)E/skin prick test or radioallergosorbent test against fungal antigen) | 15 |
| 2. Asthma | 8 |
| 3. Nasal polyposis | 15 |
| 4. Unilateral predominance | 13 |
| 5. Bone erosion on computed tomography (CT) | 12 |
| 6. Characteristic heterogeneous sinus opacification on CT | 15 |
| 7. Eosinophilic mucous without fungal invasion into sinus tissue | 15 |
| 8. Charcot Leyden crystals in mucous | 6 |
| 9. Positive fungal stain | 15 |
| 10. Positive fungal culture | 11 |
| 11. Peripheral eosinophilia | 6 |

## Conclusion

Five features were common to all as indicated in the table in Results: evidence of type 1 hypersensitivity against fungus, nasal polyposis, characteristic computed tomography findings, eosinophilic mucous without fungal invasion, and identification of fungus on stain. This set of criteria subsequently became the gold standard for the precise definition of AFRS. Interestingly all patients denied aspirin sensitivity.

## Critique

The Bent and Kuhn criteria have, subsequent to this publication, been widely accepted and used to define patients suffering with AFRS. This is remarkable given the relatively low numbers of patients in this series from a single surgical team, collected during a short study window, and without a validating control population. It was however one of the earliest attempts to unify this heterogeneous population into a discrete diagnostic entity paving the way for standardization to ensure meaningful investigation. For this reason, it is considered a landmark paper.

A number of potential problems exist with these criteria, not least that none of these criteria are unique to AFRS. In the paper, the definition of type 1 hypersensitivity to fungus was not stringent. Total IgE was elevated in six of seven patients tested, whereas only five patients were formally tested for fungal antigen-specific allergy with either skin prick or radioallergosorbent tests. Serum total IgE elevation is not specific to type 1 hypersensitivity and may be elevated in other diseases, e.g. parasite infections and autoimmune conditions. The reliance on a suggestive history to diagnose atopy as was done for the remainder of patients is open to criticism.

There is debate as to whether eosinophilic mucus is elicited by a genuine allergic type 1 hypersensitivity response to fungal antigens; furthermore, eosinophilic mucin has been described in patients without histologically detectable fungal hyphae or by conventional culture methods. These distinctions have given rise to further clinicopathological sub-categorizations such as eosinophilic fungal rhinosinusitis and eosinophilic mucinous rhinosinusitis, characterized by the absence of fungal specific IgE in both and with no identifiable fungal stigmata in the latter. Conversely with the advent of increasingly sensitive detection methods some authors contend that fungus may be found in almost all nasal cavities of patients suffering with CRS with and without polyposis and in a sizeable proportion of healthy individuals. Finally, despite the relatively unique characteristic CT and magnetic resonance imaging features, the diagnosis of fungal sinusitis solely based on radiology will be neither sensitive nor specific.

Nonetheless, despite these diagnostic uncertainties, this paper did highlight the need to be vigilant of a particularly severe variant of CRS that warrants aggressive surgical and medical management to prevent rapid postoperative recurrence; whether these cases can genuinely be categorized into a unique clinicopathologic entity still remains to be conclusively determined but the definition suggested by the paper remains the most widely used, in the absence of a true consensus for an alternative.

## Additional references

Chakrabarti A, Denning DW, Ferguson BJ, Ponikau J, Buzina W, Kita H, et al. Fungal rhinosinusitis: a categorization and definitional schema addressing current controversies. *Laryngoscope* 2009;**119**:1809–18.

Ferguson BJ. Eosinophilic mucin rhinosinusitis: a distinct clinicopathological entity. *Laryngoscope* 2000;**110**(Pt 1):799–813.

Ponikau JU, Sherris DA, Kern EB, Homburger HA, Frigas E, Gaffey TA, Roberts GD. The diagnosis and incidence of allergic fungal sinusitis. *Mayo Clin Proc* 1999;**74**:877–84.

Chapter 38

# Immunotherapy

Hesham Saleh and Jahangir Ahmed

## Details of studies

Allergic rhinitis, as one of the commonest global chronic diseases affects up to 23% of Western populations. It is a disease of the young and, untreated, has a significant impact on schooling, employment, and general quality of life. Best practice currently utilizes established diagnostic criteria, with severity and duration in turn dictating a stepwise, tailored approach to management as outlined in the latest Allergic Rhinitis and its Impact on Asthma (ARIA) guidelines, which state that allergen-specific immunotherapy should be considered for patients in whom therapy with topical and systemic antihistamines and corticosteroids have failed to alleviate symptoms, or in patients who are unwilling to comply with such treatment.

Immunotherapy usually consists of gradually increasing quantities of allergen administered in a controlled environment over a period of 6 months to 3 years depending on the mode of administration. The commonest routes of application are subcutaneous (SCIT), the gold standard, and sublingual (SLIT) and both have been associated with clinical benefit in trials, systematic reviews, and meta-analyses for seasonal 'pollen' driven allergy, with less clear-cut efficacy for 'perennial' allergen-driven disease.

Establishing the optimal dose of immunotherapy is balanced by the potential for systemic side effects, the severity of which has been reported to be higher with SCIT. The potential for anaphylaxis and bronchospasm warrants administration of SCIT in an environment with resuscitation facilities. Patients with severe asthma or irreversible airway disease are not suitable for immunotherapy for fear of eliciting bronchoconstriction. Although relatively common, the side effect profile of SLIT consists mainly of local irritant reactions such as itch and mild self-limiting oral oedema, with no reported cases of fatality from anaphylaxis. It is thus potentially safer, more tolerable and able to be administered at home. However, to date no well-designed and powered head-to-head study has been performed comparing the efficacy of SCIT with SLIT in the context of allergic rhinitis and thus a universal preference for either with due regard to safety cannot yet be made; this review aimed to use the best available evidence to indirectly compare the efficacy and side effect profiles of SCIT with SLIT.

## References

### Main study

**Durham SR, Penagos M.** Sublingual or subcutaneous immunotherapy for allergic rhinitis? *J Allergy Clin Immunol* 2016;**137**:339–49.

### Related references

**Calderon MA, Alves B, Jacobson M, Hurwitz B, Sheikh A, Durham S.** Allergen injection immunotherapy for seasonal allergic rhinitis. *Cochrane Database Syst Rev* 2007;**1**:CD001936.

**Dahl R, Kapp A, Colombo G, de Monchy JG, Rak S, Emminger W,** et al. Efficacy and safety of sublingual immunotherapy with grass allergen tablets for seasonal allergic rhinoconjunctivitis. *J Allergy Clin Immunol* 2006;**118**:434–40.

**Frew AJ, Powell RJ, Corrigan CJ, Durham SR; UK Immunotherapy Study Group.** Efficacy and safety of specific immunotherapy with SQ allergen extract in treatment-resistant seasonal allergic rhinoconjunctivitis. *J Allergy Clin Immunol* 2006;**117**:319–25.

**Radulovic S, Calderon MA, Wilson D, Durham S.** Sublingual immunotherapy for allergic *rhinitis*. *Cochrane Database Syst Rev* 2010;**12**:CD002893.

## Method

Literature review containing meta-analyses (review containing level 1a evidence).

## Results

This comprehensive review outlines the current state of evidence for use of SLIT and SCIT in AR and PAR. The key findings are reported.

A comparison of two pivotal double blinded placebo controlled randomized controlled trials using either SCIT or SLIT, using the same single aeroallergen (*Phleum pratense* extract) with similar treatment duration, outcome measures and follow up duration (Frew et al. 2006; Dahl et al. 2006). All patients had moderate to severe grass pollen seasonal allergic rhinitis (SAR) for at least 2 years.

| | No. in AIT | No. in placebo | Nasal symptoms scores | | Occular symptom score | |
|---|---|---|---|---|---|---|
| | | | Mean effect size (95% CI) | % reduction | Mean difference (95% CI) | % reduction |
| SCIT | 187 | 89 | −0.86 (−1.28 to −0.44) | −32 | −0.50 (−0.72 to −0.28) | −36 |
| SLIT | 282 | 286 | −0.60 (−0.82 to −0.38) | −26 | −0.40 (−0.52 to −0.28) | −36 |

AIT, active immunotherapy.

SLIT was associated with local reactions (oral itch (46%) and oedema (18%)) resulting in withdrawal by 4% of patients.

SCIT was associated with immediate systemic effects following injections with grade 2 and non-life threatening grade 3 reactions in 17.2% and 4.4% respectively.

The following tables are a summary of the efficacy, extrapolated from the three Cochrane meta-analyses on SCIT (one each for SAR and perennial allergic rhinitis (PAR)) and SLIT (one covering both SAR and PAR) (Calderon et al. 2007; Durham et al. 2016; Radulovic et al. 2010).

| | No. in AIT | No. in Placebo | $I^2$ (%) | Symptom scores SMD (placebo—AIT) and 95 CI | |
| --- | --- | --- | --- | --- | --- |
| | | | | Seasonal allergens | Perennial allergens |
| SCIT | 597 | 466 | 63 | −0.73 (−0.97 to −0.50) | 0.86 (−1.48 to −0.23) |
| | 187 | 189 | 86 | | |
| SLIT | 2081 | 2003 | 45 | −0.34 (−0.44 to −0.25) | −0.93 (−1.69 to −0.17) |
| | 252 | 253 | 92 | | |

AIT, active immunotherapy; SMD, standardized mean difference; CI, confidence interval.

| | No. in AIT | No. in placebo | $I^2$ (%) | Medication scores SMD (placebo—AIT) and 95 CI | |
| --- | --- | --- | --- | --- | --- |
| | | | | Seasonal allergens | Perennial allergens |
| SCIT | 549 | 414 | 64 | −0.57 (−0.82 to −0.33) | 0.05 (−0.23 to 0.32) |
| | 100 | 107 | 26 | | |
| SLIT | 1557 | 1457 | 44 | −0.30 (−0.41 to −0.19) | −0.43 (−0.89 to 0.02) |
| | 180 | 185 | 71 | | |

AIT, active immunotherapy; SMD, standardized mean difference; CI, confidence interval.

In the meta-analysis of SCIT for SAR (Calderon et al. 2007), 30 and 33 trials out of the 51 that met inclusion criteria reported local and systemic reactions respectively; most adverse events were mild and reversible.

| Reaction | SCIT (% participants) | Placebo (% participants) |
| --- | --- | --- |
| **Local** | | |
| Self-limiting | 92 | 33 |
| Requiring treatment | 10 | 4 |
| **Systemic** | | |
| Early (<30 min) G-2 | 22 | 8 |
| Early (<30 min) G-3 | 7 | 0.65 |
| Early (<30 min) G-4 | 0.72 | 0.33 |
| Late systemic | 89 | 36 |
| Adrenaline use | 3.41 | 0.25 |

G, grade.

Two patients had anaphylaxis and one had asthma exacerbation following SCIT, in comparison to one anaphylactic reaction following injection of placebo. There were no fatalities.

In the meta-analysis of SCIT for PAR (study in press, with extracts reviewed in Durham et al. 2016), all 16 included trials (n = 667) reported adverse effects as below. There were no reported fatalities.

| | SCIT (no.) | Placebo (no.) |
|---|---|---|
| Local | 65 | 27 |
| Grade 1 | 59 | 27 |
| Grade 2 | 13 | 2 |
| Grade 3 | 2 | 0 |
| Grade 4 | 8 | 0 |

In the meta-analysis of SLIT for SAR and PAR (Radulovic et al. 2010), frequencies of adverse events were reported in 54 of 60 trials analysed. Most were local and mild. The table below depicts events that are likely to occur at least once in any individual for the duration of therapy.

| Reaction | SLIT events per participant | Placebo events per participant |
|---|---|---|
| **Local** | | |
| Buccal pruritus | 1.6 | 0.46 |
| Oral (unspecified) | 2.1 | 0.34 |
| **Systemic** | | |
| Conjunctivitis | 2.95 | 3.3 |
| Rhinitis | 1.45 | 1.13 |
| Asthma/wheeze | 0.1 | 0.09 |
| Cough | 0.93 | 0.69 |

There were no episodes of anaphylaxis or adrenaline usage and the likelihood of an asthmatic exacerbation or wheeze was 0.1 and 0.09 events per participant in AIT and placebo groups respectively.

A further 28 studies were included in a more recent update on two of the aforementioned Cochrane meta-analyses (searched till April 2011) (Dretzke et al. 2013). The new data did not change the overall effect of comparisons. They estimated a standardized score difference of efficacy between SCIT and SLIT, which favoured SCIT with an effect size of 0.351 (95% credible interval 0.127 to 0.586), a statistically significant result (Dretzke et al. 2013).

| | Updated Cochrane meta-analysis | |
|---|---|---|
| | Nasal symptom scores (SMD and 95 CI) $I^2$ (%) | Medication scores (SMD and 95 CI) $I^2$ (%) |
| SCIT | −0.65 (−0.85 to −0.45) 57 | −0.55 (−0.75 to −0.34) 57 |
| SLIT | −0.33 (−0.42 to −0.25) 42 | −0.27 (−0.37 to −0.17) 49 |

SMD, standardized mean difference; CI, confidence interval.

The Durham and Penagos paper also reviewed more recent meta-analyses that incorporated more recent robustly designed studies, all of which support the Cochrane reviews that both SCIT and SLIT are effective in alleviating the symptoms of SAR. However due to the highly heterogeneous nature of the data and differences in methodology for indirect comparisons, there still remains controversy about whether the data support the apparent superiority of current SCIT treatment regimes over SLIT.

## Conclusion

A comparison of the trials conducted by Frew et al. and Dahl et al. implied relatively similar efficacies for grass pollen immunotherapy in those demonstrating seasonal allergy, when administered by either route.

The overall picture from Cochrane meta-analyses for SAR confirmed efficacious reduction of both nasal symptoms and medication usage for both routes in the context of seasonal allergy, favouring SCIT in terms of effect size.

Immunotherapy with allergens causing perennial rhinitis did not demonstrate efficacy in these meta-analyses; however, the heterogeneous nature of the relevant studies make standardization and thus comparison in this regard difficult.

Local side effects appear to be common to both routes of administration, with higher rates of systemic toxicity reported with SCIT.

## Critique and discussion

This review paper sets out an agenda to summarize important trial evidence pertaining to allergen immunotherapy for rhinitis and in particular whether the literature favours SC or SL routes of allergen administration in terms of efficacy and safety. In this regard it succeeds admirably and the reader is highly encouraged to read the full version of the article, as this chapter cannot encompass all the trials and meta-analyses discussed.

The only four double-blinded head-to-head comparison trials (also described in the review) demonstrate no clear differences in improvement in rhinitis scores or need for rescue medication between SCIT or SLIT. However, none of these was sufficiently powered, with a paucity of numbers of patients in each comparator group (ranging from 10 to 20). There is significant variability in study design and received dosage of allergen.

The paper confirms that allergen immunotherapy for SAR administered by either route is efficacious, as has been well established, and estimates a twofold effect size favouring SCIT. However, this can only be a theoretical estimate and the authors do comment that this conclusion should be treated with some degree of scepticism. In addition to the inherent problems of the validity of comparing separate trials, earlier incorporated studies were multiple, smaller in size, and conducted with less rigour with regards stringent selection criteria and outcomes. There was a high degree of heterogeneity in the data, especially apparent with studies that looked at perennial allergic rhinitis, in which populous, non-allergic factors may further confound the results.

It should be noted that five recent large double-blind randomized controlled trials of SLIT, with a combined total number of patients exceeding 4,000, have demonstrated efficacy against grass pollen allergy and against perennial mite allergy (Bergmann et al. 2014; Mosbech et al. 2015; Demoly et al. 2016; Okamoto et al. 2015; Maloney. 2014). For the latter, the three relevant trials all demonstrated a clear dose response reduction in symptom and medication scores (18–28%). There however remains a relative paucity of trials with SCIT in perennial allergic rhinitis.

In contrast to efficacy, indirect comparisons would appear to favour SLIT, with regards to tolerability and safety, during which severe systemic reactions have rarely been reported and local reactions are often self-limiting.

There thus remains an unmet need to perform double blinded adequately powered, well designed clinical trials that pitch SCIT and SLIT head to head in the context of seasonal and perennial allergic rhinitis. As discussed in the paper, these should use products that have demonstrated efficacy in placebo controlled trials, and arms should include double dummy protocols, performed according to international selection criteria, methods and outcomes analysis. Tolerability and safety should also be carefully documented. Until such studies are completed, there remains equipoise in the recommendation of SCIT versus SLIT, which at present is likely to depend on local policy and patient preference.

## References

Bergmann KC, Demoly P, Worm M, Fokkens WJ, Carrillo T, Tabar AI, et al. Efficacy and safety of sublingual tablets of house dust mite allergen extracts in adults with allergic rhinitis. *J Allergy Clin Immunol* 2014;133:1608–14

Calderon MA, Alves B, Jacobson M, Hurwitz B, Sheikh A, Durham S. Allergen injection immunotherapy for seasonal allergic rhinitis. *Cochrane Database Syst Rev* 2007;1:CD001936

Dahl R, Kapp A, Colombo G, de Monchy JG, Rak S, Emminger W, et al. Efficacy and safety of sublingual immunotherapy with grass allergen tablets for seasonal allergic rhinoconjunctivitis. *J Allergy Clin Immunol* 2006;118:434–40.

Demoly P, Emminger W, Rehm D, Backer V, Tommerup L, Kleine-Tebbe J. Effective treatment of house dust mite-induced allergic rhinitis with 2 doses of the SQ HDM SLIT-tablet: Results from a randomized, double-blind, placebo-controlled phase III trial. *J Allergy Clin Immunol* 2016;137:444–51.

Dretzke J, Meadows A, Novielli N, Huissoon A, Fry-Smith A, Meads C. Subcutaneous and sublingual immunotherapy for seasonal allergic rhinitis: a systematic review and indirect comparison. *J Allergy Clin Immunol* 2013;131:1361–6.

Durham SR, Penagos M. Sublingual or subcutaneous immunotherapy for allergic rhinitis? *J Allergy Clin Immunol* 2016;137:339–49.

Frew AJ, Powell RJ, Corrigan CJ, Durham SR; UK Immunotherapy Study Group. Efficacy and safety of specific immunotherapy with SQ allergen extract in treatment-resistant seasonal allergic rhinoconjunctivitis. *J Allergy Clin Immunol* 2006;117:319–25.

Maloney J, Bernstein DI, Nelson H, Creticos P, Hébert J, Noonan M, et al. Efficacy and safety of grass sublingual immunotherapy tablet, MK-7243: a large randomized controlled trial. *Ann Allergy Asthma Immunol* 2014;112:146–53.

Mosbech H, Canonica GW, Backer V, de Blay F, Klimek L, Broge L, Ljørring C. SQ house dust mite sublingually administered immunotherapy tablet (ALK) improves allergic rhinitis in patients with house dust mite allergic asthma and rhinitis symptoms. Ann Allergy Asthma Immunol 2015;**114**:134–40.

Okamoto Y, Okubo K, Yonekura S, Hashiguchi K, Goto M, Otsuka T, et al. Efficacy and safety of sublingual immunotherapy for two seasons in patients with Japanese cedar pollinosis. *Int Arch Allergy Immunol* 2015;**166**:177–88.

Radulovic S, Calderon MA, Wilson D, Durham S. Sublingual immunotherapy for allergic rhinitis. *Cochrane Database Syst Rev* 2010;**12**:CD002893.

# Chapter 39

# Non-infectious, non-allergic rhinitis

Luke Reid

## Details of studies

In the classification of chronic rhinitis one distinction that can be made is between syndromes that have known and unknown aetiologies. Non-infectious, non-allergic rhinitis (NINAR) falls into the latter. The NINAR symptomatology has similar hallmarks to allergic rhinitis (although with lower rates of sneezing, conjunctival symptoms, and pruritis) as well as a high prevalence of symptoms compatible with sinus disease.

Three potential functional abnormalities that may have a role to play in the pathophysiology of NINAR include

1  The ageing process of the nasal mucosa

2  Nasal hyper-reactivity

3  An imbalanced neuronal control of end organs of the nose

### Study references

#### Main study

Sanico A, Togias A. Noninfectious, nonallergic rhinitis (NINAR): considerations on possible mechanisms. *Am J Rhinol* 1998;**12**:65–72.

#### Related references

Braat J P M, Mulder P G, Fokkens W J, Gerth van Wijk R, Rijntjes E. Intranasal cold dry air is superior to histamine challenge in determining the presence and degree of nasal hyperreactivity in nonallergic noninfectious perennial rhinitis. *Am J Respir Crit Care Med* 1998;**157**:1748–55.

Lundblad L, Lundberg J M, Brodin E, Anggard A. Origin and distribution of capsaicin-sensitive substance p-immunoreactive nerves in the nasal mucosa. *Acta Otolaryngologica* 1983;**96**:485–93.

## Study design

### Type of study

♦  Level of evidence: 3a – review article

## Outcome measures

### Primary

♦  The ageing process of the nasal mucosa

♦  Nasal hyper-reactivity

♦  Imbalanced neuronal control of end organs of the nose

## Secondary

◆ Use of capsaicin for the treatment of NINAR

# Results

## NINAR is a diagnosis of exclusion

◆ The 'non-infectious' assertion in this nomenclature attempts to eliminate the obvious upper respiratory tract infections of bacterial or viral origin. The authors however state that an infective cause cannot be entirely excluded as NINAR may represent a chronic, atypical viral or other infection. As such they suggest usage of the term 'nonallergic chronic rhinitis of unknown aetiology'.

◆ The non-allergic assertion makes clear that one should be confident of the lack of an allergic/type I hypersensitivity reaction when making the diagnosis of NINAR. As such it is prudent to exclude those patients who have positive skin prick testing that has a clear temporal and /or exposure associated relationship to the symptoms of the disease indicating allergic rhinitis.

## Pathophysiological consideration

| Possible pathophysiological process implicated in NINAR | Comments |
|---|---|
| The role of mucosal ageing in non-allergic rhinitis | Non-allergic rhinitis constitutes the dominant diagnosis in rhinitis that develops in those over 40; one retrospective analysis found beyond the fifth decade of life close to 60% of patients had a diagnosis of non-allergic disease<br>It is postulated that the aging mucosa has reduced functional reserve for homeostasis and conditioning of inspired air<br>The above findings are supported by available but limited data |
| The role of nasal hyper-reactivity | This term is applied indiscriminately to describe situations where there is increased responsiveness to 'non-specific' stimuli or, in the clinical setting, any symptoms associated with a non-allergic source (smoke, strong odours)<br>This assumption is further strengthened by NINAR patients who consistently refer to such sources as at least part of the cause of their symptoms<br>Glandular, vascular and neuronal hyperactivity have all been implicated in the causation of NINAR symptoms however study data is limited<br>Neuronal hyperactivity through the activity of substance P (a histamine-like substance present in sensory nerves) has received increased attention as this response can be provoked by capsaicin<br>This observation has led treatments using capsaicin |
| The role of imbalanced neuronal control of end organs of the nose | This concept gives rise to the alternative title of NINAR as a 'vasomotor rhinitis' (considered obsolete)<br>Research into this area is limited however important differences between controls and non-allergic rhinitic patients have been shown during exercise and 'cold face/diving reflex' tests; these differences however were not striking<br>IE During exercise and cold face testing NINAR patients experienced an increase in nasal resistance (vs. a decrease or no change in nasal resistance in control patients) |

## Conclusions

The diagnosis of NINAR is one of exclusion, and research efforts are hampered by the lack of a common language to use in the study and identification of this condition. There are millions of sufferers worldwide who do not have an adequate explanation for their symptoms or effective treatments. The creation of common definitions would greatly assist researchers in this field.

There is a complex interaction between the aging mucosa, nasal hyperactivity, and neuronal control of the nose that makes study in this area fraught.

Important insights have been made into the pathophysiology of this condition that have helped to improve the management of this condition. Braat et al. (1998) used intranasal cold dry air provocation testing to measure nasal reactivity in a unique and recognisable way in patients with NINAR. Lundblad et al. (1983) identified a population of trigeminal sensory nerves in the nasal mucosa that contain substance P. The activation of these nerves with capsaisin now forms a novel therapeutic option for the treatment of patients with NINAR.

## Critique

This review article brings together the current thinking and research regarding the pathophysiology of NINAR. It was by no means exhaustive in its scope but it helped to tease out the multiple mechanisms at work that contribute to the clinical presentation of NINAR. It also proposed that non-infectious, non-allergic rhinitis was probably not a distinct entity. To date this assertion has been borne out with the sub-classifications of non-allergic rhinitis (NAR) into idiopathic NAR (formally vasomotor rhinitis), NAR with eosinophilia, atrophic rhinitis, senile rhinitis, hormonal rhinitis or rhinitis of pregnancy, drug-induced rhinitis, or rhinitis medicamentosa and gustatory rhinitis.

There continues to be a lack of consistency in the reporting of this condition in the literature as well as a lack of effective treatments. It is an area of ongoing and active research.

# Chapter 40

# Epistaxis

Rebecca Field

## Details of study

Epistaxis is one of the commonest ENT emergencies. Bleeding can be either anterior or posterior, with posterior bleeds being the more challenging to manage. Posterior packing is usually required but this can be incredibly distressing for the patient. Haemostatic agents (e.g. Floseal, Baxter Healthcare, Zurich, Switzerland) and drugs such as tranexamic acid are appealing due to their ease of delivery and/or application, but are largely ineffective at stemming brisk posterior bleeds. Endovascular embolization, another option, is not without its own complications and is not as widely available as might be assumed particularly in an emergency situation. Historically, surgical treatment of recurrent epistaxis comprised either internal maxillary artery (IMAX) ligation via the Caldwell–Luc approach or, external carotid artery (ECA) ligation via a neck incision. Sulsenti et al. (1987), however, described a novel technique for the surgical management of epistaxis that involved endonasal sphenopalatine artery (SPA) ligation.

## Study references

### Main study

Sulsenti G, Yanez C, Kadiri M. Recurrent epistaxis: microscopic endonasal clipping of the sphenopalatine artery. *Rhinology* 1987;**25**:141–2.

### Related reference

Snyderman C, Goldman S, Carrau R, Ferguson B, Grandis J. Endoscopic sphenopalatine artery ligation is an effective method of treatment for posterior epistaxis. *Am J Rhinol* 1999;**13**:137–40.

## Study design

- Retrospective review over 1 year of patients undergoing microscopic SPA ligation
- Department of Otolaryngology, Bologna, Italy

| | |
|---|---|
| Level of evidence | 4 |
| Randomization | None |
| Number of patients | 17 |

| Inclusion criteria | Posterior epistaxis of multiple aetiology (anticoagulant therapy, hypertension, iatrogenic injury, idiopathic) |
|---|---|
| Exclusion criteria | None stated |
| Follow-up | Immediate postoperative period only |

## Outcome measures

### Primary endpoint

SPA ligation utilizing an operating microscope without later recurrence of epistaxis during the immediate postoperative period.

### Secondary endpoints

None.

## Results

No further bleeding was observed in all 17 patients after microscopic SPA ligation.

## Conclusions

SPA ligation is effective in the treatment of posterior epistaxis. Although Sulsenti et al. (1987) utilized the operating microscope subsequent technological advances, of which the endoscope was one, permitted better visualization to achieve the same objective (Snyderman et al. 1999).

## Critique

Endoscopic SPA ligation (ESPAL) has now become so embedded in emergency ENT management of epistaxis that the origins of the technique are perhaps not at all appreciated. Given that the SPA is an end artery, a terminal branch of the IMAX, it is entirely logical that it would be the best candidate for intervention to treat intractable posterior epistaxis and in doing so, avoiding the complications associated with picking up the more proximal IMAX (e.g. oro-antral fistula, palatal numbness, infraorbital nerve injury, infection, or chronic sinusitis) or ECA (e.g. hypoglossal or vagus nerve injury, cerebrovascular accident or death).

Although the publication by Sulsenti et al. (1987) was only an observational retrospective review of 17 cases without (1) any long-term follow-up and without (2) any measure of comparison against the existing technique of IMAX ligation, the technique proved successful and has since been corroborated by a number of highly regarded international rhinologists. Unfortunately, a control group offering no treatment would not have been ethical although a comparison with posterior packing alone could have been deemed reasonable at the time.

The advent of the endoscope has allowed much better visualization of the anatomy and subsequent studies have identified useful surgical landmarks (crista ethmoidalis) and branching patterns of the SPA, increasing the likelihood of successful ligation. SPA ligation success may approach 98%. Today, many centres offer ESPAL as first line treatment of posterior epistaxis, thus avoiding a posterior pack, based on higher success rates, lower complication rates, cost-effectiveness and patient comfort.

## Additional references

Dedhia RC, Desai SS, Smith KJ, Lee S, Schaitkin BM, Snyderman CH, et al. Cost-effectiveness of endoscopic sphenopalatine artery ligation versus nasal packing as first-line treatment for posterior epistaxis. *Int Forum Allergy Rhinol* 2013;3:563–6.

Douglas R, Wormald PJ. Update on epistaxis. *Curr Opin Otolaryngol Head Neck Surg* 2007;15:180–3.

# Chapter 41

# Hereditary haemorrhagic telangiectasia

Claire Hopkins

## Details of studies

Hereditary haemorrhagic telangiectasia (HHT), also known as Osler Weber Rendu syndrome is a rare autosomal dominant vascular disease, characterized by telangiectasia and arterial malformations. Epistaxis is commonly the presenting feature, and reported by over 80% with HHT, resulting in a significant impact on quality of life. This landmark paper on HHT was one of the first to propose a treatment regime based on a large clinical series.

## Study references

### Main paper

Lund VJ, Howard DJ. A treatment algorithm in the management of epistaxis in hereditary haemorrhagic telangiectasia *Am J Rhinol* 1999;13:319–22.

### Other references

Faughnan ME, Palda VA, Garcia-Tsao G, Geisthoff UW, McDonald J, Proctor DD, et al; HHT Foundation International—Guidelines Working Group. International guidelines for the diagnosis and management of hereditary haemorrhagic telangiectasia. *J Med Genet* 2011;48:73–87.

Rimmer R, Lund VJ. Hereditary haemorrhagic telangiectasia. *Rhinology* 2015;53:195–203.

## Study design

Retrospective case series of patients with HHT undergoing treatment at a tertiary referral centre.

## Results

Fifty patients were included; all had epistaxis as the predominant symptom but 26% also had significant pulmonary or gastrointestinal involvement. Two patients had died of their disease.

Fourteen patients had undergone a Young's procedure (closure of the nostrils). In the 12 patients where complete closure had been achieved, all remained free of further epistaxis. Argon laser ablation of the telangiectasia reduced the frequency and severity of bleeds in 75%.

The need for blood transfusions was a good predictor of the progression to nasal closure, with 13 of the 14 patients undergoing closure having received transfusions. Transfusion requirement was therefore suggested to be a good marker of disease severity with those requiring transfusion likely to be best managed with nasal closure.

Based on this, an algorithm was suggested, with conservative options (antifibrinolytic agents, septodermoplasty, hormone therapy, selective embolization), followed by treatment with a coagulating laser, such as the Argon laser and finally nasal closure if frequent transfusions were required.

## Critique

HHT is rare and for most ENT surgeons, involvement in patients with HHT is likely to be restricted to the acute management of epistaxis. In over 25 years, little has changed in the management of HHT patents with regards to surgical intervention, and the recommendations of this landmark paper stand firm today. There are two key issues that are highlighted well by this paper and an update published in 2015. Firstly, as epistaxis is usually the presenting feature, we should consider the possibility of HHT in anyone with recurrent episodes. Secondly, during an acute bleed, it is preferable to avoid packing, as standard removable packing further traumatizes the nose. If required, absorbable packs are preferable and they can also be soaked in tranexamic acid or adrenaline.

The importance of early diagnosis, screening for associated ateriomalfomations, and identifying family members at risk are a key aspect of the management of HHT which were however not covered in this paper. Current international guidelines recommend treatment within a centre of expertise, and a clear screening protocol looking for cerebral and pulmonary arteriovenous malformation, along with genetic testing of family members.

There have been some advances in medical management of epistaxis, although all options remain far from perfect. Thirty-five per cent of the original series had undergone hormone therapy as an adjunct to care. The feminizing and prothrombotic effects of hormonal manipulation may limit use however. Interestingly, more recently, anti-oestrogen treatment with tamoxifen has also shown have benefit in a placebo-controlled trial, and may be preferable.

The elevated levels of vascular endothelial growth factor and neoangiogenesis seen in HHT have lead to trials with humanized anti-vascular endothelial growth factor monoclonal antibody (bevazicimab), both systemically and as an injectable treatment. There is limited evidence as yet, and although there is some clinical benefit, the costs and side effect profile are unlikely to make this a first-line treatment. Its place in the management of these complex patients is yet to be clearly defined.

## Conclusion

The simple treatment algorithm proposed by Lund for the surgical management of patients with HHT over 25 years ago remains relevant to this day.

# Chapter 42

# Smell and taste disorders

Sally Erskine

## Details of study

Smell and taste disorders are common and cause significant impairment in quality of life. This paper is one of the first to profile a large number of patients presenting with smell and taste impairments to otolaryngologists. Although current understanding and management of chemosensory disorders remain limited, this paper has provided much evidence supporting current practice.

## Study reference

Main study

Deems DA, Doty RL, Settle RG, Moore-Gillon V, Shaman P, Mester AF, et al. Smell and taste disorders, a study of 750 patients from the University of Pennsylvania Smell and Taste Center. *Arch Otolaryngol Head Neck Surg* 1991;117:519–28.

## Study design

A review of 750 patients attending University of Pennsylvania Smell and Taste Centre 1980–1986.

Detailed demographic, medical history, and chemosensory disturbance information were collected from 750 patients using interviews and medical examination of the head and neck. A 270-item questionnaire was completed comprising seven sections: general information, medical history, history of presenting complaint, smell symptoms, taste symptoms, endocrine information, and depression. Seven psychophysical tests were used to assess chemosensory function including the University of Pennsylvania Smell Identification Test (Deems et al. 1984). Patients were assigned to one of 28 probable aetiological categories such as head trauma, upper respiratory tract infection and exposure to toxins. Patients' disorders were classified according to whether smell or taste were affected as well as additional categories including phantosmia or subjective halitosis.

## Outcome measures

- Demographic profile of patients
- Proportions suffering from subjective and objective smell and taste disturbance including categorization of disturbance
- Likely causes of symptoms
- Impact of symptoms

## Conclusion

Chemosensory disturbance was found to affect more women than men (37.9% vs. 29.8%). Deems et al. demonstrated that chemosensory dysfunction affects quality of life (QoL) with 68% of participants stating that this was the case. Appetite, body weight, and psychological well-being were all affected. Those with dysosmia or dysgeusia experienced the greatest depression.

Taste dysfunction was found to most commonly reflect smell dysfunction rather than primary taste disturbance; most of those with olfactory disturbance reported gustatory disturbance (74%) but only 4% had had a demonstrable gustatory deficit.

Upper respiratory tract infection, head trauma, and chronic nasal/sinus disease were identified as the commonest causes of any chemosensory disturbance. Those with deficits secondary to head trauma experienced more severe nasal symptoms, those with nasal/sinus disease were more likely to experience gradual onset than those caused by upper respiratory infection.

This study suggests regional gustatory deficits are more likely to be associated with iatrogenic factors, and suggested exogenous oestrogens may protect against olfactory dysfunction in post-menopausal women.

## Critique

Deems et al. undertook a very detailed analysis of a large cohort of patients, providing subjective and objective information about their chemosensory disturbance. The study has been cited 62 times to date and remained the only indexed review of chemosensory disturbance until 2002. In more recent years it has been recognized that the fourth major group of patients with chemosensory disorders are associated with ageing or neurological illnesses such as Parkinson's disease or Alzheimer's disease. More accurate prognoses and more detailed treatment pathways have since been suggested particularly for disordered olfaction. Age-related and congenital smell disorders cannot yet be reversed or solved but up to 60% of those with post-viral loss have been found to show some recovery, compared with 10–20% of those with post-traumatic anosmia. Management tends to be stratified according to whether the cause is sinonasal or due to another cause. Sinonasal causes may be amenable to surgery; medical options included corticosteroids as topical or systemic treatment. Treatment options for non-sinogenic problems include zinc, oestrogens, vitamin A, alpha lipoeic acid and topical sodium citrate.

## Additional references

Doty RL, Shaman P, Kimmelman CP, Dann MS. University of Pennsylvania Smell Identification Test: a rapid quantitative olfactory function test for the clinic. *Laryngoscope* 1984;**94**(Pt 1):176–8.

Henkin RI, Levy LM, Fordyce A. Taste and smell function in chronic disease: a review of clinical and biochemical evaluations of taste and smell dysfunction in over 5000 patients at The Taste and Smell Clinic in Washington, DC. *Am J Otolaryngol* 2013;**34**:477–89.

Hummel T, Landis BN, Hüttenbrink KB. Smell and taste disorders. *GMS Curr Top Otorhinolaryngol Head Neck Surg* 2011;**10**:Doc04.

Chapter 43

# Facial pain

Sally Erskine

Facial pain is a common symptom in ENT clinics. Patients may present with 'sinusitis' having self-diagnosed or had a primary care diagnosis based on pain symptoms alone rather than nasal symptoms or any clinical rhinological findings. Although facial pain may have a sinonasal cause, if sinonasal examination via endoscopy and/or computed tomography (CT) is normal, then the origins of pain are unlikely to be sinonasal. Neurological diagnoses must be considered and appropriate treatment or onward referral made.

## Study reference

### Main study

West B, Jones NS. Endoscopy-negative, computed tomography-negative facial pain in a nasal clinic. *Laryngoscope* 2001;111(Pt 1):581–6.

## Study design

Retrospective analysis of case notes of 973 consecutive patients with symptoms of rhinosinusitis or facial pain presenting to a nasal clinic in a single centre in the UK. The study focuses on the 101 patients with facial pain who had normal nasal endoscopy and CT scan findings. Review of follow-up was also undertaken.

## Outcome measures

History of problem and previous treatment, type of facial pain, treatment modality used, and treatment outcome.

## Conclusion

The most common facial pain was midfacial segment pain (35/101) (Jones and Cooney 2003). This is a form of tension headache but affects the midfacial structures and forehead. First-line treatment is with low-dose amitriptyline. The next most common diagnosis was atypical facial pain (30/101): a deep, ill-defined pain, crossing dermatomes, with no obvious organic cause. It can be managed in a similar way. The next two most common diagnoses were tension-type headache (16/101) and migraine (10/101), cluster headache, temporomandibular joint dysfunction and trigeminal neuralgia were also diagnosed. Of

101 patients, eight improved with appropriate treatment for their neurological diagnosis, eight resolved spontaneously, and seven had no improvement.

## Critique

This study used retrospective analyses of all patients with symptoms of rhinosinusitis and facial pain but then focused only on those with no rhinological findings on examination. Twenty-one out of 101 patients had, despite the lack of clinical findings, undergone rhinological procedures for their pain. There has been much anecdotal literature discussing the benefit of such procedures; however, all such management lacks evidence; this study found that none of the 21 had had any benefit from surgery; in fact five had subsequently been more symptomatic. This paper reiterates the importance of making a correct diagnosis of facial pain, since correct management can then be very effective. Erroneous management of pain as though it was of sinonasal origin will have no benefit and may be harmful. A larger and more recent study of 240 patients with chronic facial pain, followed up for 36 months supports this view. In this study, the most effective long-term treatments for mid-facial pain and facial migraine were low-dose amitriptyline and triptans (Agius et al. 2014).

## Additional references

Agius AM, Jones NS, Muscat R. Prospective three-year follow up of a cohort study of 240 patients with chronic facial pain. *J Laryngol Otol* 2014;**128**:518–26.

Jones NS, Cooney TR. Facial pain and sinonasal surgery. *Rhinology* 2003;**41**:193–200.

# Chapter 44

# Body dysmorphic disorder

Rebecca Field

## Details of study

Body dysmorphic disorder (BDD) is a mental health disorder and occurs in about 5% of patients seeking cosmetic surgery (Sarwer et al. 1998). It is characterized by preoccupation with an imagined flaw or minor defect in one's appearance. The obsession causes significant distress and can impair functioning in important areas of life. Thoughts can absorb the sufferer for several hours a day. Such patients are often dissatisfied with surgery or, their symptoms may deteriorate after surgery (Veale et al. 2000). This can, therefore, become a significant problem for both the patient and their surgeon. Unfortunately, the nose is the most common preoccupation (Veale et al. 1996). It is imperative, therefore, that rhinoplasty surgeons are skilled enough to be able to recognize this disorder to avoid unnecessary angst for both parties.

## Study references

### Main study

Veale D, De Haro L, Lambrou C. Cosmetic rhinoplasty in body dysmorphic disorder. *Br Assoc Plast Surg* 2003;**56**:546–51.

### Related references

Phillips KA, Atala KD, Pope HG. Diagnostic instruments for body dysmorphic disorder. New research programs and abstracts. 57. American Psychiatric Association 148th Annual Meeting, Miami, FL: American Psychiatric Association; 1995.

Sarwer DB, Wadden TA, Pertschuk MJ, Whitaker LA. Body image dissatisfaction and body dysmorphic disorder in 100 cosmetic surgery patients. *Plast Reconstr Surg* 1998;**101**:1644–9.

## Study design

This study was completed in two stages.

### Stage 1

Screening questionnaire for BDD given to patients requesting rhinoplasty in a private setting. Prospective, multicentre, symptom-based questionnaire.

## Stage 2

Comparison of patients without BDD who had a good outcome after cosmetic rhinoplasty with BDD patients in a psychiatric clinic craving rhinoplasty. Retrospective, multicentre, case–control study.

| | |
|---|---|
| Level of evidence | 4 |
| Randomization | None |
| Number of patients | Stage 1: 29<br>Stage 2: 23 non-BDD versus 16 BDD |
| Inclusion criteria | Patients >18 years old seeking first time cosmetic rhinoplasty in the private sector. Patients in a psychiatric clinic diagnosed with BDD |
| Exclusion criteria | Nasal deformity due to trauma or medical pathology. Patients wanting to simultaneously undergo more than one cosmetic procedure. Patients with possible BDD |
| Follow-up | 3 months and 9 months |

## Outcome measures

### Primary endpoint

◆ Body dysmorphic disorder questionnaire (BDDQ) to screen for and identify patients with possible BDD (Phillips et al. 1995)

### Secondary endpoints

◆ Hospital anxiety and depression scale (HADS) to assess anxiety and depression
◆ Modified Yale Brown obsessive compulsive scale for BDD (YBOCS-BDD) to assess severity of BDD symptoms
◆ Rhinoplasty questionnaire designed specifically for the study to assess hypotheses
◆ Nose imperfection scale to assess the patient's perception of their nose
◆ Patient satisfaction questionnaire to assess satisfaction following rhinoplasty

## Results

### Stage 1

| | Preoperative | 3 months postoperative | 9 months postoperative |
|---|---|---|---|
| Possible BDD | 6/29 (20.7%) | 2/29* | 0/26 |

*Of the six patients identified as 'possible BDD' preoperatively, only two out of nine had possible BDD at 3 months postoperatively. Not included in the table is one patient who preoperatively did not have BDD, but became 'possible BDD' 3 months postoperatively.

The authors state that in these results, they believe they identified a group of patients with subclinical or very mild BDD who are satisfied by cosmetic rhinoplasty.

Secondary endpoints were analysed using the Mann–Whitney test. The possible BDD group had significantly higher severity scores than non-BDD patients, suggesting greater psychological morbidity. BDD patients were more distressed and reported much greater interference in their social and occupational functioning and relationships because of their nose. They were more socially anxious and more likely to avoid situations because of their nose. They were more likely to check their nose in mirrors or to feel it with their fingers. BDD patients were more likely to believe that cosmetic surgery would significantly alter their life (e.g. obtain a new partner or job). BDD patients were also more likely to feel misunderstood when they described what they disliked about their nose. Interestingly though, BDD patients were significantly more likely to be discouraged by their family and friends from seeking surgery.

## Stage 2

Compared to non-BDD rhinoplasty patients, psychiatric BDD patients seeking rhinoplasty were

- significantly younger
- more depressed and anxious
- more preoccupied by their nose
- likely to check their nose more frequently
- more likely to conduct 'DIY' surgery (see below)
- more likely to have multiple concerns about their body
- more likely to avoid social situations because of their nose
- more likely to be significantly handicapped in their occupation, social life, and in intimate relationships

Examples of DIY surgery included using a pair of pliers in an attempt to make the nose thinner; Sellotape to flatten the nose; or placing tissue up one side of the nose to try and make it looked more curved.

Safety behaviours were also more commonly adopted by the BDD group, such as looking down or not allowing others to see their side profile; trying to hide their nose behind their hand or their hair; or wearing large jewellery to distract others from looking at their nose.

## Conclusions

BDD is common in patients seeking rhinoplasty. It is a psychiatric condition and should be treated with selective serotonin reuptake inhibitors and cognitive behavioural therapy. There are high levels of patient dissatisfaction following cosmetic surgical intervention. Exact prevalence though seems difficult to measure.

## Critique

The use of the BDDQ was appropriate for this study and was subsequently validated by Dey et al. (2015) for use in facial plastic and reconstructive surgery patients, showing a sensitivity of 100% and specificity of 90.3%. However, using a screening tool rather than a formal psychiatric diagnosis may have identified false positives which could explain the decreased prevalence over time. Although this study was the first of its kind attempting to provide a baseline prevalence of BDD in patients undergoing rhinoplasty, there were several further faults with the methodology. These included:

◆ recruiting patients from seven independent private plastic surgical clinics in London where, it could be argued, the incidence of BDD may have artificially been higher than in the general population
◆ very small sample sizes
◆ those patients that refused to participate were not recorded
◆ the surgeons used may have been more aware of BDD

Despite these shortcomings however, a larger subsequent study by Alavi et al. (2011) identified a similar prevalence of BDD in rhinoplasty patients. This study highlights the difficulties in detecting a 'normal' level of dissatisfaction with appearance which may lead to seeking out of cosmetic procedures, as is likely in many cosmetic surgery patients, as opposed to BDD.

### Additional references

Alavi M, Kalafi Y, Dehbozorgi GR, Javadpour A. Body dysmorphic disorder and other psychiatric morbidity in aesthetic rhinoplasty candidates. *J Plast Reconstr Aesthet Surg* 2011;**64**:738–41.

Dey JK, Ishii M, Phillis M, Byrne PJ, Boahene KD, Ishii LE. Body dysmorphic disorder in a facial plastic and reconstructive surgery clinic: measuring prevalence, assessing comorbidities, and validating a feasible screening instrument. *JAMA Facial Plast Surg* 2015;**17**:137–43.

Phillips KA, Grant J, Siniscalchi J, Albertini RS. Surgical and non-psychiatric medical treatment of patients with body dysmorphic disorder. *Psychosomatics* 2001;**42**:504–10.

Veale D, Boocock A, Gournay K, Dryden W, Shah F, Willson R, et al. Body dysmorphic disorder. A survey of fifty cases. *Br J Psychiatry* 1996;**169**:196–201.

Chapter 45

# Granulomatosis with polyangiitis

Luke Reid

## Details of studies

Granulomatosis with polyangiitis (formally known as Wegener's granulomatosis) is a rare, multisystem autoimmune condition of unknown aetiology with multiple otorhinolaryngological manifestations. Many patients with this condition initially present with ENT-related symptoms and signs to either their general physician or ENT surgeon. However, due to the low prevalence of this condition and its clinical presentations being similar to many other common ENT presentations there is often

1 a delay in making a definitive diagnosis of granulomatosis with polyangiitis, and

2 once diagnosed, a variable amount of treatment directed at treating this condition

To better appreciate the scope, pattern of presentation, and management of this condition Srouji et al. (2006) performed a cross-sectional, retrospective questionnaire based study on patients with a known diagnosis of granulomatosis with polyangiitis identified through a UK based self-help group.

## Study references

### Main study

Srouji I A, Andrews P, Edwards C, Lund V J. Patterns of presentation and diagnosis of patients with Wegener's granulomatosis: ENT aspects. *J Laryngol Otol* 2006;**121**:653–8.

### Related reference

Abdou N, Kullman G, Hoffman G, Shazrp G, Specks U, McDonald T, et al. Wegener's Granulomatosis: survey of 701 patients in North America. Changes in outcome in the 1990s. *J Rheumatol* 2002;**29**:309–15.

## Study design—common template

| Type of study | Retrospective cross-sectional study |
| --- | --- |
| Intention to treat | N/A |
| Level of evidence | 4 |
| Randomization | N/A |
| Number of patients | 199 |

| Inclusion criteria | All members of the granulomatosis with polyangiitis patient's own UK self help group, the Stuart Strange Vasculitis Trust |
|---|---|
| Exclusion criteria | Returned questionnaires in which the patient's age, sex, or granulomatosis with polyangiitis diagnosis were not confirmed or if the questionnaire had been completed by somebody other than the patient (i.e. a relative) |
| Follow-up | N/A |
| Intervention(s) | Nil |

## Outcome measures

### Primary

- Time of onset of symptoms, presentation to a physician or ENT surgeon, when an actual diagnosis of granulomatosis with polyangiitis was made and delay in diagnosis
- Previous or current history of sinonasal morbidity (including a selection of relevant nasal and aural symptoms)
- Treatment regime profiles including systemic immunosuppressants, topical nasal treatments and previous nasal surgeries.

## Results

### Population, presentation, and diagnosis

| Questionnaire response rate | 25.5% (781 questionnaires sent to all members of the self help group/ 199 valid responses returned) |
|---|---|
| Male:female ratio | 35:65 |
| Mean age | 58.2 years (average age at diagnosis 50 years) |
| Time since diagnosis | 8 years (range 1 month to 23 years and 3 months) |
| ENT-related manifestations at initial presentation | 41% rhinological<br>16% otological<br>6% pharynx, larynx and trachea<br>NB: younger patients (<60 years old) had a predilection to head and neck related modes of presentation |
| Delay in diagnosis | 92% of patients reported a delay of over 1 month<br>(49% 1–6 months/20% 6–12 months/23% >12 months)<br>Overall average delay in diagnosis 7 months<br>Mean delay of 9.0 months in patients presenting initially with head and neck-related symptoms<br>Mean delay of 5.9 months in patients presenting initially with non-head and neck-related symptoms<br>There was no improvement over time in the time taken to make a diagnosis |

## ENT symptomatology and treatment

| Criteria | Results |
| --- | --- |
| Current/at time of survey ENT related symptoms specific to granulomatosis with polyangiitis | Sinonasal: 85%<br>  Crusting: 75%<br>  Excessive nose blowing: 70%<br>  Nasal obstruction: 65%<br>  Epistaxis: 59%<br>  Unhappy with nasal cosmesis: 25%<br>Aural fullness: 50%<br>Dizziness: 42%<br>Otalgia: 29% |
| Current treatment profile | Systemic immunosuppressants: 85% (53% 1+ agents)<br>Topical nasal treatments: 27%<br>  Nasal douche: 13.1%<br>  Steroid sprays: 11.1%<br>  Antibiotic creams: 9.6%<br>  Nasal douche and steroid sprays: 4.5%<br>  Nasal douche and topical cream: 1.5%<br>  All three (douche/steroids/cream): 0% |

## Conclusions

ENT manifestations of granulomatosis with polyangiitis are common. As such the otorhinolaryngologist has an important role in the initial diagnosis and ongoing treatment of these patients. However, due to the low prevalence of this condition and possibly a poor awareness of this condition within the ENT community there is often a significant delay in the diagnosis of granulomatosis with polyangiitis. These delays that have not improved over time and compared unfavourably with a US study conducted 4 years prior where 79% vs. 92% had their diagnosis delayed by >1 month. A large majority of patients present with sinonasal symptoms however there is an equally significant under treatment of granulomatosis with polyangiitis-related nasal symptoms.

## Critique

This was a cross sectional retrospective observational study that sourced patients for review from a self reported granulomatosis with polyangiitis self help support group. They were patients that had been diagnosed and were being treated for granulomatosis with polyangiitis. The response rate, although small, gave a sample size that allowed for valid conclusions to be drawn when compared with the rarity of the condition at hand (prevalence 25/100,000). The identification of patients with this rare condition would be likely difficult to do via any other avenue given that multiple clinicians, services and people involved in their care. However, as there was no clinical verification of the reported information there is a possibility of detection bias.

The findings of this study have been supported by a more recent review of the literature in 2014 by Martinez et al. that again highlighted the finding that ENT manifestations in the initial presentation of these patients is high but there are ongoing delays in making the diagnosis.

## Additional reference

Martinez Del Pedro M, McKiernan D, Jani P Presentation and initial assessment of ENT problems in patients with granulomatosis with polyangiitis (Wegener's). *J Laryngol Otol* 2014;**128**:730–7.

## Chapter 46

# The classification of orbital complications of acute rhinosinusitis

Rajiv Bhalla

## Details of studies

Orbital infection may occur as a complication of sinusitis, usually ethmoid or frontal sinus infections. The management of orbital infections should be multidisciplinary: ophthalmology, ENT, radiology, microbiology, paediatric, and haematology, or neurosurgery for more complicated cases. To permit effective communication there is a need for good classification systems which collate information from clinical assessment and performed investigations, and guide subsequent management. Chandler et al. proposed their classification for orbital infections in 1970 and, although there was one attempt at a coup by Velasco e Cruz et al. in the mid 2000s, the Chandler Classification has remained the preferred descriptor for orbital complications of sinusitis, likely due to its ease of use and clinical applicability.

## Study references

### Main study

Chandler JR, Langenbrunner DJ, Stevens ER. The pathogenesis of orbital complications in acute sinusitis. *Laryngoscope* 1970;80:1414–28.

### Related references

Smith AF, Spencer JF. Orbital complications resulting from lesions of the sinuses. *Ann Otol Rhinol Laryngol* 1948;57:5–27.

Velasco e Cruz AA, Demarco RC, Valera FC, do Santos AC, Anselmo-Lima WT, Marquezini RM. Orbital complications of acute rhinosinusitis: a new classification. *Braz J Otorhinolaryngol* 2007;73:684–8.

## Study design

### Methods

| Level of evidence | 5: descriptive paper with case reports |
| --- | --- |
| Randomization | None |
| Number of patients | 0 |

| Inclusion criteria | Classification of orbital infections, grades I–V |
|---|---|
| Exclusion criteria | n/a |
| Follow-up | n/a |

Elaborates on the embryology and anatomy of the orbit and ethmoid sinus.

## Outcome measures

### Primary endpoint

Not applicable.

### Secondary endpoints

None.

## Results

Classification of orbital infections, groups I–V

| |
|---|
| Group I inflammatory oedema–preseptal |
| Group II orbital cellulitis |
| Group III subperiosteal abscess |
| Group IV orbital abscess |
| Group V cavernous sinus thrombosis |

Reproduced from Chandler JR, Langenbrunner DJ, Stevens ER. The pathogenesis of orbital complications in acute sinusitis. Laryngoscope 1970; 80: 1414–28 with permission from Wiley.

- Impaired or worsening visual acuity is a serious sign and suggests orbital abscess formation
- Chemosis, oedema, proptosis, and ophthalmoplegia suggest orbital abscess
- Bilateral eye signs are indicative of cavernous sinus thrombosis

## Conclusions

The Chandler classification, although described in 1970, has stood the test of time in describing orbital infections and guiding multidisciplinary management. This is because it remains simple to relate clinical and radiological findings to the grading system, and descriptors remain easily transferrable between surgical and medical/paediatric disciplines involved in patient care.

## Critique

This is a descriptive paper with three brief case presentations. It elaborates on the likely routes of spread of infection between the sinuses and orbit. Suggested paths include transmission of infection through the lacrimomaxillary, lacrimoethmoidal, or sphenoethmoidal fissures, anterior or posterior ethmoidal foramina, or through con- genital dehiscences in the medial or superior orbital walls (behind the trochlear fossa or supraorbital notch, at the junction of the middle and outer thirds of the roof of the orbit, at the junction of the anterior and middle thirds of the lamina papyracea or adjacent to the posterior ethmoids). Further predisposition to orbital infection is due to the anatomy of the ophthalmic venous system, which is completely devoid of valves. Thus, there is ex- tensive two-way venous communication with the face, nasal cavity, pterygoid region, and sinuses. Both the superior and inferior ophthalmic veins drain into the cavernous sinus. Descriptions and stylized illustrations are provided for better understanding of groups/ grades I–V. To facilitate the management of orbital complications of sinusitis, there is per- haps no need for an alternative classification system to that proposed by Chandler almost 50 years ago.

# Part IV

# Malignant head and neck disease

Chapter 47

# Epidemiology of laryngeal cancer

Sally Erskine

In the USA, the incidence of laryngeal cancer has decreased from 1980s to 2000s, a decrease thought to be associated with decreasing tobacco consumption. Survival rates however, also decreased over this time. Cancer statistics reviews (Jemal et al. 2004) showed that out of 24 cancer types evaluated between 1983–1985 and 1992–1999, only laryngeal cancer showed a decrease in survival. The purpose of this study was to further evaluate this finding. Proposed hypotheses for the change included change in incidence of more advance cancers, changing demographics, and changing management strategies with increasing use of non-surgical and less aggressive surgical options.

## Study reference

### Main study

Hoffman HT, Porter K, Karnell LH, Cooper JS, Weber RS, Langer CJ, et al. Laryngeal cancer in the USA: changes in demographics, patterns of care, and survival. *Laryngoscope* 2006;**116**:1–13

## Study design

Retrospective, longitudinal study of laryngeal cancer cases taken from the National Cancer Data Base (NCDB) in the USA. All laryngeal squamous cell carcinomas (SCCs) diagnosed between 1985 and 2001 were included, excluding verrucous carcinoma. Cases included first primaries and subsequent primaries. Data submission to the NCDB was voluntary until 1996.

## Outcome measures

- Overall 5-year survival
- Evaluating whether incomplete data could account for the decrease in survival seen in previous studies
- Changes in incidence of advance stage disease
- Change in demographic (race and socioeconomic status)
- Change in management strategy over time

## Conclusion

The review confirms the trend of decreasing survival from laryngeal cancer from the mid-1980s to 1990s. No increase in incidence of advanced stage disease was identified. An increase in the proportion of a minority of patients was found, but no change in socioeconomic status. During the time of decreasing survival rates, there was an increase in the use of radiation and chemo radiation with fewer surgeries. In particular, treatment of T3M0N0 laryngeal and glottic SCC which did *not* include surgery showed poorer survival. Survival varied according to specific TNM stage; decline in survival was found to be smaller for early stage compared with advanced disease.

## Critique

This study used a very large national database to explore trends in disease and management. It is hypothesized that the decline in survival could be linked to trends in performing less aggressive surgery. Advances in clinical and translational research are constantly applied to update cancer management; modifications made during the time of decreased survival may therefore not have been beneficial, or alternatively, the poorer survival may reflect a learning curve in the particular treatment modality. Cancer trials have rigid selection criteria, treating a population with cancer is different and treatments may therefore need to be allocated more selectively. The database used, although large, was also incomplete prior to becoming compulsory in 1996. The majority of cases submitted were from community hospitals; larger facilities may have shown more favourable results.

A more recent study by Al-Gilani et al. (2016) of 487 patients with T3 glottic SCC from 1992 to 2010 in the USA showed a significant improvement in those who had surgical compared with non-surgical treatment. The study also found that adjuvant and nonsurgical treatment may result in a more dysfunctional larynx.

## Additional references

Al-Gilani M, Skillington SA, Kallogjeri D, Haughey B, Piccirillo JF. Surgical vs nonsurgical treatment modalities for T3 glottic squamous cell carcinoma. *JAMA Otolaryngol Head Neck Surg* 2016;**142**:940–6.

Jemal A, Tiwari RC, Murray T, Ghafoor A, Samuels A, Ward E, et al; **American Cancer Society.** Cancer statistics, 2004. *CA Cancer J Clin* 2004;**54**:8–29.

Chapter 48

# Smoking, alcohol, and head and neck cancer

Tom Roques

## Details of studies

By 2020 over a million people worldwide are expected to be diagnosed annually with head and neck cancers, with over half a million dying from the diseases each year. In western countries about three-quarters of cases are linked to tobacco smoking and alcohol drinking. There is also a genetic predisposition with a family history of a first-degree relative with head and neck cancer conferring a 1.7 increased risk. In recent years the role of human papilloma virus (HPV) virus infection in causing oropharyngeal cancer has also been discovered.

Public health efforts to reduce these behaviours have the possibility of saving many lives by reducing head and neck cancer incidence, not to mention the manifold other health and socioeconomic benefits. Case–control studies aim to quantify how strongly one variable is associated with another in a given population; in this study comparing smoking and drinking habits in people diagnosed with head and neck cancer with age- and gender-matched controls. This paper combines individual patient data from 18 case–control studies throughout the world with the aim of estimating the number of years of quitting required to observe a reduced risk and whether the risk declines to the level of never smokers and never drinkers. In addition, the group were interested in whether the risk reversal differs by head and neck cancer subsite, and by the frequency of tobacco or alcohol use before quitting.

## Study references

### Main study

Marron M, Boffetta P, Zhang ZF, Zaridze D, Wünsch-Filho V, Winn DM, et al. Cessation of alcohol drinking, tobacco smoking and the reversal of head and neck cancer risk. *Int J Epidemiol* 2010;39:182–96.

### Related reference

Conway DI, Hashibe M, Boffetta P, Wunsch-Filho V, Muscat J, La Vecchia C, et al. Enhancing epidemiologic research on head and neck cancer: INHANCE—the International Head and Neck Cancer Epidemiology Consortium. *Oral Oncol* 2009;45:743–6.

## Study design

◆ Level of evidence: 3a—systematic review of individual patient data from case controlled studies.

◆ Randomization: case–control studies. Subjects were matched with controls for age and gender. Individual studies also matched for some other factors, for example study centre and ethnicity

◆ Number of patients: 18 studies with 12,282 head and neck cancer case subjects and 17,189 control subjects. Fourteen of the studies were hospital based and four were population based

◆ Inclusion criteria: oral cavity, oropharynx, hypopharynx, larynx, or unspecified head and neck cancer. Some of the included studies included only squamous cell cancers. For studies which did not specify pathological type, 97% of patients with available histological information had a squamous cell cancer

◆ Exclusion criteria: cancers of the nasopharynx, salivary gland and external lip as the aetiology and risk factors for these cancers differ from other head and neck tumours.

◆ Follow-up: N/A

## Outcome measures

The paper estimated the effect of stopping smoking or drinking on the risk of developing head and neck cancer by calculating odds ratios (OR). ORs quantify how strongly one variable is associated with another in a given population. So the odds for developing head and neck cancer in never smokers and former smokers can be compared with the odds of developing head and neck cancer in current smokers. Similarly for alcohol consumption.

## Results

The risk of developing head and neck cancer was reduced by stopping smoking just 1–4 years earlier (OR = 0.70). Stopping smoking for 20 years or more reduced the odds to 0.23—the same risk as for never smokers. Current and former smokers had a higher risk of laryngeal cancer than other head and neck cancer subtypes and quitting smoking for 20 years did not reduce the risk of laryngeal cancer back to baseline levels. The benefit of stopping smoking was greater in people who had smoked more.

Ceasing alcohol consumption for 20 years or more reduced the risk of developing head and neck cancer by 40% (OR = 0.60). Stopping drinking reduced the risk in all head and neck cancer subsites but the effect was more pronounced for oral cavity and larynx cancers. The reduction in risk was less apparent and not statistically significant for stopping drinking from 1 to 19 years. The risk for never drinkers (OR = 0.55) and those who had stopped for 20 years or more (OR = 0.44) were similar. The benefit of stopping drinking was only seen in current smokers.

# Conclusions

Stopping smoking for as little as 1–4 years reduces the risk of developing head and neck cancer and stopping for 20 years reduces the risk down to non-smoking levels (77% reduction). Benefits are evident whether heavy or light smokers quit. The beneficial effects of stopping drinking were less than smoking and were not seen for 20 years after abstention from alcohol. The pattern of risk for smoking and laryngeal cancer is similar to that seen in lung cancer, suggesting that larynx and lung cancers share a common aetiology more closely than larynx and pharynx cancers.

# Critique

This study confirms the almost immediate benefits that stopping smoking confers in reducing the risk of developing head and neck cancer. Although many head and neck cancers are curable with surgery or radiotherapy (or in combination with each other or chemotherapy) there is a very significant morbidity with such treatments. Attempts to improve cancer survival usually focus on new therapies but reducing the incidence of head and neck cancer by reducing smoking rates is a much more effective and cost-effective strategy.

Worldwide there are over a billion smokers with rates continuing to increase in eastern Mediterranean region and in Africa. In the UK a consistent reduction in smoking rates since the 1970s has seen a small reduction in incidence of laryngeal cancer though the incidence of oral cavity tumours continues to rise. This may partly be due to increased numbers of people in the UK from the Indian subcontinent who chew betel nut (paan).

Though one in five UK adults still smoke, over a third tried to stop in 2014. To improve the chances of quitting successfully, smokers need a social support network, smoke-free environments, and effective therapies and services. The most effective of these are stop-smoking services, which depend on good referral routes, often from healthcare professionals. A Cochrane review has shown that even brief advice from a healthcare professional can double the chances of a person quitting smoking. ENT professionals seeing a current smoker for any symptoms or diagnosis are therefore ideally placed to influence smoking behaviours and help to reduce the incidence of head and neck cancer as well as providing other health benefits.

This study shows that stopping alcohol consumption for 20 years or more or never drinking also reduces the risk of developing head and neck cancer but it cannot provide evidence of what, if any, level of alcohol consumption is safe in this context. Although contact with health services provides an opportunity to advise those who drink more than recommended amounts to reduce consumption, asking low and moderate drinkers to abstain completely is not likely to significantly reduce their risk of head and neck cancer.

# Additional references

Cancer Research UK oral cancer incidence statistics http://www.cancerresearchuk.org/health-professional/cancer-statistics/statistics-by-cancer-type/oral-cancer/incidence#heading-Four (accessed January 2017).

McQueen J, Howe TE, Allan L, Mains D, Hardy V. Brief interventions for heavy alcohol users admitted to general hospital wards. *Cochrane Database Syst Rev* 2011;8:CD005191.

Rigotti NA. Strategies to help a smoker who is struggling to quit. *JAMA* 2012;308:1573–80.

Stead LF, Buitrago D, Preciado N, Sanchez G, Hartmann-Boyce J, Lancaster T. Physician advice for smoking cessation. *Cochrane Database Syst Rev* 2013;5:CD000165.

Winn D, Lee YC, Hashibe M, Boffetta P. The INHANCE consortium: toward a better understanding of the causes and mechanisms of head and neck cancer. *Oral Dis* 2015;21:685–93.

WHO data on prevalence of tobacco smoking http://www.who.int/gho/tobacco/use/en/ (accessed January 2017).

# Chapter 49

# Human papilloma virus

Liam Masterson

## Details of studies

RTOG 0129 was a randomized phase III trial assessing chemoradiotherapy given according to two different protocols. This study represented the largest prospective cohort of oropharyngeal squamous cell carcinoma (OPSCC) patients treated homogenously in a randomized trial setting. However, RTOG 0129 became a landmark trial for a different reason in that it demonstrated for the first time that the presence of human papilloma virus (HPV) infection in patient tumours altered disease survival.

## Study reference

### Main study

Ang KK, Harris J, Wheeler R, Weber R, Rosenthal DI, Nguyen-Tân PF, et al. Human papillomavirus and survival of patients with oropharyngeal cancer. *N Engl J Med* 2010;**363**:24–35.

## Design

- A prospective multicentre, open-label, randomized trial(with post hoc analysis of HPV status)
- Level of evidence: 1b
- Randomization: accelerated fractionation radiotherapy versus standard fractionation radiotherapy. The standard chemoradiotherapy (CRT) arm incorporated 70 Gy given over 7 weeks with three cycles of cisplatin chemotherapy at 21-day intervals. The accelerated CRT arm was given 72 Gy over 6 weeks with two cycles of cisplatin chemotherapy
- Number of patients = 720
- Inclusion criteria: age >18 years. Biopsy-proven, previously untreated stage III or IV squamous carcinoma of the oral cavity, oropharynx, hypopharynx, or larynx without distant metastases (M0)
- Exclusion criteria: inadequate hepatic, bone marrow, or renal function. Zubrod's performance status score >1
- Follow up: 4.8 years (median)

## Outcome measures

### Primary endpoint

- Overall survival (defined as the time from randomization to death)

### Secondary endpoints

- Progression-free survival (defined as the time from randomization to disease-related death or recurrence)
- Acute toxicity (evaluated weekly during the period of therapy according to the Common Terminology Criteria, version 2.0)
- HPV status—this was restricted to patients with oropharyngeal squamous-cell carcinoma because of the low prevalence of HPV among non-oropharyngeal squamous-cell carcinomas. Combined HPV cISH/p16 detection protocol

## Results

The 3-year rate of overall survival was equivocal for the group receiving standard fractionation radiotherapy versus those receiving accelerated fractionation radiotherapy (64.3% vs. 70.3% $p = 0.18$). The rate of high-grade acute and late toxic events was also similar.

Of the patients with oropharyngeal cancer, 63.8% (206 of 323) had HPV-positive tumours. This group demonstrated better 3-year rates of overall survival than the HPV-negative tumour group (82.4%, vs. 57.1%, $p < 0.001$ by the log-rank test).

The HPV-positive group had a 58% reduction in the risk of death (hazard ratio 0.42; 95% CI 0.27–0.66) after adjustment for race, age, tumour, tobacco exposure, nodal stage, and treatment assignment.

With each additional pack-year of tobacco smoking, the risk of death significantly increased.

Recursive-partitioning analysis allowed the study to classify patients into low, intermediate, or high risk of death (based on HPV status, smoking, tumour stage, and nodal stage).

## Conclusion

No significant difference was found between the two arms. As concurrent chemotherapy was utilized in both arms of the trial, the main comparison was shortening the length of radiation therapy and eliminating the third cycle of chemotherapy.

The result of the study is significant as it enabled the patient to shorten their treatment to 6 weeks instead of 7 weeks, and avoid the third cycle of chemotherapy (and the associated toxicity). Subsequent meta-analysis has confirmed that accelerated fractionation CRT does benefit patients.

RTOG 0129 allowed a definite analysis of the prognostic value of HPV infection as an aetiological agent in OPSCC. It demonstrated the presence of HPV infection in patient tumours conferred ~25% improvement in overall survival. This study was the first large randomized phase III trial (involving >700 patients) that demonstrated two different diseases constitute OPSCC (based on viral or non-viral aetiology).

## Critique

A major legacy of this study was establishing the need for separate trials for HPV+ OPSCC patients, who need similarly effective therapy with reduced intensity of chemotherapy or radiation therapy. Specifically, this led to the RTOG 1016 trial, which replaced cisplatin with cetuximab, using 70 Gy of radiation in both arms.

The finding of reduced survival of smokers within the HPV+ OPSCC cohort is of interest and may be related to genetic alterations induced by tobacco-associated carcinogens making HPV-positive tumours less responsive to therapy.

Of interest, tumour p16 over expression by immunohistochemistry (IHC) conferred a better prognostic impact than HPV DNA positivity itself.

In this study, HPV-positive but p16-negative tumours occurred 4% of the time, whereas, p16-positive but HPV-negative tumours occurred 19% of the time. Thus, concordance with HPV DNA in situ hybridization and the p16 IHC diagnostic test was strong (~95%).

RTOG 0129 also demonstrated that HPV16 subtype was responsible for the overwhelming majority of HPV+ OPSCC (96% of the HPV-positive patients that were also p16 positive).

This study suggests that collection of tissue and other specimens from prospective clinical trials (to establish a biobank) is of fundamental importance. Even when a trials primary endpoint is not met, new technology or other information (e.g. HPV data as above) may shed light on the biology of carcinogenesis and/or response to therapy.

### Additional references

Bourhis J, Overgaard J, Audry H, Ang KK, Saunders M, Bernier J, et al. Hyperfractionated or accelerated radiotherapy in head and neck cancer: a meta-analysis. *Lancet* 2006;**368**:843–54.

D'Souza G, Kreimer AR, Viscidi R, Pawlita M, Fakhry C, Koch WM, et al. Case-control study of human papillomavirus and oropharyngeal cancer. *N Engl J Med* 2007;**356**:1944–56.

Gillison ML, Koch WM, Capone RB, Spafford M, Westra WH, Wu L, Zahurak ML, et al. Evidence for a causal association between human papillomavirus and a subset of head and neck cancers. *J Natl Cancer Inst* 2000;**92**:709–20.

Masterson L, Moualed D, Liu ZW, Howard J, Dwivedi R, Benson R, et al. De-escalation treatment protocols for HPV associated oropharyngeal squamous cell carcinoma: a systematic review and meta-analysis of current clinical trials. *Eur J Cancer* 2014;**50**:2636–48.

Chapter 50

# Laser microsurgery for laryngeal cancer

## Vinidh Paleri and Hannah Fox

## Details of studies

Endoscopic techniques for the resection of laryngeal cancer had been described as far back as the late part of the nineteenth century. However it is only since the 1970s that the technique of transoral surgery using the $CO_2$ laser has come into widespread use. In Europe, the work of Wolfgang Steiner was dominant in establishing the viability of laser microsurgery and the technique. His first case series of 240 patients with early-stage glottic cancer was a landmark in the evolution of our current practice.

## Study references

### Main study

Steiner W. Results of curative laser microsurgery of laryngeal carcinomas. *Am J Otolaryngol* 1993;**14**:116–21.

### Related references

Steiner W, Ambrosch P. $CO_2$ laser microsurgery for laryngeal cancer: In Smee R, Bridger P. (eds). Proceedings of the second world congress on laryngeal cancer. Amsterdam; Elsevier, 1994;369–72.

Steiner W, Ambrosch P. Endoscopic laser surgery of the upper aerodigestive tract: with special emphasis on cancer surgery. New York: Theime, 2000.

## Study design

◆ An observational case series detailing the author's patients treated between 1979 and 1985 at Erlangen otorhinolaryngology department

◆ During the study period the author's technique evolved from treating early stage cancer to also include more advanced resectable disease

◆ The study reports group A (early stage) and group B (advanced stage) cancers separately

| | |
|---|---|
| Level of evidence | 4 |
| Randomization | None |
| Number of patients | 240 |

| Inclusion criteria | All patients with early stage glottic cancer (pTiS-pT2N0, M0/UICC 1987)—group A |
| --- | --- |
| | Patients with resectable cancer pT2-pT4, pN0-N2c/UJCC 1987)—group B |
| | Patients in whom pre-operative laryngeal function could be preserved |
| Exclusion criteria | Synchronous second primary |
| | Distant metastasis |
| Follow up | 5 years (median 78 months) |

## Outcome measures

### Primary endpoints

- 5-year overall survival
- Locoregional recurrence

### Secondary endpoints

- Postoperative complications
- Voice outcomes
- Requirement for tracheostomy

## Results

### Overall survival

| | Overall survival at 5 years |
| --- | --- |
| Total | 59% |
| Group A (n = 159) | 86.5% (adjusted 5-year survival rate 100%) |
| TiS | 97% |
| T1 | 87% |
| T2 | 78% |
| Group B (n = 81) | 59% (adjusted 5-year survival rate 89%) |

### Local recurrence rate

- Group A: 6%
- Group B: 22%

### Laryngectomy rate

- 9% patients needed total laryngectomy
- Six patients for oncological reasons and one for functional reasons

## Conclusion

This study confirms the usefulness of laser microsurgery for laryngeal carcinoma. Surgery is individualized and adapted to the size of the tumour. Multi-institutional studies are needed to compare laser microsurgery with radiation therapy.

## Critique

This seminal study had a significant impact on clinical practice across the world. The study is a case series, and as such is subject to the usual criticisms of being prone to bias as a non-randomized study without a control group. The technique was a significant departure from the norm, espousing trans-tumoral cuts to define tumour depth and a mosaic resection, going against the convention of en bloc resection in oncologic surgery. The rigorous data collection, robust, and didactic description of the technique, excellent outcomes, lively debates on the radically new treatment paradigm at global meetings in the 80s and 90s, combined with the charismatic personality of the lead surgeon led to slow, but steady dissemination of this practice. The current National Institute of Clinical Excellence guidelines recommend that all patients with newly diagnosed T1a squamous cell carcinoma are offered transoral laser microsurgery, and that those with T1b disease are offered a choice between transoral laser microsurgery and radiotherapy. Transoral laser surgery is widely available across the UK.

The principles laid down by transoral laser surgery for glottic cancer have been validated at other tumour sites in the upper aerodigestive tract, and contributed to the evolution of transoral robotic surgery. The treatment paradigm for early head and neck cancers has shifted towards minimally invasive surgery, with an emphasis on functional outcomes.

### Additional references

National Institute of Clinical Excellence. Cancer of the upper aerodigestive tract: assessment and management in people aged 16 and over; 2016; https://www.nice.org.uk/guidance/ng36 (accessed February 2018).

Prettyjohns M, Winter S, Kerawala C, Paleri V; the NICE cancer of the upper aerodigestive tract guideline committee. Transoral laser microsurgery versus radiation therapy in the management of T1 and T2 laryngeal glottic carcinoma: which modality is cost-effective within the UK? *Clin Otolaryngol* 2017;**42**:404–15.

# Chapter 51

# Oncological management of head and neck cancer I

Liam Masterson

## Detail of studies

For many decades, the management of local advanced laryngeal carcinoma was based on two different approaches: definitive irradiation with salvage surgery if required, or total laryngectomy with postoperative irradiation. With no available randomized controlled trial (RCT) data, the utilization of either option was influenced by local institution or national policies, e.g. southern Europe favoured upfront surgery whereas northern Europe favoured primary radiotherapy.

In 1991, the Department of Veterans Affairs Laryngeal Study Group, published the first RCT on laryngeal preservation. This trial had an important impact on clinical practice and influenced the design of subsequent clinical trials.

The concept of this randomized trial was to compare the conventional treatment (total laryngectomy versus postoperative irradiation) and an experimental arm starting with induction chemotherapy followed in good responders by irradiation or by surgery and postoperative irradiation in poor responders.

## Study reference

### Main study

The Department of Veterans Affairs Laryngeal Cancer Study Group. Induction chemotherapy plus radiation compared with surgery plus radiation in patients with advanced laryngeal cancer. *N Engl J Med* 1991;324:1685–90.

## Design

- A prospective multicentre, open-label, randomized trial
- Level of evidence: 1b
- Randomization: surgery and adjuvant radiation therapy versus induction chemotherapy (cisplatin and fluorouracil) and primary radiation therapy
- Number of patients: 332
- Inclusion criteria: biopsy-proven, previously untreated stage III or IV squamous carcinoma of the larynx, according to the 1985 classification system of the American Joint

Committee on Cancer. Adequate auditory, nutritional, pulmonary, renal, and cardiac status. White cell count > 4 × 10$^9$/L, platelets >100 × 10$^9$/L

◆ Exclusion criteria: patients with T1N1 carcinomas, unresectable cancers, distant metastases, previous radiation therapy to the head or neck, or previous cancer were excluded

◆ Follow up: 33 months (median)

## Outcome measures

### Primary endpoint

◆ Overall survival

### Secondary endpoints

◆ Toxicity (surgery-related deaths; chemotherapy-related death; mucositis)
◆ Locoregional recurrence
◆ Preservation of the larynx
◆ Tumour response to chemotherapy

## Results

The estimated 2-year survival was 68% (95% CI 60–76%) for both treatment groups (p = 0.9846).

The disease recurrence rate differed between the two groups with more local recurrences (p = 0.0005) and fewer distant metastases (p = 0.016) in the induction chemotherapy group than in the surgical group.

After induction chemotherapy, tumour response was complete in 31% of the patients and partial in 54%. Approximately one-third of the chemotherapy patients required total laryngectomy.

## Critique

This study recruited a large number of patients (332 in total, 166 patients in each arm), allowing valid statistical comparison tests. The larynx could be preserved in nearly two-thirds of the experimental arm (induction chemotherapy) and there was no significant difference in overall survival.

A subsequent European trial (EORTC 24954) confirmed the laryngeal preservation rate but could not find any difference between concurrent chemoradiotherapy and induction chemotherapy before irradiation. A North American trial (RTOG 91-11) showed improved larynx preservation with concurrent chemoradiotherapy but not in overall survival.

A comparison between these studies is also challenging due to different inclusion criteria. In the Veterans trial, 'stage III or IV disease according to the 1985 AJCC staging system' was the main inclusion criteria for total laryngectomy and one in ten patients had T1 or T2 disease. In the EORTC trial, eligibility comprised simply 'larynx cancer patients for whom a total laryngectomy is indicated'. Owing to such discrepancies, comparisons of published results may be misleading.

The question of laryngeal function also remains unsolved as the definition of larynx preservation varies in different trials. In addition, the side effects of non-surgical treatments may improve or worsen over time, and the quality of function may subsequently change with time. Quality of life after laryngeal preservation remains a much-debated issue.

The study generated discussion surrounding the applicability of study protocols applicable to daily practice, i.e. these randomized trials are conducted on highly selected groups of patients with precise treatment and follow up protocols which may not be replicable.

## References

Forastiere AA, Zhang Q, Weber RS, Maor MH, Goepfert H, Pajak TF, et al. Long-term results of RTOG 91-11: a comparison of three nonsurgical treatment strategies to preserve the larynx in patients with locally advanced larynx cancer. *J Clin Oncol* 2013;**31**:845–52.

Lefebvre JL, Rolland F, Tesselaar M, Bardet E, Leemans CR, Geoffrois L, et al. Phase 3 randomized trial on larynx preservation comparing sequential vs alternating chemotherapy and radiotherapy. *J Natl Cancer Inst* 2009;**101**:142–52.

## Chapter 52

# Oncological management of head and neck cancer II

Tom Roques

## Details of studies

In 2004, the standard of care for resectable locally advanced or high-risk head and cancer was surgery with postoperative radiotherapy, but the relatively high (>50%) chances of recurrence prompted trials to look at intensifying treatment. Two papers published in the *New England Journal of Medicine* looked at the addition of concomitant 3-weekly cisplatin chemotherapy to postoperative radiotherapy for these patients. One trial was run by the RTOG and carried out in North America, the other designed by the EORTC recruited in Europe. While the results of the two studies were broadly concordant, showing improved locoregional control and progression-free survival for the addition of chemotherapy, only the European trial reported improved overall survival. Important differences in inclusion criteria (what constituted high risk for recurrence) and in reported endpoints may explain this difference. Authors from both papers combined their datasets and analysed them to assess the effect of adding chemotherapy on outcomes for patients with different risk factors.

## Study references

### Main study

Bernier J, Cooper JS, Pajak TF, van Glabbeke M, Bourhis J, Forastiere A, et al. Defining risk levels in locally advanced head and neck cancers: a comparative analysis of concurrent postoperative radiation plus chemotherapy trials of the EORTC (#22931) and RTOG (#9501). *Head Neck* 2005;**27**:843–50.

### Related references

Benier J, Domenge C, Ozsahin M, et al. Postoperative irradiation with or without concomitant chemotherapy for locally advanced head and neck cancer. *N Engl J Med* 2004;**350**:1945–52.

Cooper JS, Pajak TF, Forastiere AA, Jacobs J, Campbell BH, Saxman SB, et al. Postoperative concurrent radiotherapy and chemotherapy for high-risk squamous-cell carcinoma of the head and neck. *N Engl J Med* 2004;**350**:1937–44.

## Study design

- Level of evidence: 1b: pooled individual patient data from RCTs

◆ Randomization: radiotherapy (60–66 Gy) with or without cisplatin 100 mg/m², given on days 1, 22, and 43

◆ Number of patients: 748. All 334 patients from the EORTC trial and 414 out of 459 from the RTOG trial. The paper does not explain the reasons for excluding the other 45 patients

## Inclusion criteria

◆ EORTC: age <70, resected oral cavity, oropharynx, larynx, or hypopharynx cancer, pT3, pT4, pN2, or pN3. Or T1-2, N0-1 cancer with a positive resection margin, extracapsular nodal extension, perineural invasion (PNI), or vascular invasion (VI). Or with level IV or V nodes from an oral or oropharynx cancer

◆ RTOG: resected oral cavity, oropharynx, larynx, or hypopharynx cancer with any of positive resection margin, extracapsular nodal extension, or more than one lymph node involved

The differences in inclusion criteria are key to the discussion as shown in Figure 52.1

## Exclusion criteria

◆ Patients not well enough to consider concomitant chemotherapy—in particular with respect to renal function

## Follow-up

◆ Differed slightly in each study but in both groups was indefinite for the life of the study

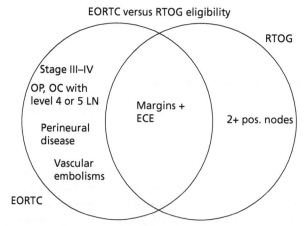

**Figure 52.1** Eligibility criteria in EORTC 22931 and RTOG 9501 trials. OP, oropharynx; OC, oral cavity; LN, lymph node; ECE, extracapsular extension.

Reproduced from Bernier J, Cooper JS, Pajak TF et al. Defining risk levels in locally advanced head and neck cancers: a comparative analysis of concurrent postoperative radiation plus chemotherapy trials of the EORTC (#22931) and RTOG (# 9501). *Head Neck* 2005;27(10):843–50 with permission from Wiley.

## Outcome measures

|  | RTOG | EORTC |
|---|---|---|
| Primary | Local and regional disease control | Progression-free survival |
| Secondary | Overall survival<br>Disease free survival<br>Adverse effects | Overall survival<br>Relapse<br>Acute and late toxicity |
| Time of analysis | 3 years | 5 years |

In the pooled analysis hazard ratios are presented, but it is not clear if the pooled data has been analysed at 3 years or 5 years.

## Results

Adding chemotherapy improved outcomes for patients with positive resection margins and/or extracapsular nodal extension. Hazard ratios showed a 48% reduction in risk of locoregional relapse, 30% reduction in risk of recurrence, 30% reduction in risk of death. The absolute benefits were not stated. There was a trend towards a benefit of adding chemotherapy in patients with PNI, VI, stage III or IV disease, or low neck nodes—i.e. those who would have been eligible for the EORTC study. Patients with two or more in- volved nodes as their only risk factor have no benefit from the addition of chemotherapy.

## Critique

The addition of chemotherapy to radiotherapy in high-risk patients was shown in the two individual trials here to improve disease free survival from 36% to 47% (measured at 5 years in the EORTC paper and 3 years in RTOG) though only the EORTC trial showed an improvement in overall survival—from 40% to 53% at 5 years. The benefit of con- comitant chemotherapy comes with a cost—increased acute side effects such as mucositis, vomiting and neutropenic sepsis, and increased late effects such as dysphagia and fibrosis. Importantly, neither study measured patient-reported outcomes or quality of life, which would be seen as standard data items in a more modern trial. Trying to decide which pa- tients might benefit from the addition of chemotherapy to what is already a potentially toxic combination of surgery and radiotherapy is therefore important.

By pooling the data, the authors were able to conclude that there is 30% reduction in the risk of death in patients with the addition of chemotherapy to radiotherapy for either posi- tive resection margins, extracapsular nodal spread or both (the high-risk group). There is no statistically significant improvement in overall survival, local control, or disease- specific survival in other groups of patients eligible for either study. This has had a direct bearing on multidisciplinary team discussions and recommendations for patients in that concomitant chemotherapy is routinely offered if there are positive resection margins or extracapsular nodal spread but debated more keenly in patients with other risk factors. For these intermediate-risk patients the number of risk factors, the patient fitness for combined treatment, and individual patient preferences all need to be taken into account when deciding whether to add chemotherapy to postoperative radiotherapy.

It is important to note that the radiation dose was not the same in the two papers. In the EORTC study, 91% received 66 Gy, 5% received 60 Gy, and 4% less than 60 Gy. In the RTOG study only 13% had 66 Gy with the majority receiving 60 Gy. Though these differences may seem small, an increase in dose of 6 Gy would be expected to improve locoregional control as the dose–response curve for radiotherapy at these doses is steep. The two studies aimed for radiotherapy to start 6 and 8 weeks after surgery and there is consensus that 6 weeks is an appropriate target, though one that can be hard to achieve if recovery from surgery is slow.

The authors acknowledge the perils of pooled data analyses such as this that are unplanned and rely on analysis of subsets of patients for which neither trial was initially powered. But their conclusions support previous data-driven hypotheses in which pathological risk factors are most important in predicting recurrence and therefore the added benefit of more intense treatment.

Looking back at this paper from a 2017 viewpoint, the biggest challenge is perhaps factoring in changes to adjuvant radiotherapy technique. Most patients in the study were treated in the 1990s when radiotherapy target volumes were defined on lateral X-rays or crudely derived body contours and the delivery of treatment often involved matching different types of radiation beam at locations at risk of recurrence, hence risking under- (or over-) dosing. Now these patients would have treatment volumes meticulously defined on cross-sectional imaging and would have intensity-modulated radiotherapy (IMRT) enabling the targeting of different risk levels to different doses and allowing relative preservation of uninvolved organs. Surgery, too, has changed over this time. It is logical to assume that risks of recurrence after modern surgery and radiotherapy are lower even in patients with adverse pathological findings and that the 30% reduction in the risk of death may be lower with modern day treatments. Equally improvements in supportive treatment—for example better chemotherapy anti-emetics—should ameliorate the toxicity of combined modality therapy more effectively.

The other major change in 2017 is the recognition that not all head and neck cancers have the same biology. In particular 42% of the RTOG patients had oropharynx cancer compared with 30% in the EORTC study and some of these may have had human papilloma virus (HPV)-related disease which has higher cure rates regardless of the treatment modalities used. Studies that pool many subsites of head and neck cancers together, perhaps necessarily to allow them to be adequately powered, risk hiding specific data about different head and neck cancers which we know have different biology and treatment outcomes. Advances in tumour genetics will hopefully define characteristics predictive of recurrence that are more accurate than current histopathological criteria.

Nonetheless, this paper and its two constituent studies remain practice-defining. No approach to patients at high risk of recurrence following resection has been found to be superior to radiation and concomitant chemotherapy, with a phase 3 trial testing the addition of cetuximab to radiotherapy and concomitant chemotherapy failing to show any extra benefit. All patients should be risk stratified after potentially curative surgery according to the pathological criteria defined in this paper. Those at highest risk of recurrence (involved margins and/or extracapsular nodal extension) should be offered adjuvant radiotherapy and chemotherapy. The intermediate risk group should be offered adjuvant radiotherapy with or without chemotherapy depending on the balance of the potential benefits and risks for each individual. Most other patients with lowest risk disease (i.e. not eligible for either trial) should not have adjuvant therapy.

## Additional references

Ang KK, Trotti A, Brown BW, Garden AS, Foote RL, Morrison WH, et al. Randomized trial addressing risk features and time factors of surgery plus radiotherapy in advanced head-and-neck cancer. *Int J Radiat Oncol Biol Phys* 2001;**51**:571–8.

Ang KK, Zhang Q, Rosenthal DI, Nguyen-Tan PF, Sherman EJ, Weber RS, et al. Randomized phase III trial of concurrent accelerated radiation plus cisplatin with or without cetuximab for stage III to IV head and neck carcinoma: RTOG 0522. *J Clin Oncol* 2014;**32**:2940–50.

Harari PM, Harris J, Kies MS, et al. Postoperative chemoradiotherapy and cetuximab for high-risk squamous cell carcinoma of the head and neck: radiation therapy oncology group RTOG-0234. *J Clin Oncol* 2014;**32**:2486–95.

Lavaf A, Genden EM, Cesaretti JA, Packer S, Kao J. Adjuvant radiotherapy improves overall survival for patients with lymph node-positive head and neck squamous cell carcinoma. *Cancer* 2008;**112**:535–43.

Machtay M, Moughan J, Trotti A, Garden AS, Weber RS, Cooper JS, et al. Factors associated with severe late toxicity after concurrent chemoradiation for locally advanced head and neck cancer: an RTOG analysis. *J Clin Oncol* 2008;**26**:3582–9.

# Chapter 53

# Oncological management of head and neck cancer III

Tom Roques

## Details of studies

Large-scale adequately powered randomized clinical trials are a challenge to conduct well in less common cancers such as head and neck cancer. Heterogeneity in inclusion criteria make meta-analysis challenging, not least because head and neck cancer is a mix of several quite different subtypes of cancer. The epidemiology of head and neck cancer has changed over recent years so large-scale studies are required to ensure treatment stays up to date.

In this context the MACH-NC analysis is a superb achievement—an individual patient data meta-analysis of thousands of patients to estimate the additional benefit of chemotherapy either before or during radiotherapy. Analysing individual patient data rather than just pooling the results of similar studies provides more validity for the results whilst the size of the dataset allows meaningful subset and subgroup analyses to be conducted—exploring the value of different chemotherapy regimes or of chemotherapy in different subsites. The authors include unpublished trials too—identified from clinical trial registries—to reduce publication bias. This version of the analysis updates the original paper from 2000 with data from 24 trials reported in the intervening time and with updated outcomes data from patients in all studies. The two papers combined and analysed in the previous chapter are both included. A similar analysis of different radiotherapy fractionation regimes has also been published.

## Study references

### Main study

Pignon JP, le Maître A, Maillard E, Bourhis J on behalf of the MACH-NC Collaborative Group. Meta-analysis of chemotherapy in head and neck cancer (MACH-NC): an update on 93 randomised trials and 17,346 patients. *Radiother Oncol* 2009;**92**:4–14.

### Related references

Bourhis J, Overgaard J, Audry H, Ang KK, Saunders M, Bernier J, et al. Hyperfractionated or accelerated radiotherapy in head and neck cancer: an individual patient data metaanalysis of 15 randomized trials. *Lancet* 2006;**368**:843–54.

Pignon J-P, Bourhis J, Domenge C, Désigné L on behalf of the MACH-NC Collaborative Group. Chemotherapy added to locoregional treatment for head and neck squamous-cell carcinoma: three meta-analyses of updated individual data. *Lancet* 2000;255:949–55.

## Study design

♦ Level of evidence: 1a

♦ Randomization: all patients were part of randomized controlled trials. In all trials, the physician could not know in advance of randomization which treatment and individual would receive (reducing the possibility of allocation bias)

♦ Number of patients: 16,485 patients from 87 trials

♦ Inclusion criteria: randomized controlled trials comparing localized treatment alone to localized treatment plus chemotherapy in previously untreated head and neck cancer from 1963 to 2000.

♦ Exclusion criteria: trials of only nasopharyngeal cancer were not included. Six studies that were initially identified were excluded for various methodological reasons

♦ Follow-up: median follow-up 5.6 years

♦ Outcome measures: overall survival was the main endpoint. Secondary endpoints were event-free survival and cumulative loco-regional and distant failure

## Results

Concomitant chemotherapy improved overall survival at 5 years by 6.5%, hazard ratio (HR) = 0.81. This benefit is due to a reduction in head and neck cancer deaths with no effect on non-cancer deaths. This magnitude of benefit is smaller with increasing patient age with no benefit found for those aged 71 and over. Cisplatin was more effective than other single-agent chemotherapy regimes. Most patients had radiotherapy as locoregional treatment and had stage III or IV disease

Induction (neo-adjuvant) chemotherapy did not improve overall survival to a statistically significant degree. Five-year survival increased by 2.4% but the confidence intervals of the hazard ratio include 1.

There was no benefit to adding adjuvant chemotherapy to standard treatment. Data on compliance with therapy and on toxicity were not analysed.

## Conclusions

Concomitant chemotherapy with cisplatin is a standard of care for head and neck cancer, improving local control and overall survival. The benefit is lower in older patients where, given toxicity, it should be used cautiously. Induction chemotherapy may have a small benefit in reducing distant metastases but has no convincing effect on overall survival, suggesting that the two approaches may be complementary to a degree.

# Critique

This paper has established concomitant chemotherapy (chemotherapy given during a radiotherapy course, often called chemoradiation) as a standard of care in stage III and IV head and neck cancer. It is now the internationally recognized gold standard but comes with toxicity, which is not covered in this analysis. Acute side effects are increased but are usually self-limiting and can be helped with good supportive care. The absolute benefit of chemotherapy is relatively small and its use must not compromise delivery of radiotherapy, for example by making patients too ill to have radiation according to the prescribed schedule. But there are also concerns that long-term functions such as swallowing are not as good after combination treatment. Only if the therapeutic ratio is enhanced by concomitant chemotherapy (a greater effect on tumour cells than on normal tissues) will it be a more effective strategy than just increasing the dose of radiotherapy.

Many questions remain about concomitant chemotherapy. Are regimes such as weekly lower dose cisplatin as effective but with reduced toxicity compared with larger doses? What is the optimal treatment for older people with head and neck cancer, given that the added benefit of concomitant chemotherapy declines with age? What is the role of cetuximab as an alternative or addition to concomitant chemotherapy? What about newer molecular agents or immunotherapy combined with radiotherapy? And how should the data on patients treated before 2000 with two-dimensional radiotherapy be interpreted in the intensity-modulated radiotherapy (IMRT) era when side effects are reduced by the sparing of critical structures?

Induction or neoadjuvant chemotherapy is given before locoregional therapy (usually radiotherapy). Although this paper shows any benefit to be small there are still proponents of this approach, particularly in very poor prognosis disease as a form of treatment escalation or as a way to select out tumours with better biology which may also respond to radiation. The excellent response rates with chemotherapy are seductive but the failure to translate into a survival benefit cannot be ignored. There are three trials that show a survival benefit of induction TPF (docetaxel, cisplatin, and 5-fluorouracil) over PF (cisplatin and 5-fluorouracil) but no data supporting TPF over no induction chemotherapy. A recent meta-analysis of five trials of variable quality suggests there is no added benefit from adding induction TPF to radiation and concomitant chemotherapy.

The strengths of a very large dataset also create weaknesses. Trials reporting radiotherapy in the two-dimensional era cannot necessarily be extrapolated to the era of targeted, organ-sparing IMRT. Amalgamating data on each head and neck subsite adds to the statistical power but removes the subtlety of needing to differentiate between oral and laryngeal cancers for example. Although the Blanchard subgroup analysis confirms a benefit of concomitant chemotherapy in all subsites, the magnitude of that benefit varies (largest for oropharynx, smallest for hypopharynx).

Perhaps the key lies in more adroit patient selection. For excellent prognosis human papilloma virus (HPV)-associated oropharyngeal cancer, many trials are now looking to de-intensify standard radiotherapy and concomitant chemotherapy approaches, for example using radiation alone or lower dose radiation after transoral laser resection. (Some of these trials are also adding in more induction chemotherapy in spite of the lack of data to support this approach.) For patients with locally advanced HPV-negative oropharynx cancer or other head and neck tumours, the prognosis remains poor. In this paper the 5-year survival of patients receiving radiotherapy and concomitant chemotherapy was only 33.7% and although improvements in surgery and radiotherapy mean this figure in 2017 will be a little higher, it is not likely to be more than 50%. So there is a real need to investigate more effective treatments for this cohort including adding molecularly targeted drugs or immunotherapy as well as improving current surgical and radiotherapy techniques.

## Additional references

Ang KK, Harris J, Wheeler R, Weber R, Rosenthal DI, Nguyen-Tân PF, et al. Human papillomavirus and survival of patients with oropharyngeal cancer. *N Engl J Med* 2010;**363**:24–35.

Blanchard P, Baujat B, Holostenco V, Bourredjem A, Baey C, Bourhis J, et al. Meta-analysis of chemotherapy in head and neck cancer (MACH-NC): a comprehensive analysis by tumour site. *Radiother Oncol* 2011;**100**:33–40.

Blanchard P, Bourhis J, Lacas B, Posner MR, Vermorken JB, Cruz Hernandez JJ, et al. Taxane-cisplatin-fluorouracil as induction chemotherapy in locally advanced head and neck cancers: an individual patient data meta-analysis of the meta-analysis of chemotherapy in head and neck cancer group. *J Clin Oncol* 2013;**31**:2854–60.

Bonner JA, Harari PM, Giralt J, Cohen RB, Jones CU, Sur RK, et al. Radiotherapy plus cetuximab for locoregionally advanced head and neck cancer: 5-year survival data from a phase 3 randomised trial, and relation between cetuximab-induced rash and survival. *Lancet Oncol* 2010;**11**:21–8.

Budach W, Bölke E, Kammers K, Gerber PA, Orth K, Gripp S, Matuschek C. Induction chemotherapy followed by concurrent radio-chemotherapy versus concurrent radio-chemotherapy alone as treatment of locally advanced squamous cell carcinoma of the head and neck (HNSCC): a meta-analysis of randomized trials. *Radiother Oncol* 2016;**118**:238–43.

Department of Veterans Affairs Laryngeal Cancer Study Group. Induction chemotherapy plus radiation compared with surgery plus radiation in patients with advanced laryngeal cancer. *N Engl J Med* 1991:**324**:1685–90.

# Chapter 54

# PET-CT as a method of surveillance for head and neck cancer

Liam Masterson

## Details of studies

Patients with squamous cell carcinoma of the head and neck are frequently managed with primary chemoradiotherapy. For those with advanced nodal disease (N2 and N3) there is widespread variation in management of the neck following treatment. Options include planned neck dissection or surveillance with cross-sectional imaging. Historically, planned neck dissection was felt to offer a significant survival benefit to patients. However, this has remained controversial. Image guided approaches have been increasingly used without good quality evidence. Integration of $^{18}$F-fluorodeoxyglucose (FDG) positron emission tomography and computed tomography (PET-CT) has become increasingly available, and studies have shown a high negative-predictive value.

Mehanna et al. (2016) performed 'a prospective, randomised controlled trial, to compare the clinical usefulness and health economic outcomes of planned neck dissection versus PET-CT guided surveillance in patients with nodal stage N2 or N3, metastasis stage M0 disease'.

## Study reference

### Main study

Mehanna H, Wong W, McConkey CC, Rahman JK, Robinson M, Hartley AGJ, et al. for the PET-NECK Trial Management Group. PET-CT surveillance versus neck dissection in advanced head and neck cancer. *N Engl J Med* 2016;**374**:1444–54.

### Related references

Isles MG, McConkey C, Mehanna HM. A systematic review and meta-analysis of the role of positron emission tomography in the follow up of head and neck squamous cell carcinoma following radiotherapy or chemoradiotherapy. *Clin Otolaryngol* 2008;**33**:210–22.

## Study design

- A prospective, multicentre, randomized, unblinded, controlled trial
- Intention to treat design
- Non-inferiority trial

| Level of evidence | 1b |
| --- | --- |
| Randomization | Planned neck dissection versus PET-CT 12 weeks after completion of chemoradiotherapy |
| Number of patients | 564 |
| Inclusion criteria | Adults (18 years of age or older) |
| | Histologically confirmed diagnosis of squamous-cell carcinoma of the oropharynx, hypopharynx, larynx, oral cavity, or an unknown primary site in the head or neck |
| | Clinical and radiologic (CT or magnetic resonance imaging) stage N2 or N3 nodal metastasis |
| | Suitable candidate for chemoradiotherapy |
| | No contraindications to neck dissection |
| Exclusion criteria | Pregnancy |
| | Distant metastasis |
| | Other cancer diagnosis within the last 5 years (excluding basal cell carcinoma or cervical carcinoma *in situ*) |
| | Prior treatment for head and neck squamous cell carcinoma |
| Follow up | Up to 5 years |
| | Quality of life measures at 2 weeks (following chemoradiotherapy), 6 months, 12 months, 24 months |

- PET-CT was performed 12 weeks after the last radiotherapy fraction was delivered
- PET-CT findings were interpreted locally by PET-CT specialty radiologists and nuclear medicine physicians
- Patients with incomplete or equivocal response in the lymph nodes in the neck and who had a complete response in the primary site underwent neck dissection within 4 weeks after PET-CT
- Modified radical and selective neck dissection were permitted in both groups, with the decision made by the treating surgeon

## Outcome measures

### Primary endpoints

- Overall survival at 24 months
- Health economics using quality-adjusted life years

### Secondary endpoints

- Disease specific survival at 24 months
- Recurrence and local control in neck at 24 months

- Surgical complication rates for 30 days post surgery
- Serious adverse event rates for 3 months after last treatment (chemoradiotherapy or surgery)

## Results

Two-year survival was equivocal among patients who underwent PET-CT-guided surveillance and those who underwent planned neck dissection (84.9%, 95% CI 80.7–89.1, versus 81.5%, 95% CI 76.9–86.3).

Considerably fewer operations were required in the PET-CT group (54 versus 221) which resulted in a more cost effective outcome (£1,492 per person over the duration of the trial).

## Conclusion

Survival was similar among patients who underwent PET-CT-guided surveillance and those who underwent planned neck dissection. Surveillance resulted in considerably fewer operations and was more cost-effective.

## Critique

This was a multicentre UK-based trial, and had the distinction of being the largest head and neck surgical trial to date. It was conducted to high standard with low levels of bias, and as such these results have significant implications for clinical practice.

This study recognizes in its discussion that while patients with N3 nodal disease were recruited into the study, the numbers were small, only nine patients were included in the PET-CT surveillance group, of whom five demonstrated a complete response. Caution should therefore be used when extrapolating the results to clinical practice in this group.

There is a high proportion of human papilloma virus (HPV)-positive oropharyngeal cancers in both arms of the study (representative of current UK clinical practice), which could impact the relevance of the findings to HPV-negative disease, or disease at other subsites. Non-HPV-related head and neck squamous cell carcinoma patients may demonstrate a complete metabolic response but have residual cervical lymph node enlargement on PET-CT. If metabolically inactive residual lymph node tissue can be safely observed, this would significantly improve overall morbidity, quality of life, and health economic outcomes. Grading systems for lymph node metabolic response are now routinely applied to patients with lymphoma.

The study also recognizes that it was not possible to calibrate the scanning systems across the centres at the time of the study, and therefore this may lead to variability in results. While many across the UK have been keen to implement the recommendations of this study (and indeed many undertook a similar policy prior to the study results being published), there is wide variability in the availability of access to PET-CT, and subsequently the quality of expertise of those interpreting the imaging. This should be considered and monitored closely within centres to ensure safety and applicability to local populations.

## Additional references

Brizel DM, Prosnitz RG, Hunter S, Fisher SR, Clough RL, Downey MA, Scher RL. Necessity for adjuvant neck dissection in setting of concurrent chemoradiation for advanced head-and-neck cancer. *Int J Radiat Oncol Biol Phys* 2004;**58**:1418–23.

Gupta T, Master Z, Kannan S, Agarwal JP, Ghsoh-Laskar S, Rangarajan V, et al. Diagnostic performance of post-treatment FDG PET or FDG PET/CT imaging in head and neck cancer: a systematic review and meta-analysis. *Eur J Nucl Med Mol Imaging* 2011;**38**:2083–95.

Marcus C, Ciarallo A, Tahari AK, et al. Head and neck PET/CT: therapy response interpretation criteria (Hopkins Criteria) inter-reader reliability, accuracy, and survival outcomes. *J Nucl Med* 2014;**55**:1411–6.

Rabalais A, Walvekar RR, Johnson JT, Smith KJ. A cost-effectiveness analysis of positron emission tomography-computed tomography surveillance versus up-front neck dissection for management of the neck for N2 disease after chemoradiotherapy. *Laryngoscope* 2012;**122**:311–4.

Chapter 55

# Quality of life for patients with laryngeal cancer

Sally Erskine

## Details of study

The treatment of head and neck cancer, particularly when in more advanced stages, often involves sacrificing basic daily functioning, including speech, swallow, sense of taste and smell, and the need for permanent or temporary tracheal airway, as well as readily visible physical scars. Much research in cancer management has focused on survival rates, and although increasingly quality of life is taken into account, quantitating the trade-off between quantity and quality of life is very challenging. It is particularly pertinent in head and neck cancer when both disease and treatment can be very disabling, and when perceptions of such disability vary greatly between individuals. One of the first papers to consider this challenge is a study by McNeil et al. (1981), who presented 37 healthy participants with various management scenarios for a T3 laryngeal tumour and used expected-utility theory to analyse the degree of importance based on both quantity and quality of life in each scenario.

## Study references

### Main study

McNeil BJ, Weichselbaum R, Pauker SG. Speech and survival: tradeoffs between quality and quantity of life in laryngeal cancer. *N Engl J Med* 1981;**305**:982–7.

### Related reference

Hamilton DW, Bins JE, McMeekin P, Pedersen A, Steen N, De Soyza A, et al. Quality compared to quantity of life in laryngeal cancer: a time trade-off study. *Head Neck* 2016;**38**(Suppl. 1):E631–7.

## Study design

Interviews with 37 healthy subjects, including 12 firefighters and 25 middle- and upper-management executives with an average age of 40 years. Interviews lasted 30–45 minutes, using hypothetical management and survival options to determine treatment preferences for localized but advanced laryngeal cancer. The three types of data collected were attitudes towards survival in early compared with later years after diagnosis, attitudes towards artificial or oesophageal speech, and survival associated with different treatment strategies, with a choice of surgery (survival 60% at 3 years, speech lost) or radiation (survival 30% at 3 years, speech preserved), to determine relative importance placed on quality vs. quantity of life. Participants were played recordings of oesophageal speech and were asked questions on their attitudes to treatment modalities and outcomes to help quantify views.

## Outcome measures

Utility curves for survival with normal speech and artificial speech.

## Conclusion

Most participants were prepared to trade some decrease in long-term survival to maintain normal speech but few would accept any decrease below 5 years of survival; survival alone may not be the priority for all patients treated.

## Critique

McNeil et al. attempted to integrate attitudes towards survival and quality of life at a time when medical care and treatment options were handled in a more paternalistic manner. The first study of its kind in head and neck cancer management, it has subsequently been cited over 600 times. Quality of life is now considered an important outcome measure in trials of new therapies with differing preferences of individuals with regards to quality and quantity of life recognized.

McNeil et al. do not fully explain recruitment beyond participants being of a similar age to those with laryngeal cancer. They do not clearly define the content of the questions used in their interviews but do explain the construction of utility curves in detail.

In 1981, total laryngectomy was the most common procedure for locally advanced laryngeal cancer, and was associated with poorer voice outcomes than today. Radical courses of chemoradiotherapy now appear to offer equivalent survival to total laryngectomy;

Hamilton et al. (2016) have repeated the study with modern management choices and with study participants demographically matched to new attenders at a head and neck cancer clinic.

They conclude that laryngeal preservation (which has been assumed to be of great importance) may *not* be the priority of all patients, with quality of treatment outcome more important than modality. Utility value therefore remains an important tool in the evaluation of treatment options both for affected individuals and in signposting important avenues of research.

## Additional references

Laccourreye O, Malinvaud D, Holsinger FC, Consoli S, Menard M, Bonfils P. Trade-off between survival and laryngeal preservation in advanced laryngeal cancer: the otorhinolaryngology patient's perspective. *Ann Otol Rhinol Laryngol* 2012;**121**:570–5.

# Chapter 56

# Incidence of thyroid cancer

Tom Roques

## Details of studies

Papillary thyroid cancer is increasing in incidence in many developed countries including the UK and USA. The authors of this American study wanted to examine whether this was due to a change in risk factors such as radiation exposure or due to better diagnostic techniques including ultrasound and fine needle aspiration (FNA). They realized the importance of several autopsy studies that had suggested that so called micropapillary cancers (<10 mm) were detectable in a large percentage of the population at post-mortem examination with some authors even suggesting that micropapillary cancers are so common as to be normal. They analysed data on changing thyroid cancer incidence over 30 years from the National Cancer Institute's Surveillance, Epidemiology and End Results (SEER) programme, which covers 10% of the USA population. This was compared to changes in mortality from thyroid cancer analysed from a US national database of causes of death from death certificates.

## Study references

### Main study

Davies l, Welch HG. Increasing incidence of thyroid cancer in the United States, 1973-2002. *JAMA* 2006;**295**:2164–7

### Related reference

Harach HR, Franssila KO, Wasenius VM. Occult papillary carcinoma of the thyroid: a "normal" finding in Finland. *Cancer* 1985;**56**:531–8.

## Study design

- Level of evidence: 2c—national database analyses
- Randomization: N/A
- Number of patients: SEER covers 10% of the USA population and contains data from five states and six metropolitan areas. In 2002, the final year analysed, there was data for 2,400 thyroid cancers
- Inclusion criteria: N/A
- Exclusion criteria: N/A
- Follow-up: N/A

## Outcome measures

Data obtained from SEER included pathological subtype of thyroid cancer, grouped as papillary vs. follicular vs. medullary and anaplastic combined. From 1988 there was also pathology report data available for thyroid cancer size.

## Results

Thyroid cancer incidence rose from 3.6 per 100,000 in 1973 to 8.7 per 100,000 in 2002. This increase was almost entirely due to more papillary thyroid cancer diagnoses. Thyroid cancer mortality did not change significantly over the same time period, remaining at 0.5 per 100,000. In the period 1988–2002 when size data were available, papillary thyroid cancer incidence increased by 4.1 per 100,000. Most of this increase was due to small cancers—49% were less than 1 cm and 87% were less than 2 cm in maximum diameter.

## Conclusions

The increased incidence of thyroid cancer in the USA over 30 years is predominantly due to an increase in the detection of small papillary cancers. This has had no effect on overall mortality from thyroid cancer over the same time period.

## Critique

Treatment for papillary thyroid cancer has usually consisted of a total thyroidectomy followed by radioactive iodine therapy to ablate any remaining thyroid tissue and make long term monitoring with serum thyroglobulin more accurate. This approach has excellent long-term cure rates but there are risks of a thyroidectomy, including damage to the recurrent laryngeal nerve and parathyroid glands. Radioactive iodine also has short- and long-term risks including xerostomia. Some patients report never feeling as well on thyroid hormone replacement as they did with an intact thyroid. A cancer diagnosis also adds to psychological morbidity and commits patients to the anxiety of lifelong follow-up.

This paper makes use of large datasets on diagnosis and mortality to propose that asymptomatic thyroid cancers are being diagnosed that do not need treatment. Cancer incidence is increasing rapidly but mortality is unchanged over 30 years. The authors explore and refute other possible explanations for these data. They argue that no new cause for thyroid cancer has been found: in fact radiation exposure has decreased over the same period with fewer nuclear tests and therapeutic radiation of the head and neck for common benign diseases such as tine capitis and acne no longer used. It seems unlikely that treatment for thyroid cancer has improved at exactly the same rate as detection, hence keeping mortality completely unchanged. The explanation that there is a new category of symptomatic but non-life-threatening cancers is not plausible as the excess cancers are almost all small and therefore very likely to be asymptomatic. The pathological diagnostic criteria for papillary thyroid cancer did not change from 1988 to 2002 whereas the incidence of the disease almost doubled. The most logical explanation of the data is that improvements in diagnostic tests, ultrasound and in particular FNA, and an increase number of these tests being performed, have led to more papillary cancers being detected. The treatment of these cancers does not improve mortality as they rarely shorten life when not treated. This presents real challenges to the diagnostician and the surgeon. Palpable thyroid swellings or discrete lumps are very common. They often prompt thyroid ultrasounds, which may reveal other small suspicious nodules which are then biopsied by FNA. This leads to surgery and a cancer diagnosis in a small nodule which was originally asymptomatic. Alternatively, a thyroid lobectomy for a symptomatic benign nodule may reveal a tiny hidden cancer which would otherwise never have caused symptoms.

It seems relatively easy to recommend treatment for a cancer, but to tell someone they have cancer and to then suggest no treatment is required is difficult for healthcare professionals and patients alike, particularly when cancer is so feared. Current guidelines suggest a risk-stratified personal decision-making approach to treatment taking factors such as patient age and histological subtype into account before deciding on the extent of surgery, the need for I-131 therapy and the extent and duration of thyroid-stimulating hormone suppression. Molecular diagnostics may make the very small number of tiny but higher risk cancers easier to identify. If a category of papillary thyroid cancer that behaves so indolently that it does not need treatment can be agreed, then perhaps we can reduce the number of ultrasounds where the risk of cancer is minimal and stop performing FNAs of small nodules, leading to a reduction in the number of cancer diagnoses with no change in mortality. It may also be appropriate to rename very low-risk lesions, as has been done for encapsulated follicular variant of papillary thyroid carcinoma, so that they are not described as a cancer.

In South Korea in the early 2000s the practice of ultrasound screening of the thyroid glands became part of a regime of cancer-screening tests paid for by government. As a result the incidence of thyroid cancer increased between 1999 and 2008 from 6.4 per 100,000 to 40.7 per 100,000. As in the US study, this increase was almost all accounted for by papillary tumours less than 20 mm diameter and was not reflected in any increase in mortality from thyroid cancer. In more recent years guidelines and public campaigns in South Korea have seen this tide change so that fewer thyroidectomies are now performed each year. But the individual physical and psychological consequences of a cancer over diagnosis and subsequent treatment and added healthcare costs of this overdiagnosis (estimated to be $1.3 billion in the USA in 2013) are considerable. This paper heralded a better appreciation of the realities and dangers of overdiagnosis of thyroid cancer— something all endocrinologists, oncologists, and ENT surgeons need to consider carefully before investigating and treating thyroid disease.

## Additional references

**Ahn HS, Kim HJ, Welch HG.** Korea's thyroid cancer 'epidemic'—screening and overdiagnosis. *N Engl J Med* 2014;**371**:1765–7.

**Fagin JA, Wells SA.** Biologic and clinical perspectives on thyroid cancer. *N Engl J Med* 2016;**375**:1054–67.

Mallick U, Harmer C, Yap B, Wadsley J, Clarke S, Moss L et al. Ablation with low-dose radioiodine and thyrotropin alfa in thyroid cancer. *N Engl J Med* 2012;**366**:1674–85

Nikiforov, YE, Seethala RR, Tallini G, Baloch ZW, Basolo F, Thompson LD, et al. Nomenclature revision for encapsulated follicular variant of papillary thyroid carcinoma: a paradigm shift to reduce overtreatment of indolent tumors *JAMA Oncol* 2016;**2**:1023–9.

Park S, Oh C-M, Cho H, Lee JY, Jung K-W, Jun JK, et al. Association between screening and the thyroid cancer 'epidemic' in South Korea: evidence from a nationwide study. *BMJ* 2016;**355**:i5745.

Perros P, Boelaert K, Colley S, Evans C, Evans RM, Gerrard Ba G, et al; British Thyroid Association. Guidelines for the management of thyroid cancer. *Clin Endocrinol (Oxf)* 2014;**81**(Suppl. 1):1–122.

Chapter 57

# Radiological assessment of thyroid nodules

Vinidh Paleri and Hannah Fox

## Details of current knowledge

The incidence of detectable thyroid nodules on ultrasound is between 30% and 70% and increases progressively with age. The investigation and management of thyroid nodules has evolved and changed significantly over the last decade. This is reflected in the most recent British Thyroid Association document 'Guidelines for the management of thyroid cancer', third edition February 2014. This is an evidence-based document produced after studying the latest literature, and chapter 4 of this document involves the ultrasound assessment of thyroid nodules.

## Study references

### Main study

Moon WJ, Jung SL, Lee JH, Na DG, Baek JH, Lee YH, et al. Benign and malignant thyroid nodules: us differentiation—multicenter retrospective study. *Radiology* 2008;**247**:762–70.

### Related reference

Perros P, Boelaert K, Colley S, Evans C, Evans RM, Ba G, et al; British Thyroid Association. Guidelines for the management of thyroid cancer. *Clin Endocrinol (Oxf)* 2014;**81**(Suppl. 1):1–122.

## Study design

Prospective, single blind review of retrospective multicentre data

| | |
|---|---|
| Level of evidence | 2b |
| Number of patients | 831 |
| Inclusion criteria | Patients who underwent surgery or gun biopsy after thyroid ultrasound, patients with benign nodules who underwent at least two cytological assessments within a 1-year period, patients who underwent cytological assessment and then ultrasound after at least a 12-month period |
| Exclusion criteria | Patients with Hurtle cell or follicular lesions without a final definitive diagnosis |

## Outcome measures

### Primary endpoint

Assessment of recognized ultrasound findings as predictors of malignancy in thyroid nodules.

### Secondly outcome measure

Assessment of interobserver agreement when interpreting static use images of thyroid nodules. This study provides one of the benchmark pieces of research underpinning the current guidelines that demonstrate a significant shift from the need for cytological/histological confirmation of nodular benignity to ultrasonographic demonstration of benignity and the use of the 'U' classification. The study comprises a prospective review of retrospective ultrasound images by three blinded senior head and neck radiologists to assess which ultrasonographic features of thyroid nodules are indicative of benignity versus malignancy.

## Results

Results of multiple logistic regression analysis for detection of malignant thyroid nodules

| Characteristic | Odds ratio | p |
|---|---|---|
| Marked hypoechogenicity | 8.463 | 0.014 |
| Microcalcification | 4.599 | <0.001 |
| Macrocalcification | 2.792 | <0.001 |
| Taller than wide shape | 2.787 | <0.001 |
| Speculated margin | 2.749 | <0.001 |
| Spongiform appearance | 0.032 | <0.001 |

## Conclusion

Using specific descriptive criteria to characterize thyroid nodules, notably shape (taller than wide), margin (spiculated), echogenicity (marked hypoechogenicity), and the presence of calcifications (micro- or macro-) with ultrasound will accurately predict malignancy in up to 78% of nodules with reasonable interviewer reliability.

## Critique

This paper provides one of the benchmark pieces of evidence underpinning the current way we assess and manage thyroid nodules. It has led to a shift away from fine needle aspiration and more towards ultrasound evaluation as the main assessment tool used to optimize our likelihood of differentiating benign from malignant thyroid nodules.

The strengths of the paper include the large number of patients included, from nine university-affiliated institutions, the fact that reviewers were blinded to previous ultrasound findings, were experienced head and neck radiologists with a minimum of 6 years' experience, and were initially trained to establish baseline consensus. In addition, the cohort only included patients who had undergone at least a biopsy with two separate assessments spaced at least 12 months apart to establish the nature of the lesion.

However, there were significant weaknesses. The study was retrospective, hence the reviewers were reviewing static images, and ultrasound is a dynamic investigation. In addition, as only subjects with histological confirmation were included and many ultrasonographically benign nodules did not undergo biopsy there is significant selection bias.

## Additional references

Hambly NM, Gonen M, Gerst SR. Implementation of evidence-based guidelines for thyroid nodule biopsy: a model for establishment of practice standards. *Am J Roentgenol* 2011;**196**:655–60.

Kwak JY, Han KH, Yoon JH, Moon HJ, Son EJ, Park SH, et al. Thyroid imaging reporting and data system for US features of nodules: a step in establishing better stratification of cancer risk. *Radiology* 2011;**260**:892–9.

Lee YH, Kim DW, In HS, Park JS, Kim SH, Eom JW, et al. Differentiation between benign and malignant solid thyroid nodules using an US classification system. *Korean J Radiol* 2011;**12**:559–67.

# Chapter 58

# Predicting outcome in thyroid cancer

## James England

## Details of studies

Papillary thyroid carcinoma (PTC) is the commonest type of thyroid cancer and its prognosis is dependent on various risk factors. This has led to development of various scoring systems to assess prognosis led by the EORTC in 1979. The Mayo Clinic series of thyroid cancer patients contains patient details from 1940 onwards therefore providing a large and valuable patient cohort from which outcomes can be studied and conclusions drawn. Using this cohort, Hay et al. (1993) have studied disease specific mortality with relation to patient and tumour characteristics and have derived a scoring system using multivariate analysis to be used as a prognostic tool for survival prediction.

## Study references

### Main study

Hay ID, Bergstralh EJ, Goellner JR, Ebersold JR, Grant CS. Predicting outcome in papillary thyroid carcinoma: development of a reliable prognostic scoring system in a cohort of 1779 patients surgically treated at one institution during 1940 through 1989. *Surgery* 1993;**114**:1050–7.

### Related reference

Byar DP, Green SB, Dor P, Williams ED, Colon J, van Gilse HA, et al. A prognostic index for thyroid carcinoma. A study of the E.O.R.T.C. thyroid cancer cooperative group. *Eur J Cancer* 1979;**15**:1033–41.

## Study design

Prospectively collected single institution observational cohort study including all patients who underwent surgery for the management of PTC.

| | |
|---|---|
| Level of evidence | 4 |
| Randomization | No |
| Number of patients | 1,779 |
| Inclusion criteria | All patients treated surgically for PTC in the Mayo Clinic between 1940 and 1989 inclusive |
| Exclusion criteria | Patients with a diagnosis of PTC who were not treated within 60 days of initial diagnosis |
| Follow-up | From date of treatment to death over the time of the study |

All patients treated with curative intent from 1940 to 1989 within 60 days of diagnosis were included. To develop the scoring system the patients were divided into two groups: those treated from 1940 to 1965 and those treated from 1965 to 1989. The first group were used to develop the prognostic score and the second group for external validation of the system developed. This study includes a large cohort of patients arguably making its findings and conclusions more compelling.

## Outcome measures

This study attempted to define a reliable prognostic scoring system for predicting mortality from PTC by assessing 15 potential variable factors.

## Results

The final model included five variables abbreviated by metastasis, age, completeness of resection, invasion, and size (MACIS).

The final prognostic score was defined as MACIS = 3.1 (if aged ≤39 years) or $0.08 \times$ age (if aged ≥40 years), + 0.3 × tumour size (in centimetres), + 1 (if incompletely resected), + 1 (if locally invasive), + 3 (if distant metastases present).

Twenty-year cause-specific survival rates for patients with MACIS less than 6, 6–6.99, 7–7.99, and 8+ were 99%, 89%, 56%, and 24%, respectively ($p < 0.0001$).

## Critique

The aim of the study is to develop a scoring system for assessment of disease-specific mortality from PTC derived from individual patient and tumour variables and it led to MACIS.

The study has major weaknesses. The study is single centred and there is no differentiation for the extent of thyroid resection which tended to be more conservative in the older section of the cohort.

In addition, follow-up length varied due to the retrospective nature of the information gathering. The 20-year follow-up rate was 32% with the 40-year follow-up percentage only 2%, a potentially significant weakness given the tendency of late recurrence in PTC which may or may not influence mortality. However, this paper, along with others, has led to the widespread acceptance of risk stratification in the management of differentiated thyroid cancer and MACIS is still in use. Interestingly, the series scrutinized were solely patients with PTC, although the same conclusions have been made regarding the management of patients with follicular thyroid cancer.

Chapter 59

# Radioiodine for thyroid cancer

Vinidh Paleri and Hannah Fox

## Details of studies

Thyroid cancer is common, with most cases being differentiated thyroid cancer. Radioiodine ablation is a commonly used adjuvant treatment following surgery. There is uncertainty over whether low-dose (1.1 GBq) or high-dose (3.7 GBq) radioiodine ablation is associated with similar success rates. A systematic review by Hackshaw et al. (2007) of randomized and observational studies on the topic was inconclusive. Additionally, many patients undergo thyroid hormone withdrawal prior to ablation, which can have a significant impact of their ability to work and quality of life. There is uncertainty as to whether recombinant human thyrotropin (thyrotropin alpha) reduces the rate of ablation success, particularly with low-dose radioiodine. The HiLo trial by Mallick et al. (2012) aimed to determine whether low-dose radioiodine could be used instead of high-dose radioiodine, and whether patients could receive thyrotropin alpha before ablation instead of thyroid hormone withdrawal.

## Study references

### Main study

Mallick U, Harmer C, Yap B, Wadsley J, Clarke S, Moss L, et al. Ablation with low-dose radioiodine and thyrotropin alfa in thyroid cancer. *N Engl J Med* 2012;**366**:1674–85.

### Related reference

Hackshaw A, Harmer C, Mallick U, Haq M, Franklyn JA. [131]I activity for remnant ablation in patients with differentiated thyroid cancer: a systematic review. *J Clin Endocrinol Metab* 2007;**92**:28–38.

## Study design

♦ A prospective, multicentre, randomized, unblinded, controlled trial

♦ Non-inferiority trial

| Level of evidence | 1b |
| --- | --- |
| Randomization | One of four groups: low-dose or high-dose radioiodine each combined with thyrotropin alpha or thyroid hormone withdrawal |

| | |
|---|---|
| Number of patients | 438 |
| Inclusion criteria | Adults 16-80 years old |
| | Performance status 0–2 |
| | Histological confirmation of differentiated thyroid cancer (including Hurthle cell carcinoma) requiring radioiodine ablation |
| | Tumour stage T1–T3 with the possibility of lymph-node involvement |
| | No microscopic residual disease |
| | One- or two-stage total thyroidectomy with or without central lymph node dissection |
| Exclusion criteria | Metastasis |
| | Aggressive malignant variants |
| | Pregnancy |
| | Severe co-existing conditions |
| | Previous cancer with limited life expectancy |
| | Previous iodine-131 or iodine-123 pre-ablation scanning |
| | Previous treatment for thyroid cancer except surgery |
| Follow-up | 6–9 months |

- Successful ablation was defined as either a negative scan (<0.1% uptake on the basis of the region of interest method drawn over the thyroid bed), or a thyroglobulin level of less than 2.0 ng per millilitre at 6–9 months

## Outcome measures

### Primary endpoints

- Success of ablation at 6 to 9 months

### Secondary endpoints

- Adverse events during ablation and 3 months after ablation
- Quality of life
- Length of hospital stay
- Tumour recurrence
- Socioeconomic factors

# Results

| | Comparison 1 | | Comparison 2 | |
|---|---|---|---|---|
| | Low-dose radioiodine | High-dose radioiodine | Thyrotropin alpha | Thyroid hormone withdrawal |
| Ablation success | 85% | 88.9% | 87.1% | 86.7% |
| Risk difference (95% CI)—percentage points | −3.8 (−10.2 to 2.6) | | 0.4 (−6.0 to 6.8) | |
| p value | 0.24 | | 0.90 | |

| | Comparison 3 | | Comparison 4 | |
|---|---|---|---|---|
| | Low-dose radioiodine plus thyrotropin alpha | High-dose radioiodine plus thyroid hormone withdrawal | Low-dose radioiodine plus thyrotropin alpha | High-dose radioiodine plus thyrotropin alpha |
| Ablation success | 84.3% | 87.6% | 84.3% | 90.2% |
| Risk difference (95% CI)—percentage points | −3.3 (−12.7 to 6.0) | | −5.9 (14.9 to 3.0) | |
| p value | 0.48 | | 0.20 | |

## Adverse events

The rate was lower for patients receiving low-dose radioiodine plus thyrotropin alpha (16%) than for those receiving either high-dose radioiodine plus thyroid hormone withdrawal (35%, p = 0.001) or high-dose radioiodine plus thyrotropin alpha (30%, p = 0.01).

## Conclusion

Low-dose radioiodine plus thyrotropin alpha was as effective as high-dose radioiodine with a lower rate of adverse events.

## Critique

This was a large, multicentre UK-based trial. It was conducted to a high standard with low levels of bias, and as such these results have significant implications for clinical practice, and have already reached mainstream practice throughout the UK.

In particular, the study deliberately tried to avoid design limitations of previous studies:

◆ Histopathological findings were reviewed by central independent evaluators
◆ Only specialist surgeons were involved to reduce variation in the extent of surgery

- Pre-ablation scanning was performed with technetium-99m to assess remnant size by central review
- Thyroglobulin levels were measured in two central laboratories by mean of imunometric assay with thyroglobulin antibody levels in one laboratory and radioimmunoassay in the other
- Thyroid-specific symptoms and economic indicators were assessed on the basis of a fixed timeline after ablation, using a specific definition of ablation success
- Tumour blocks were collected for translational research

Following publication of this study Mallick has commenced a new randomized, controlled trial asking the question 'Is ablative radio-iodine necessary for low risk differentiated thyroid cancer?': the IoN trial (NCT01398085). This study aims to complete data collection in 2020 and its results are eagerly awaited.

## Additional references

Schlumberger M, Catargi B, Borget I, Deandreis D, Zerdoud S, Brikji B, et al. for the Tumeurs de la thyroide refractaires network for the essai stimulation ablation equivalence trial; strategies of radioiodine ablation in patients with low-risk thyroid cancer. *N Engl J Med* 2012;**366**:1663–73.

Part V

# Benign head and neck disease, laryngology, and sleep medicine

Chapter 60

# Pharyngeal pouch surgery

James England

## Details of studies

Pharyngeal pouches, or Zenker's diverticula, are relatively rare with an annual incidence of two cases per 100,000, occurring most frequently in elderly men. The transoral approach in their management was first described by Mosher et al. (1917) using a knife a century ago. Other techniques using electrocautery and laser have also been advocated, in particular by Dolman and Mattsson in 1960 and van Overbeek (1994), but have failed to gain popularity due to the relatively high perforation risk. As a result, in 1993, Collard et al. from Brussels presented a case series of six patients with Zenker's diverticula treated endoscopically using an Endo-GIA 30 stapler (US Surgical Corp, Norwalk, CT).

## Study references

### Main study

Collard J-M, Otte J-B, Kastens PJ. Endoscopic stapling technique of esophagodiverticulostomy for Zenker's diverticulum. *Ann Thorac Surg* 1993;**56**:573–6.

### Related references

Dolman G, Mattsson O. The endoscopic operation for hypo pharyngeal diverticula. *Arch Otolaryngol* 1960;**71**:744–52.

Mosher H. Webs and pouches of the oesophagus, their diagnosis and management. *Sure Gynecol Obstet* 1917;**25**:175–87.

van Overbeek JJM. Meditation on the pathogenesis of hypo pharyngeal (Zenkers) diverticulum and a report of endoscopic treatment in 545 patients. *Ann Otol Rhinol Laryngol* 1994;**103**:178–85.

## Study design

A single-centre, non-randomized case series.

| | |
|---|---|
| Level of evidence | 4 |
| Randomization | No |
| Inclusion criteria | Presence of a pharyngeal pouch |
| Exclusion criteria | A small diverticulum (1 or 2 cm) mentioned as a contraindication |
| Follow-up | 2–16 months |

## Outcome measures

### Primary endpoint

Relief of cervical dysphagia.

## Results

Five of the series of six experienced 'relief of cervical dysphagia', one experienced 'improvement'.

## Conclusion

Endoscopic stapling was predicted from this case series to be likely to challenge other methods of management of hypopharyngeal diverticula because it was a quick procedure requiring a short anaesthetic in often critically ill patients with aspiration related pneumonitis. However, it was recognized that further experience was required, and that there was potential for residual regurgitation from the diverticular remnant.

## Critique

Although the technique of endoscopic stapling for management of hypopharyngeal diverticula was first described one month earlier by Martin-Hirsch et al. (1993), this paper contains the first series of patients who have undergone the technique. As with most new techniques, the study is not well controlled and therefore constitutes low-level evidence. However, the original paper and this initial case series have led to a sea change in the surgical management of the pharyngeal pouch. A recent meta analysis comparing open pharyngeal pouch surgery to the endoscopic approach identified 358 articles on the subject. Only 11 met eligibility criteria. Currently there are no randomized controlled trials comparing the two approaches, but from the 596 patients included in the 11 studies, the endoscopic approach was found to be quicker, resulted in a shorter hospital stay, and is associated with fewer side effects. The open approach leads to lower recurrence rates due to the ability to perform a complete myotomy, and is also an option in patients with small pouches not amenable to endoscopic stapling, and those with adverse anatomical proportions (Albers et al. 2016).

### Additional references

Martin-Hirsch DP, Newbegin CJ. Autosuture GIA gun: a new application in the treatment of hypo pharyngeal diverticula. *J Laryngal Otol* 1993;107:723–5.

Albers DV, Kondo A, Bernardo WM, Sakai P, Moura RN, Silva GL, et al. Endoscopic versus surgical approach in the treatment of Zenker's diverticulum: systematic review and meta-analysis. *Endosc Int Open* 2016;4:E678–86.

# Chapter 61

# Thyroglossal duct cyst surgery

James England

## Details of studies

Thyroglossal duct cysts are the commonest congenital midline neck lumps presenting in children, making up approximately 55% of the total. They are frequently excised because of cosmetic concerns, cancer concerns, and recurrent infections. Embryological development of the thyroid involves descent of tissue from the tongue to the normal infracricoid position during the fourth and seventh weeks of development. During this process the middle portion the gland remains attached to the tongue at the foramen caecum by the thyroglossal duct. The hyoid bone develops from the second branchial arch at the same time and hence is intimately associated with the thyroglossal tract. The duct is intimately associated with the hyoid bone and can pass anterior, posterior, or through the hyoid. The duct usually atrophies by the tenth week of gestation.

## Study reference

### Main study

Sistrunk WE. The surgical treatment of cysts of the thyroglossal tract. *Ann Surg* 1920:71:121–4.

## Study design

A non-randomized report of a single surgeons case series.

| | |
|---|---|
| Level of evidence | 4 |
| Randomization | No |
| Number of patients | Not mentioned |
| Inclusion/exclusion criteria | Not mentioned |
| Follow-up | Not mentioned |

## Critique

The definitive surgical procedure to remove a thyroglossal cyst is eponymously named Sistrunk's operation after Walter Ellis Sistrunk, who described the procedure in the main paper in 1920. Interestingly, Sistrunk is generally attributed with the first description of the necessity of removal of the mid-portion of the hyoid bone in addition to simple cyst-ectomy and it is generally accepted that this reduces recurrence rates from 50% to be-tween 2% and 4%. However, this is historically inaccurate. In fact Schlange first described removal of the mid-portion of the hyoid bone in 1893 and Sistrunk's modification in-volved the additional removal of a core of tissue

> for a distance of about one-eighth of an inch on all sides, coring out, as it were, the tissues between
> the hyoid bone and the foramen caecum in a line, which the tract almost invariably follows, drawn
> at an angle of 45 degrees from the upper surface of the centre of the hyoid bone in the midline of
> the neck, backward and upward, toward the base of the tongue.[1]

Sistrunk's description involves creating an opening within the mouth to remove the for-amen caecum and then closing the defect. Additionally, methylene blue usage is advocated to identify any lateral branches, and suturing together the remaining hyoid remnants and use of a drain are also described.

The original paper states that the incidence of thyroglossal cyst found in the Mayo Clinic patients was 31 in 86,000. The surgical procedure is described in some detail with accompanying medical diagrams. No mention is made of cure and/or recurrence rates and no complications are reported although no mention is made of the number of cases performed.

As with many innovations in surgical management, a change in practice was bought about in this case by low level evidence comprising the opinion and experience of a single surgeon's practice.

## Additional references

Gioacchini FM, Alicandri-Ciufelli M, Kaleci S, Magliulo G, Presutti L, Re M. Clinical presentation and treatment outcomes of thyroglossal duct cysts: a systematic review. *J Oral Maxillofac Surg* 2015;44:119–26.

Kepertis C, Anastasiadis K, Lambropoulos V, Mouravas V, Spyridakis I. Diagnostic and surgical approach of thyroglossal duct cyst in children: ten years data review. *Diagn Res* 2015;9:13–5

Schlange H. Ueber die Fistula Colli Congenita. *Arch Klin Chir* 1893;46:390–2.

Smith CD. Cysts and sinuses of the neck. Paediatric surgery. St. Louis: Mosby 1998, pp. 757–71.

---

1 Reproduced from Sistrunk WE. The surgical treatment of cysts of the thyroglossal tract. Ann Surg 1920:71:121–4 with permission from Wolters Kluwer.

# Chapter 62

# The physiology of vocal cord movement

Stephanie Cooper

## Details of studies

Vocal fold vibration is interesting because unlike a simple oscillator (such as a pendulum), oscillation is sustained over time. Although a number of theoretical and computer models have been put forward to explain the nature of sustained vocal fold oscillation, these have proven to be incomplete or difficult to relate to vocal fold morphology. In this paper, Titze develops a theory of vocal fold oscillation based on a body-cover concept of vocal fold morphology. The aim of the paper is to present a framework of basic principles by which the mechanics of vocal fold oscillation can be understood in limited mathematical terms, with parameters that relate to vocal fold anatomy.

## Study reference

Main study

Titze IR. The physics of small-amplitude oscillation of the vocal folds. *J Acoust Soc Am* 1988;**83**:1536–52.

## Level of evidence

Level 5.

## Methods

Titze adopted the 'body-cover' concept of vocal fold morphology to represent the basic characteristics of vocal fold vibration. In this concept, the *body* represents the deep muscle layer of the vocal fold and the *cover* represents the vocal fold mucosa. For the purpose of the concept, the body is assumed to be static and the cover mobile. The mobile cover propagates a surface wave along the vocal fold from the bottom to the top edges of the glottis. On the basis of this upward propagating surface wave, Titze derived a series of equations for oscillatory motion. These equations were subjected to further processing (linearization) that allowed statements concerning the conditions of vocal fold oscillation to be obtained.

According to the theory, the driving force for oscillation comes from a time delayed movement between upper and lower edges of the vocal folds. Such tissue movement causes a delay in the build-up and collapse of airflow in the glottal duct resulting in a greater driving force pressure existing during opening than closing. This asymmetry of driving force supplies energy to the vocal folds and sustains oscillation.

## Critique

One of the first models that attempted to explain the process of self-sustained vocal fold oscillation was the 'myoelastic-aerodynamic theory of voice production' (Van den Berg 1958). This theory described vocal fold oscillation in terms of tissue elasticity and the Bernoulli effect. As a result of negative pressure (Bernoulli forces), the vocal folds are drawn together creating a closed subglottic space. Air pressure from the lungs builds up below the closed glottis until it reaches a point where the folds are forced apart. The vocal folds continue to open until tissue elasticity overrides and they start to close. Once the folds have returned to their original closed position, the cycle repeats. However, Titze's theory shows the myoelastic–aerodynamic theory to be incomplete and too simplistic. Assigning a secondary role to the Bernoulli effect, Titze demonstrated that vocal fold oscillation is not dependent upon glottal pressure being negative. Instead, to sustain oscillation, it is necessary that more energy is imparted by flow than is lost by friction in the tissue.

Unlike previous work in this area, the body-cover concept adopted by Titze relates well to vocal fold morphology. The anatomical and functional division between the body and cover reduces analytical complexity and allows the theory statements to be visualized and understood more easily. However, this does not mean that the paper is an easy read. Titze's theory is developed via a number of mathematical equations that for many readers will prove difficult to follow.

This paper is important both clinically and theoretically. From a clinical perspective the body-cover theory of vocal fold oscillation is used by many clinicians to explain to patients how factors such as vocal fold stiffness, lung pressure, and dehydration affect vocal fold oscillation and consequently voice quality. From a theoretical perspective Titze's paper has contributed significantly to the current view of vocal fold oscillation and thus remains influential to the present day.

### Additional reference

**Van de Berg J.** Myoelastic-aerodynamic theory of voice production. *J Speech Hearing Res* 1958;1:227–43.

# Chapter 63

# Evaluation of dysphonia

Stephanie Cooper

## Details of study

A standardized perceptual description of voice quality is important for both clinical practice and research. One of the most widely used perceptual voice evaluation measures is
the GRBAS scale (Hirano 1981). This scale is simple and easy to use and aims to describe
and quantify pathological voice quality in terms of overall grade, roughness, breathiness,
aesthenicity, and strain. In addition to being easy to use, a perceptual scale must also be
reliable and clinically relevant. However, until recently, there was little information available regarding the reliability and clinical relevance of the GRBAS scale. Dejonckere et al.'s
(1993) study was one of the first to address this gap in the literature by aiming to investigate the reliability and clinical relevance of a number of perceptual voice parameters,
including those that form the GRBAS scale.

## Study references

### Main study

Dejonckere PH, Obbens C, de Moor GM, Wieneke GH. Perceptual evaluation of dysphonia: reliability
and relevance. *Folia Phoniatr Logop* 1993;**45**:76–83.

### Related reference

Hirano M. Clinical examination of voice. New York: Springer, 1981.

## Study design

Level of evidence: 3b—correlational study.

### The study consisted of two experiments

#### Experiment 1

On two separate occasions, six experienced judges scored 12 clearly dissimilar pathological voice recordings for 15 perceptual parameters. The aim of this experiment was to
select the most reliable and clinically relevant parameters for use in the second experiment.

#### Experiment 2

Using the selected parameters from experiment 1, two experienced judges assessed the
voices of 54 patients with a vocal pathology. The aim of this experiment was to investigate

the relationship between the perceptual parameters and to compare scale profiles of different vocal pathologies.

## Outcome measures

### Experiment 1

Magnitude estimation (normal to extremely pathological) for each of the following perceptual parameters: overall severity of dysphonia, pitch, intonation, diplophonia, tremor, pitch breaks, loudness, breathiness, roughness, vibration stops, resonance, nasality, voice tonicity, voice onsets, and speech rate.

### Experiment 2

Magnitude estimation (minimum to maximum) for each of the following perceptual parameters: overall grade of dysphonia, breathiness, roughness, strain, and aesthenicity. For computations, strain and aesthenicity were combined in the single parameter of voice tonicity.

## Results

### Experiment 1

The perceptual parameters found to be most reliable (low intrajudge and interjudge variance) and clinically relevant (high intervoice variance) were those that the authors stated make up the GRBAS scale: overall severity of dysphonia, breathiness, roughness, and voice tonicity (hypotonus = aesthenicity and hypertonus = strain).

### Experiment 2

- Significant correlation between level of aesthenicity and grade ($r = 0.53$; $p < 0.05$)
- Significant differences in grade ($p = 0.004$), breathiness ($p = 0.04$), roughness ($p = 0.001$), and level of dystonia ($p = 0.008$) between the groups of primarily functional and primarily organic voice pathology

## Conclusions

- GRBAS scale parameters are reliable and clinically relevant for evaluating the severity of hoarseness
- Interjudge reliability is highest for the overall grade of severity and lowest for voice tonicity (aesthenicity/strain)
- The overall grade of severity is mainly determined by breathiness. Breathiness and roughness are scored antagonistically
- GRBAS profiles differ between the different vocal pathologies, especially between organic and functional voice disorders

## Critique

Perceptual evaluation of voice is considered by many as the gold standard for voice disorder documentation. The GRBAS scale is very widely used and Dejonckere et al. were first to assess its reliability and clinical relevance. The study's conclusions are supported by the findings of more recent studies in this area.

The study is not without its limitations. Demographic detail regarding the voice recordings is sketchy and the number of voice recordings and judges is small. Of concern is the use of the 'aesthenicity' and 'strain' parameters in the second experiment based on the results of the 'voice tonicity' parameter in the first experiment. While aesthenicity and strain are clearly facets of voice tonicity, it would have perhaps been more robust in the first experiment to ascertain the reliability and relevance of these parameters individually. Also of concern is that in clinical practice, the parameters forming the GRBAS scale are scored using a simple 0–3 ordinal scale. However, this study scored each parameter as a continuous variable. While such a scoring system facilitates statistical computations, it is also likely to have increased sensitivity. Thus in the clinical setting, the GRBAS parameters may not be as reliable and clinically relevant as this paper suggests.

## Additional references

Carding PN, Wilson JA, MacKenzie K, Dreary IJ. Measuring voice outcomes: state of the science review. *J Laryngol Otol* 2009;**123**:823–9.

Oates J. Auditory-perceptual evaluation of disordered voice quality: pros, cons and future directions. *Folia Phoniatr Logopaed* 2009;**61**:49–56.

## Chapter 64

# Laryngopharyngeal reflux disease

Stephanie Cooper

## Details of study

Gastroesophageal reflux disease (GERD) is typically associated with the symptoms of heartburn and acid regurgitation. It has been proposed that otolaryngology patients with GERD are atypical in that these symptoms are frequently absent and gastro-oesophageal reflux is 'silent'. The link between overt gastro-oesophageal reflux and upper aerodigestive conditions has been well documented for many years. However, none of the early studies in this area suggested that these conditions may also result from silent or intermittent GERD. In this paper, Kaufman (1991) investigates via human and animal studies, the hypothesis that silent (and sometimes intermittent) GERD is associated with the development of inflammatory and neoplastic disorders of the upper aerodigestive tract.

## Study reference

### Main study

Koufman JA. The otolaryngologic manifestations of gastroesophageal reflux disease (GERD): a clinical investigation of 225 patients using ambulatory 24-hour pH monitoring and an experimental investigation of the role of acid and pepsin in the development of laryngeal injury. *Laryngoscope* 1991;**101**:1–78.

## Study design

Level of evidence: 2b.
The study consists of two investigations: one human study and one animal experiment.

### Human study

- A total of 225 consecutive patients with otolaryngologic disorders having suspected GERD were evaluated over a 4-year period
- Each patient was assigned to one of seven diagnostic subgroups: carcinoma of the larynx, laryngeal and tracheal stenosis, reflux laryngitis, globus pharyngeus, dysphagia, chronic cough, and miscellaneous disorders
- All patients were referred for ambulatory 24-hour intraoesophageal pH monitoring. Of those that underwent this procedure, 148 also underwent barium oesophagography with videofluoroscopy

♦ All of the study patients were treated with antireflux therapy. This consisted of a regimen of specific lifestyle advice, liquid antacid taken after meals and before bed, and a twice daily H2 blocker (ranitidine). Patients were re-evaluated 6 months following treatment

## Animal study

The aim of this study was to investigate the role of gastroesophageal reflux in the development of subglottic injury in the canine model. A series of laboratory experiments mimicked the effects of intermittent reflux (acid and pepsin) on the canine larynx.

## Results

A summary of the main results is displayed in Table 64.1

♦ Of the patients undergoing diagnostic pH monitoring, 62% had abnormal oesophageal pH studies and 30% demonstrated reflux into the pharynx

♦ Compared to pH monitoring, diagnostic barium oesophagogram with videofluoroscopy was frequently negative

♦ After 6 months of treatment, symptoms had resolved in 85% of participants

♦ There was a higher degree of laryngeal mucosal inflammation and slower healing in animals subjected to acid and pepsin compared with those subjected to acid only

♦ Inflammatory damage occurred at pH 1.5, 2.5 and 4.0 in animals subjected to acid and pepsin

## Conclusions

♦ Many otolaryngology patients have a different pattern of GERD than gastroenterology patients. Importantly, reflux is often silent in otolaryngology patients

♦ The results suggest a possible aetiological role for GERD in the pathogenesis of laryngeal carcinoma

♦ Three episodes of reflux per week can result in severe laryngeal damage if a mucosal injury is present

♦ Pepsin and not hydrochloric acid is the principle injurious agent of the refluxate

♦ Threshold for injury is lower in the upper aerodigestive tract than in the oesophagus

♦ Severe laryngeal damage can occur even when the pH of the refluxate is 4.0

**Table 64.1** Diagnostic pH monitoring: percentage of abnormal studies for each subgroup

| Diagnostic pH monitoring | Carcinoma | Stenosis | Reflux laryngitis | Globus | Dysphagia | Chronic cough | Misc. |
|---|---|---|---|---|---|---|---|
| Percentage of abnormal studies | 71 | 78 | 60 | 58 | 45 | 52 | 13 |

## Critique

The relationship between overt gastro-oesophageal reflux and upper aerodigestive conditions, including laryngeal carcinoma, is well established. However, it was not until the publication of this paper that a link between silent reflux and laryngeal damage was documented.

In terms of the effect of reflux on the upper aerodigestive tract, Koufman demonstrated that just three episodes of reflux per week can result in severe laryngeal damage when a mucosal injury is present. Furthermore, the paper was pioneering in that it highlighted the injurious nature of pepsin in refluxate. Such findings emphasize the importance of diagnosing and treating silent reflux in the otolaryngology patient. Concerning this, a key recommendation of this paper was the use of a second pharyngeal probe for otolaryngology patients undergoing pH studies. Koufman also advocated perioperative antireflux treatment for otolaryngology surgery in which the laryngeal mucosa is compromised.

Koufman's paper can be considered landmark, in that it emphasizes the differences between overt and silent gastro-oesophageal reflux and makes a number of recommendations that underpin present-day diagnostic and treatment practices. This paper is essential reading for any clinician working in the field of otolaryngology. Despite being more than 20 years old, its findings are frequently put forward as supporting evidence for the existence of silent reflux. They also form the evidence base for many clinicians' recommendations regarding the diagnosis and treatment of this condition.

# Chapter 65

# Assessing daytime sleepiness

Olivier Vanderveken

## Details of studies

Together with loud socially disturbing snoring, excessive daytime sleepiness (EDS) is a cardinal symptom in patients with sleep-disordered breathing (SDB). Daytime sleepiness can be assessed either through objective testing or using self-report.

Johns first described the Epworth Sleepiness Scale (ESS) in 1991. The ESS is a self-administered questionnaire that measures how likely patients are to fall asleep in eight different situations. Since its first description the ESS has become a widely used scoring system for the self-reported assessment of the degree of daytime sleepiness or hypersomnolence. In addition, ESS has become a widely used and accepted method of reporting outcomes in clinical trials in order to report on changes in subjective symptoms of daytime somnolence during therapy for sleep disorders such as obstructive sleep apnoea syndrome (OSAS).

The mean sleep latency test (MSLT) and the maintenance of wakefulness test (MWT) are the two most commonly used objective, sleep laboratory-based methods for the assessment of the ability to fall asleep and stay awake, respectively (Littner et al. 2005).

The MSLT is an objective assessment of the tendency to fall asleep, and requires electro-encephalogram (EEG) evaluation of the participants. The day after a polysomnographic evaluation, the patient is invited to lie on a bed in a quiet, darkened room and is instructed to fall asleep. The time required to reach a sleeping phase is determined in a 20-minute period every 2 hours during the day for a total of four sessions. The mean sleep latency is then calculated and is considered pathological if it is less than 8 minutes and normal if it is longer than 10 minutes.

The MWT is a validated objective measure of the ability to stay awake for a defined time. The MWT also requires EEG monitoring and, ideally, consists of four 40-minutes trials performed at 2-hour intervals, with the first trial starting about 1.5–3 hours after the patient's usual wake-up time. The subject will be instructed to sit still in a dimly lit, warm, quiet room and to remain awake for as long as possible while the patient is not allowed to use other measures to stay awake. If the patient is able to stay awake on all MWT trials that would provide the strongest objective data available to support an individual's ability to stay awake. A mean sleep latency less than 8 minutes on the 40-minute MWT is considered abnormal.

Both MSLT and MWT are regarded as being cumbersome, time-consuming, and expensive to perform. The tests take a whole day, both for the subject and the sleep laboratory staff. Therefore, the use of a simple questionnaire to assess the degree of daytime sleepiness is appealing.

## Study references

### Main study

Johns MW. A new method for measuring daytime sleepiness: the Epworth sleepiness scale. *Sleep* 1991;14:540–5.

### Related references

Lim PV, Curry AR. The role of history, Epworth Sleepiness Scale Score and body mass index in identifying non-apnoeic snorers. *Clin Otolaryngol Allied Sci* 2000;25:244–8.

Osman EZ, Osborne J, Hill PD, Lee BW. The Epworth Sleepiness Scale: can it be used for sleep apnoea screening among snorers? *Clin Otolaryngol Allied Sci* 1999;24:239–41.

## Study design

In the main study Johns (1991) describes the development and use of the new ESS designed to measure sleep propensity in a simple, standardized way.

| | |
|---|---|
| Level of evidence | 2b |
| Randomization | N/A |
| Number of patients | 180 |
| Inclusion criteria | Adult controls (n = 30) <br> Adult patients with a range of sleep disorders (n = 150) |
| Exclusion criteria | Patients suffering from insomnia with mood disorders or drug effects. <br> Patients suffering from both OSA and periodic limb movement disorder |
| Follow-up | N/A |

The ESS is a simple, self-administered questionnaire which aims at providing a measurement of the subject's general level of daytime sleepiness. The ESS rates the chances that a patient would doze off or fall asleep when in eight different situations commonly encountered in daily life. Subjects are asked to rate on a scale of 0 to 3 how likely they would be to doze or fall asleep in these eight everyday situations based on their usual way of life in recent times. The ESS as described originally is reproduced here,

How likely are you to doze off or fall asleep in the following situations, in contrast to feeling just tired? This refers to your usual way of life in recent times. Even if you have not done some of these things recently try to work out how they would have affected you.

Use the following scale to choose the most appropriate number for each situation:

0 = would never doze; 1 = slight chance of dozing; 2 = moderate change of dozing; 3 = high chance of dozing

| Situation | Chance of dozing |
| --- | --- |
| Sitting and reading | |
| Watching TV | |
| Sitting, inactive in a public place (e.g. a theatre or a meeting) | |
| As a passenger in a car for an hour without a break | |
| Lying down to rest in the afternoon when circumstances permit | |
| Sitting and talking to someone | |
| Sitting quietly after a lunch without alcohol | |
| In a car, while stopped for a few minutes in the traffic | |
| As a result, total ESS scores range from 0 to 24. Scores of 11 or 16 are indicative of EDS or severe EDS, respectively | |

Reproduced from Johns MW. A new method for measuring daytime sleepiness: the Epworth sleepiness scale. *Sleep.* 1991;14(6):540–5 with permission from Oxford University Press.

## Results

The ESS scores for primary snorers were not statistically significant different from the controls. Scores for patients suffering from OSAS and other included sleep disorders were significantly higher than controls or primary snorers.

ESS scores were significantly correlated with sleep latency measured during MSLT and during overnight polysomnography. In patients with OSAS the ESS scores were significantly correlated with the respiratory disturbance index (RDI) and the minimum oxygen saturation recorded overnight.

## Conclusion

The results of the main study would support the use of the ESS as a simple, self-administered questionnaire assessing the degree of daytime sleepiness. The ESS clearly is less cumbersome, less time-consuming, and less expensive to perform than MSLT or MWT. The results also indicate that the ESS is able to distinguish normal patients from patients suffering from sleep disorders such as OSAS. In addition, significant relations were noted between ESS and both sleep latency and the severity of OSAS in terms of RDI and the minimum oxygen saturation.

## Discussion and critique

The ESS is the most widely used scale for the subjective measurement of the degree of daytime sleepiness worldwide. Despite its widespread acceptance and use, the ESS has not been without its critics and limitations.

In contrast to the results of the main study, Osman et al. (1999) were not able to find an obvious correlation between ESS and RDI. Consequently, these authors do not recommend the ESS to be used as their study demonstrates that the ESS is an unreliable tool for diagnosing OSA.

In their study, Lim and Curry (2000) were able to compare clinical assessment including history, ESS, and body mass index (BMI) with the results of polysomnography in identifying the OSAS patients out of a cohort of snorers . The results indicate that the applied method comes with a high sensitivity and lower specificity.

The ESS has the obvious advantage of being a simple, quick and inexpensive test and it also shows a high test–retest reliability. On the other hand, the ESS has the possible disadvantage of exhibiting a poor correlation with the severity of OSAS and to rely on subjective reporting by patients who may underestimate or intentionally underreport the severity of EDS (Chervin and Aldrich 1999). Objective tests as the MSLT and the MWT overcome this problem but are expensive and time consuming (Johns 2000).

## Additional references

Chervin RD, Aldrich MS. The Epworth Sleepiness Scale may not reflect objective measures of sleepiness or sleep apnea. *Neurology* 1999;**52**:125–31.

Johns MW. Sensitivity and specificity of the multiple sleep latency test (MSLT), the maintenance of wakefulness test and the Epworth Sleepiness Scale: failure of the MSLT as a gold standard. *J Sleep Res* 2000;**9**:5–11.

Littner MR, Kushida C, Wise M, Davila DG, Morgenthaler T, Lee-Chiong T, et al; Standards of Practice Committee of the American Academy of Sleep Medicine. Practice parameters for clinical use of the multiple sleep latency test and the maintenance of wakefulness test. *Sleep* 2005;**281**:113–21.

# Chapter 66

# Sleep nasendoscopy

Olivier Vanderveken

## Details of studies

Sleep-disordered breathing (SDB) constitutes a spectrum of diseases going from simple snoring to full-blown obstructive sleep apnoea (OSA). OSA is a highly prevalent disorder with a range of harmful sequelae. The most recent prevalence estimates of moderate to severe OSA are 10% among middle-aged men. The cardinal symptoms of OSA constitute of socially disturbing snoring and excessive daytime sleepiness. The golden standard method to objectively confirm the diagnosis of OSA is a full-night attended polysomnography (PSG).

Continuous positive airway pressure (CPAP) is the gold standard for the treatment of moderate to severe OSA. Unfortunately, only approximately 50% of patients tolerate CPAP therapy. Therefore, a high need for successful non-CPAP therapies exists. These therapeutic options include oral appliance therapy using mandibular advancement device (MAD), upper airway surgery including electrical neurostimulation of the hypoglossal nerve, skeletal surgical modifications, and tracheotomy. In unselected patients, however, non-CPAP therapies are inconsistently effective with unpredictable results. In order to improve patient selection information about the pharyngeal site(s) of collapse during sleep should be obtained. For this purpose, natural sleep endoscopy would be regarded the gold standard for upper airway evaluation in OSA patients, but like other investigations during sleep this technique has a highly labour-intensive nature. Therefore, the technique of sleep nasendoscopy (SNE) or sleep endoscopy as first described by Croft and Pringle (1991) has emerged as an alternative method to dynamically investigate the upper airway in patients with OSA. Nowadays the technique is referred to as drug-induced sedation endoscopy (DISE).

## Study references

### Main study

Croft CB, Pringle M. Sleep nasendoscopy: a technique of assessment in snoring and obstructive sleep apnoea. *Clin Otolaryngol Allied Sci* 1991;16:504–9.

### Related references

Berry S, Roblin G, Williams A, Watkins A, Whittet HB. Validity of sleep nasendoscopy in the investigation of sleep related breathing disorders. *Laryngoscope* 2005;115:538–40.

Connolly AA, Martin J, White P. Sedation with a target-controlled propofol infusion system during assessment of the upper airway in snorers. *J Laryngol Otol* 1994;108:865–7.

De Vito A, Carrasco Llatas M, Vanni A, Bosi M, Braghiroli A, Campanini A, et al. European position paper on drug-induced sedation endoscopy (DISE). *Sleep Breath* 2014;**18**:453–65.

## Study design

A single-centre observational study with prospective inclusion.

| | |
|---|---|
| Level of evidence | 2b |
| Randomization | N/A |
| Number of patients | 71 |
| Inclusion criteria | Patients who had failed uvulopalatopharyngoplasty (UPPP) (group 1) |
| | Patients with a history of snoring or OSA that already underwent portable sleep monitoring (group 2) |
| Exclusion criteria | History of cardiac and respiratory disease |
| Follow-up | N/A |

In the main study the authors first described the technique of SNE that was developed with the aim to distinguish the SDB patients who would have a high probability to benefit from surgical management, e.g. palatal surgery.

The participating patients were pharmacologically induced into a light phase of sleep while a direct and dynamic visualization of the upper airway was obtained using a flexible, fibreoptic nasopharyngo-endoscope.

## Results

In 56 of the 71 included patients (79%) the authors were able to successfully demonstrate the site of the problem. SNE in these patients did allow them to divide the participants into three broad groups.

### Group A: simple palatal snorers (n = 7)

No obstructive respiratory events were observed in this group. Palatal vibration would be the most obvious finding with possibly associated narrowing, usually circumferential, at the velopharyngeal (VP) level in this group. The oro- and hypopharyngeal area would be normal.

The authors suggest that these patients should benefit from UPPP.

### Group B: single level palatal obstruction (n = 18)

In these patients both palatal vibration and episodes of obstruction at the VP level were observed. The pattern of VP closure was usually circumferential and associated with apnoea. The oro- and hypopharyngeal area as well as the laryngeal inlet would remain open.

Croft and Pringle argue that the upper airway obstruction demonstrated during SNE in this group B patients should be correctable by UPPP.

## Group C: multisegment involvement (n = 31)

These patients would also exhibit snoring and obstructive episodes but in contrast to group B the observations at the level of the upper airway would not be limited to palatal vibration and circumferential closure at the VP level. In this group an associated involvement of the oro- and/or hypopharyngeal area was seen.

All participants who failed UPPP (n = 3) were among the group C patients and all showed complete multisegment collapse during SNE.

As there was a marked variation in the degree of oro/hypopharyngeal involvement seen regarding the degree of narrowing and collapse, the authors suggested a further subdivision of group C.

## Conclusion

The results of the main study support the theory of a wide spectrum of upper airway narrowing and obstruction among SDB patients. The authors could describe a technique allowing to classify the patients into three main groups in which the patients could roughly be divided. In both groups A and B the authors feel that the vibration, narrowing, and obstruction should have been correctable by UPPP. On the other hand, all UPPP failures were classified to be in group C as they clearly exhibited a sustained multilevel collapse as documented using SNE. As such, the results of the main study by Croft and Pringle illustrate that the use of SNE as a preoperative assessment is able to improve outcomes for palatal surgery. The technique of SNE overcomes some of the problems of evaluation and is quick, simple to perform, and allows a direct and accurate visualization of the site(s) of vibration, narrowing, and/or collapse.

## Discussion

This study was the first to describe the systematic assessment of the upper airway in SDB patients under pharmacologically induced sleep. The technique of SNE allows a direct and dynamic documentation of the site(s) of pharyngeal vibration leading to snoring, and narrowing or obstruction leading to hypopnoea or apnoea. Since the first description of SNE by Croft and Pringle the technique has progressively gained popularity. A recent European Position Paper suggests the technique to be referred to as drug-induced sedation endoscopy or DISE (De Vito et al. 2014).

In their original paper Croft and Pringle suggested a grading scheme describing the level(s) of partial or complete pharyngeal collapse. In this specific grading system upper airway narrowing and obstruction was designated as palatal, multilevel, or tongue based. Eventually, a grading scale was devised (see Table 66.1).

One year after the introduction of SNE into the field of the diagnosis and treatment of SDB, Connolly et al. (1994) presented the ability of a target-controlled infusion (TCI) system for the use of propofol in order to provide sedation for patients with snoring and/ or OSA undergoing assessment of the upper airway. These authors advocated the use of

**Table 66.1** Pringle and Croft's 1993 grading system*

| Grade 1 | Palatal level snoring |
|---------|----------------------|
| Grade 2 | Palatal level obstruction |
| Grade 3 | Multisegmental involvement—intermittent oro- and hypopharyngeal collapse |
| Grade 4 | Sustained multilevel collapse |
| Grade 5 | Tongue base obstruction |

*Reproduced from Pringle MB, Croft CB. A grading system for patients with obstructive sleep apnoea—based on sleep nasendoscopy. *Clin Otolaryngol Allied Sci.* 1993;18(6):480-4 with permission from Wiley.

TCI for SNE as the technique allows one to provide the desired level of sedation, is short acting, and allows control readily. In their prospective study, Berry et al. (2005) were able to validate SNE in a total group of 107 patients of which half had no documented history of SDB . In this validation study sedation was also administered using TCI with propofol.

The main study (Pringle and Croft 1993) has suggested that a large majority of SDB patients exhibit at least a palatal involvement and that in more than half of the participants a multilevel involvement could be documented (31 out of 56 patients; 56%). These results are in line with the findings of a recent observational study that describes DISE findings in a total of 1,249 SDB patients (Vroegop et al. 2014). In that study by Vroegop and colleagues, palatal collapse was seen most frequently (81%) and multilevel collapse was noted in 68% of all patients.

The fact that the use of SNE or DISE is valuable as a preoperative assessment to improve outcomes for palatal surgery was confirmed in later studies (Hessel and de Vries 2003). In addition, in his cross-sectional study, Kezirian (2011) could clearly illustrate that DISE is able to enhance to understand the residual upper airway obstruction in non-responders to pharyngeal surgery for OSA. Almost all of the non-responders demonstrated hypopharyngeal obstruction and a majority also exhibited residual palatal obstruction.

Instead of the original grading as proposed by Croft and Pringle nowadays DISE findings would be categorized to the following pharyngeal levels: palate, oropharynx, tongue base, and hypopharynx including the epiglottis and the lateral walls. For each pharyngeal level the degree of collapse will be reported as complete, partial, or none, and, the pattern of the obstruction would be described as anteroposterior, lateral, or concentric (Vroegop et al. 2014).

## Additional references

Hessel NS, de Vries N. Results of uvulopalatopharyngoplasty after diagnostic workup with polysomnography and sleep endoscopy: a report of 136 snoring patients. *Eur Arch Otorhinolaryngol* 2003;**260**:91–5.

Kezirian EJ. Nonresponders to pharyngeal surgery for obstructive sleep apnea: insights from drug-induced sleep endoscopy. *Laryngoscope* 2011;**121**:1320–6.

Pringle MB, Croft CB. A grading system for patients with obstructive sleep apnoea--based on sleep nasendoscopy. *Clin Otolaryngol Allied Sci* 1993;**18**:480–4.

Vroegop AV, Vanderveken OM, Boudewyns AN, Scholman J, Saldien V, Wouters K, et al. Drug-induced sleep endoscopy in sleep-disordered breathing: report on 1,249 cases. *Laryngoscope* 2014;**124**:797–802.

Chapter 67

# Snoring surgery

Olivier Vanderveken

## Details of studies

The classical uvulopalatopharyngoplasty (UPPP), first introduced in 1981, is still the most well-known and commonly performed surgical procedure for sleep-disordered breathing (SDB). The surgical procedure consists of a tonsillectomy, if not previously performed, trimming, and reorientation of the anterior and posterior tonsillar pillars, together with reduction in size of the uvula and the postero-inferior part of the palate (Fujita et al. 1981). During the UPPP procedure the underlying muscular structure is left intact.

Different modifications on this technique have been described with the aim to improve effectiveness, reduce surgical morbidity, and target specific collapse patterns. Examples are the Z-palatoplasty, expansion sphincter pharyngoplasty, transpalatal advancement pharyngoplasty, and lateral pharyngoplasty.

In their landmark review of the literature Sher et al. (1996) could demonstrate that UPPP came with an overall success rate, defined as a reduction of apnea/hypopnea index (AHI) by at least 50% and AHI being less than 20 events per hour of sleep, of only 40% in unselected OSA patients.

In well-selected patients, however, UPPP has been proven to be effective both as a stand-alone therapy and as part of a multilevel approach in SDB patients with multisegmental involvement of their upper airway collapse during sleep.

## Study references

### Main study

Fujita S, Conway WA, Zorick FJ, Sicklesteel JM, Roehrs TA, Wittig RM, et al. Evaluation of the effectiveness of uvulopharyngoplasty. *Laryngoscope* 1985;**95**:70–4.

### Related references

Fujita S, Conway W, Zorick F, Roth T. Surgical correction of anatomic abnormalities in obstructive sleep apnea syndrome: uvulopalatopharyngoplasty. *Otolaryngol Head Neck Surg* 1981;**89**:923–34.

Hessel NS, de Vries N. Results of uvulopalatopharyngoplasty after diagnostic workup with polysomnography and sleep endoscopy: a report of 136 snoring patients. *Eur Arch Otorhinolaryngol* 2003;**260**:91–5.

Sher AE, Schechtman KB, Piccirillo JF. The efficacy of surgical modifications of the upper airway in adults with obstructive sleep apnea syndrome. *Sleep* 1996;**19**:156–77.

Sher AE, Thorpy MJ, Shprintzen RJ, Spielman AJ, Burack B, McGregor PA. Predictive value of Müller maneuver in selection of patients for uvulopalatopharyngoplasty. *Laryngoscope* 1985;**95**:1483–7.

## Study design

A single-centre observational study with prospective inclusion.

| | |
|---|---|
| Level of evidence | 2b |
| Randomization | N/A |
| Number of patients | 66 |
| Inclusion criteria | Patients undergoing UPPP for the treatment of objectively documented sleep apnea syndrome |
| Exclusion criteria | None |
| Follow-up | Polysomnography (PSG), multiple sleep latency test (MSLT), and assessment of symptoms of apnea, 6 week after surgery |

In the main study the authors report on the first thorough evaluation of the effect of surgical removal of redundant tissue in the oropharynx with UPPP on obstructive sleep apnoea (OSAS) and its signs and symptoms. The pre- and postoperative outcomes included polysomnographic parameters and measures of daytime sleepiness including a multiple sleep latency test (MSLT) and the Epworth sleepiness scale (ESS).

## Results

Subjectively, 85% of the participating patients experienced an improvement in their excessive daytime sleepiness and almost all patients (98%) experienced a decrease in their snoring. Following UPPP the mean latency on MSLT increased significantly to 6.6 minutes compared with baseline (3.9 minutes; $p < 0.02$). Significant post-UPPP improvement was also noted for the apnoea index including a 84% reduction regarding this key parameter in the responders group being the patients in whom a reduction by at least 50% in apnoea index was observed. Half of the patients fulfilled the criterion of being a responder. The only difference found between responders and non-responders was in body weight. The authors suggested that the variable probably discriminating responders from non-responders most significantly could have been the location of the principal site(s) of upper airway obstruction.

## Conclusion

The results of the main study indicate that UPPP is able to significantly affect the signs and symptoms of OSAS including a decrease in the degree of daytime sleepiness and a reduction of the apnoea index as a marker of OSAS severity. Exactly half of the participants could be classified as responders to treatment with a reduction of at least 50% in apnoea index after UPPP as compared to baseline. The authors discussed that two variables seem to discriminate responders from non-responders: body weight and the anatomical site(s) of upper airway narrowing (Fujita et al. 1985).

## Discussion

Based on the reported series the number of responders to UPPP in unselected OSAS patients is only about 40 to 50% (Fujita et al. 1985; Sher et al. 1996).

For the purpose of proper preoperative selection of those OSAS patients that might benefit from UPPP, whose locus of pharyngeal obstruction is at the level of the velo- and oropharynx, fibreoptic nasopharyngoscopy with Müller manoeuvre (FNMM) can be used. The Müller manoeuvre consists of a forced inspiratory effort with the mouth and nose closed. In a series reported by Sher et al. (1985) 87% of the patients undergoing UPPP with prior preoperative selection using FNMM had at least 50% decrease in apnoea index.

Alternatively, sleep nasendoscopy or drug-induced sedation endoscopy (DISE) can be applied preoperatively for the assessment of the site(s) of upper airway collapse in OSAS patients. In their study Croft and Pringle (1991) were able to demonstrate that the use of DISE as a preoperative assessment is able to improve outcomes of UPPP in OSAS patients. The fact that the use of DISE provides an added value in the preoperative assessment to improve outcomes for UPPP was confirmed in later studies (Hessel and de Vries 2003).

In a recent systematic review, studies were included that reported on direct comparison between awake examination data and DISE outcome data in terms of surgical decision making and treatment success for OSAS. The review emphasized the impact of DISE on the changes in decision making compared with awake examinations of the upper airway such as FNMM. The published literature, however, lacks evidence on the association between this impact and the surgical outcomes (Certal et al. 2015).

In conclusion, information about the pharyngeal site(s) of collapse during sleep should be obtained preoperatively in OSAS patients in order to improve the success of UPPP in particular and upper airway surgery in general. Further studies are needed that evaluate the value of the different techniques for pre-operative assessment of the site(s) of upper airway collapse and their impact on UPPP success rates.

## Additional references

Certal VF, Pratas R, Guimarães L, Lugo R, Tsou Y, Camacho M, Capasso R. Awake examination versus DISE for surgical decision making in patients with OSA: A systematic review. *Laryngoscope* 2016;**126**:768–74.

Croft CB, Pringle M. Sleep nasendoscopy: a technique of assessment in snoring and obstructive sleep apnoea. *Clin Otolaryngol Allied Sci* 1991;**16**:504–9.

# Paediatrics

# Chapter 68

# Tonsillitis

Andy Bath

## Details of studies

Recurrent sore throats and recurrent tonsillitis are common in primary care and a common cause of referral to ENT. They cause significant morbidity, and decrease school and work attendance. Surgical removal of the tonsils, with or without adenoidectomy (adeno-/tonsillectomy), is a common ENT operation, but the indications for surgery due to recurrent tonsillitis are controversial.

## Study references

### Main study

Paradise JL, Bluestone CD, Bachman RZ, Colborn DK, Bernard BS, Taylor FH, et al. Efficacy of tonsillectomy for recurrent throat infection in severely affected children. Results of parallel randomized and nonrandomized clinical trials. *N Engl J Med* 1984;310:674–83.

### Related reference

Burton MJ, Glasziou PP, Chong LY, Venekamp RP. Tonsillectomy or adenotonsillectomy versus non-surgical treatment for chronic/recurrent acute tonsillitis. *Cochrane Database Syst Rev* 2014:CD001802.

## Study design

| | |
|---|---|
| Level of evidence | 1c |
| Randomization | Intervention group 1: tonsillectomy; n = 27 |
| | Intervention group 2: adenotonsillectomy; n = 16 |
| | Comparator group 1: non-surgical treatment; n = 29 |
| | Comparator group 2: non-surgical treatment; n = 19 |
| | The trial data were pooled in the publication: intervention group, tonsillectomy or adenotonsillectomy, n = 43; comparator group, non-surgical treatment; n = 48 |
| | Cultures were done for group A streptococci in case of suspected or diagnosed throat infections and treated with antibiotics |
| N | 91 children from 2,043 screened |

| | |
|---|---|
| Inclusion | Age 3–15 years |
| | History of recurrent episodes of throat infection (i.e. tonsillitis, pharyngitis or tonsillopharyngitis) |
| | The episodes had to meet four categories: (1) frequency: seven or more episodes in the preceding year, five or more in each of the 2 preceding years, or three or more in each of the preceding 3 years; (2) clinical features, each episode one or more of: oral temperature of at least 38.3°C, cervical lymphadenopathy (enlarged (>2 cm) or tender cervical lymph nodes), tonsillar or pharyngeal exudate, or positive culture for group A beta-haemolytic *Streptococcus*; (3) treatment, antibiotics administered at conventional dosage for proven or suspected streptococcal episodes; (4) documentation, each episode documented in clinical record |
| Exclusion | Judged to require prompt removal of large tonsils or adenoids because of alveolar hypoventilation, severe difficulty in swallowing or breathing; prior tonsil or adenoid surgery; major physical or mental disease; structural middle-ear damage or sensorineural hearing loss; hypogammaglobulinaemia; enrolment of a sibling in the study |
| Follow-up | Biweekly symptom assessment and 6-weekly clinical assessment, and during respiratory infections for 4 years |

## Outcomes

### Primary

Observed episodes of throat infections.

### Secondary outcomes

+ Proportion of visits with isolated cervical lymphadenopathy
+ Number of parent-reported sore throat days
+ Number of days of sore throat-associated school absence

## Results

+ Episodes of sore throat of any severity at 12 months: tonsillo-adenoidectomy n = 38 mean 2.2 episodes; no surgery 3.1
+ Episodes of moderately bad sore throat including post-surgical as one episode: tonsillo-adenoidectomy 1.08; 1.17 no surgery

## Systematic review (Burton et al.)

This Cochrane review included seven trials: five in children (n = 987 participants) and two in adults (n = 156). Five trials included 'severely affected' children (based on the 'Paradise' criteria) and less severely affected. Children who had an adeno-/tonsillectomy had three episodes of sore throats in 12 months compared to 3.6 episodes in the control group (difference 0.6 episodes, 95% CI –1 to –0.1), one of which in the surgical group was the 'predictable' one immediately postoperative. For *moderate/severe* sore throats among more severely affected children there were 1.1 vs. 1.2 episodes respectively. Among less severely affected children there were more episodes of moderate/severe sore throat after surgery 1.2 vs. 0.4. In 12 months there were on average fewer days of sore throat 18 vs. 23 days.

In the two adult studies there were 3.6 fewer episodes, and 10.6 fewer days in the group receiving surgery within 6 months post surgery, but there was significant statistical heterogeneity for both analyses.

## Conclusion

Both in the original Paradise trial, and in the systematic review which included subsequent trials in more severely affected children, there is very little evidence of benefit. Among trials which included less severely affected children there is also no clear evidence of benefit: although there may be fewer days of sore throat, there are apparently more severe episodes. There may be significantly more benefit among adults but the trial data is very limited indeed, with high heterogeneity, making robust conclusions difficult. An advantage of the sore throats that occur in surgically treated individuals is that one of the episodes is predictable in the immediate postoperative period.

## Critique

The original Paradise trial was limited in its description (unclear what mechanism of random allocation was used), as in all trials blinding of intervention is impossible in such open trials. Of more concern is that blinding of outcome assessment was not achieved in any trial, and although not easy it should be possible. There was also high attrition after 12 months in both the Paradise trial and other trials so we have very little robust information about the extent of benefit after 12 months. An important problem is that neither the trials nor the Cochrane review were able to document the level of major harm with surgery—which can include life threatening secondary haemorrhage.

The 'Paradise' criteria for recurrent tonsillitis are still used today, most notably in the Scottish Intercollegiate Guidelines Network (SIGN) and the American Academy (AAO-NHS) guidelines for tonsillectomy.

### Related references

**Scottish Intercollegiate Guidelines Network**. Management of sore throat and indications for tonsillectomy. A national clinical guideline 2010;117. http://www.sign.ac.uk/sign-117-management-of-sore-throat-and-indications-for-tonsillectomy.html

**Randel A**. AAO–HNS guidelines for tonsillectomy in children and adolescents. *Am Fam Physician* 2011;**84**:566–73.

# Chapter 69

# Tonsillectomy

Paul Little

## Details of study

Tonsillectomy is one of the most frequently performed operations in the UK. Numerous techniques have evolved from the 'cold steel' dissection initially performed, to diathermy and coblation—so called 'hot techniques', which are often employed either for the whole procedure or to deal with intraoperative haemorrhage. Among the ENT community, there was some concern whether these techniques caused a higher incidence of secondary haemorrhage or if they may be preferable to cold steel dissection. To address this issue, Lowe et al. (2004) performed a national prospective audit to compare the rates of postoperative haemorrhage for seven tonsillectomy techniques commonly performed in the UK.

## Study references

### Main reference

Lowe D, van der Meulen J; National Prospective Tonsillectomy Audit. Tonsillectomy technique as a risk factor for postoperative haemorrhage. *Lancet* 2004;**364**:697–702.

### Related reference

National Prospective Tonsillectomy Audit Final Report of an audit carried out in England and Northern Ireland between July 2003 and September 2004. On behalf of the British Association of Otorhinolaryngologists—Head and Neck Surgeons Comparative Audit Group and the Clinical Effectiveness Unit, The Royal College of Surgeons of England. London: Royal College of Surgeons.

## Study design

A prospective multicentre audit of tonsillectomy technique and associated postoperative haemorrhage in the UK.

| Level of evidence | 2b: observational study |
|---|---|
| Randomization | None |
| Number of patients | 13,554 |
| Inclusion criteria | All patients undergoing tonsillectomy in the UK |
| Exclusion criteria | Unilateral tonsillectomy |

| | |
|---|---|
| | Tonsillar biopsy |
| | Tonsillectomy for cancer |
| | Tonsillectomy performed in conjunction with palatal surgery |
| Follow-up | 28 days |

Data were collected by operating surgeon including surgical technique, instruments used, and grade of surgeon.

## Outcome measures

- Primary haemorrhage: bleeding that led to delayed hospital discharge, blood transfusion, or return to theatre during initial stay.
- Secondary haemorrhage: bleeding that led to re-admission within 28 days of surgery.
- Patients who returned to theatre were judged to have had a severe haemorrhage.

## Results

About 60% of the tonsillectomy patients were female, and about 60% were under 16 years. Haemorrhage occurred in 389 patients (3.3%). Fifty-nine patients (0.5%) had a primary haemorrhage (during initial stay), 337 (2.9%) a secondary haemorrhage (after discharge), and seven had both. Adults had higher haemorrhage rates than children.

| Surgical technique | Haemorrhage rate | Primary | Secondary | Relative risk of secondary haemorrhage compared to cold steel | p value for RR |
|---|---|---|---|---|---|
| Cold steel | 1.28 | 0.60 | 0.75 | – | – |
| Cold steel and monopolar | 2.94 | 0.82 | 2.12 | 2.29 | 0.01 |
| Cold steel and bipolar | 2.85 | 0.37 | 2.48 | 2.22 | 0.0001 |
| Monopolar forceps | 6.06 | 0.51 | 5.56 | 4.73 | <0.0001 |
| Bipolar forceps | 3.92 | 0.37 | 3.63 | 3.06 | <0.0001 |
| Bipolar scissors | 4.03 | 0.78 | 3.36 | 4.03 | <0.0001 |
| Coblation | 4.39 | 1.02 | 3.36 | 3.42 | <0.0001 |

# Conclusion

Tonsillectomy using hot techniques caused significantly higher rates of secondary haemorrhage with diathermy and coblation tonsillectomy leading to a postoperative haemorrhage rate that was at least three times as high as cold steel tonsillectomy without the use of a hot technique.

# Critique

There is recognition of potential bias within this study:

◆ Only 60% of tonsillectomies performed in the UK during this period of this study were included

◆ It was not randomized

◆ There is a possibility that individual departments may have under-reported haemorrhages, especially those not returning to theatre

Differences in postoperative haemorrhage rates between the tonsillectomy techniques might truly vary and depend not just on the tonsillectomy technique but on many other patient-, surgeon-, and equipment-related factors which would be almost impossible to assess or quantify. However, the size of the study reduces this likelihood. One important question that was missing from this study was 'Did the surgeon use bipolar diathermy to deal with excessive bleeding?'

Despite limitations, this is an extremely large study with similar postoperative haemorrhage rates to other large studies and has become a landmark paper. This study has guided surgeons to perform tonsillectomy with cold steel as the gold standard technique and to use any bipolar diathermy sparingly in view of the increased risk of causing secondary haemorrhage.

Coblation tonsillectomy is being increasingly popular, despite the audit results. Coblation involves passing a radiofrequency bipolar electrical current through a medium of normal saline, producing a plasma field of sodium ions that dissects the tissue by disrupting intercellular bonds leading to tissue vaporization. It is increasingly popular due to reduction of intraoperative bleeding and is particularly favoured in very young children for this reason. Specific guidance following the NPTA stated that those using coblation techniques should be specifically trained and the practice audited. A recent study of 500 children undergoing coblation tonsillectomy identified no primary haemorrhages and only two secondary haemorrhages (rate 0.4%). The debate surrounding optimal tonsillectomy technique is likely to continue.

## Additional reference

Hoey AW, Foden NM, Hadjisymeou Andreou S, Noonan F, Chowdhury AK, Greig SR, et al. Coblation® intracapsular tonsillectomy (tonsillotomy) in children: a prospective study of 500 consecutive cases with long term follow up. *Clin Otolaryngol* 2017;**42**:1211–17.

# Chapter 70

# Acute otitis media

Paul Little

## Details of studies

Acute otitis media (AOM) is a very common childhood infection, leading to frequent doctors' consultations, and the most frequent reason for children to take antibiotics. Prescribing antibiotics affects future health-related behaviours by encouraging visits for further episodes and ultimately promoting antibiotic resistance. Many children with AOM require only symptomatic relief. Individual trials to test effectiveness of antibiotics for AOM have been too small for valid subgroup analyses. The purpose of this review was to identify subgroups of children who would and would not benefit from treatment with antibiotics.

## Study references

### Main reference

Rovers MM, Glasziou P, Appelman CL, Burke P, McCormick DP, Damoiseaux RA, et al. Antibiotics for acute otitis media: a meta-analysis with individual patient data. *Lancet* 2006;**368**:1429–35.

### Related reference

Venekamp RP, Sanders S, Glasziou PP, Del Mar CB, Rovers MM. Antibiotics for acute otitis media in children. *Cochrane Database Syst Rev* 2013;**1**:CD000219.

## Study design

| | |
|---|---|
| Level of evidence | 1a |
| Studies | meta-analysis of data from six randomized trials of the effects of antibiotics in children with AOM. Individual patient data from 1,643 children aged from 6 months to 12 years were validated and re-analysed. The primary outcome was an extended course of AOM (pain, fever, or both at 3–7 days). |
| N | 1,643 children aged 6 months to 12 years |
| Inclusion | Trials had to be (1) randomized, (2) include children aged 0 to 12 years with AOM , (3) the comparison between antibiotics and placebo or no treatment, and (4) documenting pain and fever as an outcome |

| Key subgroups | Independent baseline predictors, age (< 2 years vs. ≥ 2 years), fever (yes vs. no), and bilateral AOM (yes vs. no), were used to study whether those at risk of a prolonged course also benefited more from treatment with antibiotics. In addition, otorrhoea (yes vs. no) at baseline was assessed (both alone and in combination with the identified predictors) |
| --- | --- |
| Follow-up | Symptoms during the week after randomization |

## Outcomes

### Primary

The primary outcome was defined as pain and/or fever at 3–7 days, justified by stating that both factors are relevant from a clinical and patients' (parental) perspective. Fever was defined as a temperature equal or greater than 38°C, and pain (yes vs. no) was measured by diaries filled out by the parents. Both outcome measures had to be dichotomized as several trials only measured them in this way.

### Secondary outcomes

Pain and fever separately.

## Results of independent patient data meta-analysis

Significant effect modifications were found for otorrhoea, and for age and bilateral AOM. In children younger than 2 years of age with bilateral AOM, 55% of controls and 30% on antibiotics still had pain, fever, or both at 3–7 days, with a rate difference between these groups of –25% (95% CI –36% to –14%), resulting in a number-needed-to-treat (NNT) of four children. There was no significant effect for age alone. In children with otorrhoea the rate difference and NNT, respectively, were –36% (–53% to –19%) and three, whereas in children without otorrhoea the equivalent values were –14% (–23% to –5%) and eight.

## Results of Cochrane systematic review

Thirteen trials of antibiotics against placebo (3,401 children and 3,938 AOM episodes) documented that by 24 hours from the start of treatment, 60% of the children had recovered whether or not they had placebo or antibiotics. Pain was not significantly reduced by antibiotics at 24 hours (risk ratio (RR) 0.89, 95% CI 0.78–1.01) but fewer had residual pain at 2–3 days (NNT 20), and at 4–7 days (NNT 16), and 10–12 days (NNT 7) compared with placebo. Antibiotics reduced the number of children with tympanic membrane perforations (NNT 33) and halved contralateral otitis episodes (NNT 11) compared with placebo. However, antibiotics neither reduced the number of children with abnormal tympanometry findings at 3 months nor the number of children with late AOM recurrences. Severe complications were rare and did not differ between groups. Adverse events (such as vomiting, diarrhoea, or rash) occurred more often in children taking antibiotics (RR 1.38, 95% CI 1.19–1.59; number needed to treat for an additional harmful outcome

(NNTH) 14). For immediate antibiotics against expectant observation, four trials (959 children) found no difference in: pain at 3–7 days (RR 0.75, 95% CI 0.50–1.12); abnormal tympanometry findings at 4 weeks; tympanic membrane perforations; and AOM recurrence. No serious complications occurred. Immediate antibiotics were associated with more vomiting, diarrhoea, or rash than expectant observation (NNTH 9).

## Conclusion

The independent patient data (IPD) meta-analysis suggests targeting antibiotics: antibiotics seem to be most beneficial in children younger than 2 years of age with bilateral AOM, and in children with both AOM and otorrhoea. The Cochrane review suggests that overall there is limited benefit of antibiotics on average for most children with otitis media, and modest harms.

## Critique

The IPD meta-analysis was good quality and demonstrated no evidence of selection bias using funnel plots. However, it was limited by the range of outcomes and predictors available that were common between papers, and thus could not address outcomes of great importance to parents such as disturbed night's sleep or distress. The primary outcome of pain or fever on days 3–7 seems on the face of it important but by day 3 the pain is very much milder for the children who still have some discomfort, and so the relatively low NNTs must be seen in that context and so do not necessarily mean that the child needs to be treated. The IPD meta-analysis could also not assess longer term outcomes. Whether restrictive antibiotic use increases acute mastoiditis at the population level is still unresolved, but the potential increase is only two cases per 100,000 person-years and must be weighed against potential adverse effects.

# Chapter 71

# Ventilation tubes

Veronica Kennedy

## Details of studies

Insertion of ventilation tubes, otherwise known as tympanostomy tubes or grommets, is one of the commonest surgical procedures in the otolaryngology field. First introduced in 1954 by Beverly Armstrong in the case series discussed here, ventilation tubes have become the predominant surgical treatment for persistent otitis media with effusion (OME). OME is a common condition of childhood affecting approximately 80% of children by the age of 4 years (Browning et al. 2010). While for most children OME resolves spontaneously, it can recur and in some cases can be persistent. Untreated persistent OME can lead to educational, language, and behavioural problems. The American Academy of Otolaryngology-Head and Neck Surgery Foundation (AAO-HNSF) (Rosenfield et al. 2016) produced guidelines which recommend diagnostic criteria and management options for the treatment of OME. The National Institute for Health and Clinical Excellence produced guidelines on the surgical management of OME (NICE 2008).

## Study references

### Main study

Armstrong BW. A new treatment for chronic secretory otitis media. *Arch Otolaryngol Head Neck Surg* 1954;**59**:653–5

### Related references

Rosenfeld RM, Shin JJ, Schwartz SR, Coggins R, Gagnon L, Hackell JM et al. Clinical practice guideline: otitis media with effusion (update). *Otolaryngol Head Neck Surg* 2016;**154**(Suppl.):S1–S41.

National Institute for Health and Clinical Excellence 2008 Otitis media with effusion in under 12s: surgery. NICE Clinical Guideline 60. https://www.nice.org.uk/guidance/cg60 (accessed March 2018).

## Study design

Case series illustrating the first use of ventilation tubes in secretory otitis media in five children.

## Outcome measures

◆ Hearing assessment

◆ Valsalva inflation to assess the presence of middle ear effusion

## Results

◆ There was a reported improvement in hearing of 17.9% after insertion of ventilation tube

◆ There was no re-accumulation of middle ear fluid after removal of the ventilation tube. The ventilation tubes were reported to have been left in place between 1 and 4 weeks depending on the duration of the disease and clinical response

## Conclusion

◆ Ventilation tubes are a successful short-term treatment of secretory otitis media

## Critique

Untreated hearing loss in children, e.g. due to persistent otitis media, can result in a delay in speech and language development and have a subsequent impact on educational and social development.

In this case series, the innovative ventilation tube was used for a persistent unilateral secretory otitis media in five patients after accepted treatments at the time were unsuccessful. Only one patient was discussed in detail. The treatments administered included repeated inflation of the ear, myringotomy, nose drops, antihistamines, and cortisone. The procedure is described in only one patient in whom the ventilation tube was removed after 15 days but symptoms recurred. The ventilation tube was reinserted with good effect and removed after 1 month with no recurrence of symptoms. There was an acknowledgement that there could be a risk of perforation with prolonged use. It is a short paper which is more focused on the technique than on the presenting symptoms or outcomes. There is understandably little mention of the possible impact of the use of the ventilation tube in a child both on hearing levels and the wider impact of communication, education and social development.

Sixty years later the use of ventilation tubes remains an established surgical treatment for children with persistent OME and a significant hearing loss, with guidelines giving indications and contraindications for their use. As OME in children often resolves without intervention, it is only if OME and hearing loss persists over a period of 3 months that intervention should be considered. Both AAO-HNSF and NICE guidelines recommend that during this period, support should be offered in terms of advice on listening, behavioural, and school strategies. However there are some differences between the guidelines. The AAO-HNSF guidelines include an extensive section on diagnostic assessment. These guidelines recommend the insertion of ventilation tubes where there is bilateral hearing loss and OME, and also recommend consideration of ventilation tubes where there is uni- or bilateral OME in the presence of symptoms of behavioural or educational difficulties, balance problems, or ear discomfort, or, generally, a reduced quality of life. The NICE guidelines recommend the insertion of ventilation tubes where there is bilateral hearing loss and OME. Both guidelines recommend against the use of nose drops, antihistamines and cortisone as well as routine adenoidectomy in the absence of upper respiratory tract symptoms.

There is a need for research into the long-term benefits and adverse effects of ventilation tubes. Long-term effects of the ventilation tubes on the tympanic membrane have been noted including tympanosclerosis, retraction, atrophy, and perforation (Barfoed 1980). Otorrhoea is a common finding in infants with ventilation tubes. A systematic review of randomized controlled trials (Browning et al. 2010) showed only a small effect of ventilation tubes compared with the improvement in hearing with natural resolution of the otitis media with effusion. However as neither speech and language outcomes nor social or educational outcomes were routinely included in the trials, the wider impact of using ventilations tubes to treat hearing loss due to OME could not be established.

## Additional references

Barfoed C, Rosborg J. Secretory otitis media long-term observations after treatment with grommets. Arch Otolaryngol 1980;**106**:553–6.

Browning GG, Rovers MM, Williamson I, Lous J, Burton MJ. Grommets (ventilation tubes) for hearing loss associated with otitis media with effusion in children. *Cochrane Database Syst Rev* 2010;**10**:CD001801.

Chapter 72

# Otitis media with effusion

Paul Little

## Details of studies

Otitis media with effusion is responsible for the majority of hearing loss cases in early and middle childhood with high associated healthcare expenditure. The condition is ultimately largely self-limiting, and there has been much debate over management strategies. Affected children may be given temporary hearing aids while they grow out of the condition, or they may have ventilation tubes (VTs) or grommets placed. Concurrently with VTs they may have adjuvant adenoidectomy (+ad). The adjuvant role of adenoidectomy was one of the main reasons why the TARGET trial was funded; previous trials had presented conflicting evidence of benefit.

## Study references

### Main study

MRC Multicentre Otitis Media Study Group. Adjuvant adenoidectomy in persistent bilateral otitis media with effusion: hearing and revision surgery outcomes through 2 years in the TARGET randomised trial. *Clin Otolaryngol* 2012;**37**:107–16.

### Related references

Maw R, Bawden R. Spontaneous resolution of severe chronic glue ear in children and the effect of adenoidectomy, tonsillectomy, and insertion of ventilation tubes (grommets). *BMJ* 1993;**306**:756–60.

Medical Research Council Multicentre Otitis Media Study Group. Surgery for persistent otitis media with effusion: generalizability of results from the UK trial (TARGET). Trial of Alternative Regimens in Glue Ear Treatment. *Clin Otolaryngol Allied Sci* 2001;**26**:417–24.

Van den Aardweg MTA, Schilder AGM, Herkert E, Boonacker CWB, Rovers MM. Adenoidectomy for otitis media in children. *Cochrane Database Syst Rev* 2010;**1**:CD007810.

## Study design

| Level of evidence | 1b |
|---|---|
| Randomization | Medical management (n = 122)<br>VTs only (n = 126)<br>VTs+ adenoidectomy (n = 128) |
| N | 376 from 571 children assessed at second visit from 3,828 originally referred |

| Inclusion | Children aged 3–7 years with bilateral otitis media with persistent effusion and better ear hearing level (HL) ≥20 dB |
|---|---|
| Exclusion | Children not having B+B or B+C2 tympanograms 3 months apart<br>At the discretion of the physician children with HL >40 dB could be treated and not randomized |
| Follow-up | 3,12, and 24 months |

## Outcomes

### Primary

Pure tone air conduction thresholds at 0.5, 1.0, 2.0, and 4.0 kHz in each ear averaged over all the visits, summarized as the four-frequency average binaural hearing thresholds.

### Secondary

Revision surgery rates, complications, otoscopic abnormalities (discharge, infections, tympanosclerosis).

### Results of main TARGET paper

Fifty-seven per cent of children in the control group transferred to other groups. On an intention-to-treat basis VTs had a benefit of 8.8 dB in the 3–6 months postoperatively, during which time there was no additional benefit from adenoidectomy. In later follow-up (averaged over 12, 18, and 24 months) there was no benefit from VTs but 4.2 dB of benefit (CI 2.6–5.7) from adenoidectomy. Adenoidectomy reduced the numbers of those eligible for repeat tube surgery (a 25 dB HL bilateral cut-off) from 33% to 15% at 18 months, and for actual surgery performed an absolute risk difference of 21%. In VT-managed ears but not in control ears, tympanosclerosis occurred in 27% but other abnormalities rarely (otorrhoea <2%; permanent perforations <1%). One child in the adenoidectomy group (0.6%) had haemorrhage requiring return to theatre.

### Results of the related papers

Three trials in the Cochrane review demonstrated that adenoidectomy for OME provides significant benefit in resolving fluid by 1 year (a risk difference of 29%) comparing the operated with the non-operated ears. The Maw and Bawden trial randomized 228 children with ≥25 dB pure audiometric or free field hearing loss in each ear at one or more frequencies to adenotonsillectomy +VT, adenoidectomy +VT, VT alone, or no surgery and followed them up for more than 5 years annually, although with lower numbers after 5 years. Comparison was made between operated and non-operated ears, and the survival curves for fluid resolution suggested significant benefit from VTs or adenoidectomy during the first year, and separation of the curves at 5 years—albeit not statistically significant by 5 years. A statistically significant benefit from adenoidectomy in addition to VTs was sustained throughout follow-up. However, although the authors report hearing benefit for children if fluid had resolved, the average HLs were very similar in the whole trial groups.

The second TARGET cohort paper demonstrated the likely generalizability of the results—with no important differences between the eligible children who were recruited or not recruited at the first visit, or randomized or not randomized at visit 2.

## Conclusion

Adjuvant adenoidectomy probably increases benefit of VTs for both fluid resolution and hearing by lasting into the second year, even allowing for the fact that a large proportion of children in the control group switched to surgical intervention. Although the absolute magnitude of hearing benefit is not large, 21% fewer children are likely to required repeat VT surgery.

## Critique

From the Cochrane review the clinical importance of fluid resolution at 1 year is unclear; comparison between ears may not be reliable given the variability between ears; and for a child the overall impact on functioning is probably more important than what is happening to fluid in individual ears. The Maw trial also compared fluid resolution ears, and although finding additional benefit from adenoidectomy the trial was not adequately powered to compare between all the trial groups in the longer term. Although follow-up was creditable in the Maw trial (nearly 70% by 5 years) attrition bias is likely (more than 30% missing data) and analysis did not impute missing data. Thus the estimates from the TARGET trial which both assessed overall hearing and imputed missing data are likely to be more robust, and also are likely to be generalizable. However, the extent of clinically meaningful benefit is still not very clear beyond 1 year—is 4 dB HL really clinically important, what level of impaired functioning does this mean for the child, and is such a benefit worth the modest harms? Harms are mostly modest and uncommon—modest local complications, and rare serious events (<1% requiring repeat trip to theatre), but there is also the inconvenience of time in hospital and recuperating afterwards. The lack of an economic analysis also make it more difficult to assess whether commissioners of services should invest in VTs and/or adenoidectomy operation for OME.

Chapter 73

# Brainstem-evoked response audiometry

Veronica Kennedy

## Details of study

This is certainly a landmark paper, presenting brainstem-evoked response audiometry (BERA) for the first time as an objective newborn hearing screening test. As the early years of childhood are critical periods for the plasticity of the auditory system (Moore 2002) with the foundation for hearing, language, and speech being laid down in the first 6 months of age (Yoshinaga-Itano et al. 1998), the need for early intervention is now well recognized. Universal newborn hearing screening (JCIH 2007) is in place in many countries with BERA or auditory brainstem response audiometry as one of the key tests used. It is considered an effective test both as a screening and diagnostic test for hearing loss in universal hearing screening programmes (Stevens et al. 2013). While Jewett and Williston were the first to report its use in 1971, Schulman-Galambos and Galambos (1979) were the first to use this method in infants as a newborn hearing screening test. Up to that point, they reported that there was no 'acceptably objective and reliable technique for newborn screening'. In order to demonstrate the feasibility of this test for newborn screening, this study assesses this test in different groups of infants.

## Study references

### Main study

Schulman-Galambos C, Galambos R. Brainstem evoked response audiometry in newborn hearing screening. *Arch Otolaryngol Head Neck Surg* 1979;**105**:86–90.

### Related references

Joint Committee on Infant Hearing (JCIH). Year 2007 position statement: principles and guidelines for early hearing detection and intervention programs. *Pediatric* 2007;**120**:898–921.

Stevens J, Boul A, Lear S, Parker G, Ashall-Kelly K, Gratton D. Predictive value of hearing assessment by the auditory brainstem response following universal newborn hearing screening. *Int J Audiol* 2013;**52**:500–6.

## Study design

- ◆ Comparative study of BERA findings in three groups of infants
  - • Group 1: healthy normal-term newborns; n = 220
  - • Group 2: high-risk newborns, i.e. those treated in an intensive care unit; n = 75
  - • Group 3: high-risk follow up group aged ≥ 1 year; n = 325
- ◆ Three protocols were used
  - • A screening protocol using a click stimulus at 60 dB HL and 30 dB HL for one ear with the second ear tested if time allowed
  - • Threshold measurement protocol measuring thresholds at 60, 30, 20, and 10 dB HL
  - • Threshold measurement protocol measuring responses to 10 dB HL decrements from 60 to 10 dB HL
- ◆ The electrical activity of the brain was reported to be amplified ×10$^4$, filtered between 150 and 1,500 Hz and responses to auditory stimuli of 1,000, 2,000, and 4,000 Hz clicks averaged
- ◆ Impedance audiometry was used to assess middle ear function

## Outcome measures

- ◆ Threshold of hearing as judged by the presence and latency of wave V of the recorded brainstem evoked response
- ◆ Conventional audiometric measures: all abnormalities that were identified by BERA were subsequently confirmed by conventional audiometric measures

## Results

- ◆ Group 1: no hearing abnormalities were uncovered (386 ears)
- ◆ Group 2: four cases of severe sensorineural hearing loss (seven ears)
- ◆ Group 3: additional four cases of severe sensorineural hearing loss

The incidence of hearing loss in the normal newborn group was 0% and 2.14% in the high-risk newborn group. When the efficacy of the protocols were reviewed, reliable responses were obtained at the screening levels. A clearly defined wave V shape and latency appropriate for age at 30 dB HL was considered to indicate essentially normal cochlear function.

Threshold responses were not always obtained at low intensity thresholds, e.g. 10 or 20 dB HL. Responses for threshold assessment were reported as small, relatively unstable and time-consuming.

## Conclusions

The authors suggest that BERA is an effective and reliable test for screening newborn hearing. It is an expensive test as it requires expensive equipment and trained personnel. Its effectiveness as a screening test was considered to justify its cost.

# Critique

Overall the paper provided a good account of why BERA/ABR should be used for neonatal screening and has shown itself to be the start of what is now well accepted practice. BERA, or ABR, is now one of the key tests in detecting hearing loss in neonates, with an automated version available for the screening assessment which removes the need for operator interpretation (Jacobson et al. 1990). It is usually paired with an otoacoustic emissions (OAEs) test to assess the integrity of outer hair cell function.

Click-evoked BERA or ABR correlates well with hearing thresholds between 1,000 and 4,000 Hz. However, as the paper acknowledges, click auditory stimuli are not optimal for testing low-frequency hearing sensitivity. Equally, as the responses were averaged, a ski slope high-frequency loss can also be overlooked. It is now accepted practice to use frequency specific tone pip stimuli.

The latencies of the recorded wave V in this study were noted to increase as the intensity of the stimulus decreased there was a maturational decrease of the latency of this wave noted between the premature babies and the full-term newborns. We know that the latencies can also increase with a conductive hearing loss. It is now recommended practice to use air- and bone-conduction ABR for diagnostic hearing assessment.

There was one area where the paper is unclear. This was on how group 3 were tested: while this group were reported to have a BERA, no mention was made whether this was done under general anaesthetic/sedation. This age group (>1 year old) is unlikely to allow testing under the natural sleep conditions of groups 1 and 2 but, in the absence of developmental delay, should be able to perform behavioural audiometry.

As this paper is on the early use of BERA/ABR, the knowledge of the time would not include the awareness of auditory neuropathy/dys-synchrony disorder (Hood 2015). This is a condition which may be found in some high-risk babies often related to central insults, e.g. severe hyperbilinrubinaemia, hypoxic ischaemic encephalopathy. OAEs are present indicating normal cochlear function but the waveform configuration on BERA/ABR is generally absent or distorted beyond the wave I of the cochlear microphonics.

## Additional references

Jewett DL, Williston JS. Auditory-evoked far fields averaged from the scalp of humans *Brain* 1971;94:681–96.

Hood LJ. auditory neuropathy/dys-synchrony disorder: diagnosis and management. Otolaryngol Clin North Am 2015;48:1027–40

Jacobson JT, Jacobson CA, Spahr RC. Automated and conventional ABR screening techniques in high-risk infants. *J Am Acad Audiol* 1990;1:187–95.

Moore DR. Auditory development and the role of experience. *Br Med Bull* 2002;63:1171–81.

Yoshinaga-Itano C, Sedey AL, Coulter DK, Mehl AL. Language of early- and later-identified children with hearing loss. *Pediatrics* 1998;102:1161–71.

Chapter 74

# Paediatric sensorineural hearing loss

Veronica Kennedy

## Details of studies

It is important to investigate the aetiology of sensorineural hearing loss (SNHL) in children. Identification of the aetiology may allow treatment of the causative factor, determination, and counselling the family about the prognosis of the hearing loss in the individual child, identification of associated conditions, and development of appropriate multimodal management (audiological, medical, education, communication support). Zakzouk and Al-Anazy (2002) reported that, after investigation, aetiology could be established in 44% of cases of SNHL of unknown cause with the remaining 56% attributable to genetic causes. Taking into account the costs, risks, and yield of investigations, the studies here look at an evidence-based approach to this investigation.

## Study references

### Main studies

British Association of Audiovestibular Physicians (BAAP). Guidelines for aetiological investigation into severe to profound bilateral permanent childhood hearing impairment. *Hearing, Balance Commun* 2016;**14**:135–45.

Morzaria S, Westerberg BD, Kozak FK. Evidence-based algorithm for the evaluation of a child with bilateral sensorineural hearing loss. *Otolaryngology* 2005;**34**:297–303.

### Related references

British Association of Audiovestibular Physicians (BAAP) Guidelines for aetiological investigation into mild to moderate bilateral permanent childhood hearing impairment. *Hearing, Balance Commun* 2016;**14**:125–34.

British Association of Audiovestibular Physicians (BAAP). Guidelines for aetiological investigation into unilateral permanent childhood hearing impairment. *Hearing, Balance Commun* 2016;**14**:146–55.

Morzaria S, Westerberg BD, Kozak FK. Systematic review of the etiology of bilateral sensorineural hearing loss in children. *Int J Pediatr Otorhinolaryngol* 2004;**68**:1193–8.

## Study design

| | |
|---|---|
| Morzaria et al. 2004 | Systematic review of the literature between 1940 and January 2003 for studies providing information on the diagnosis of each aetiology related to hearing loss relevant to its clinical presentation |
| BAAP 2016 | Systematic review of the literature between January 2008 and March 2014 for articles relevant to the investigations into the aetiology of SNHL in children |

## Results

The literature for the diagnostic yield of the individual investigations into SNHL in children was reviewed but will not be listed in this overview.

## Conclusion

Morzaria at al. (2004) proposed the following diagnostic algorithm:

- Careful history and physical examination by a clinician familiar with the causes of SNHL in children
- Full audiometric evaluation, including assessment for auditory neuropathy if indicated
- Ophthalmological assessment for visual abnormalities and abnormalities associated with syndromes, e.g. retinitis pigmentosa with Usher's syndrome
- If no cause identified from the above assessments, high-resolution computed tomography (CT) scan of temporal bones
- Genetic testing for connexin 26 mutation, probably in conjunction with a genetics consultation
- Electrocardiogram (ECG) for all children with a bilateral profound SNHL

The British Association of Audiovestibular Physicians (2016) produced evidence-based guidelines for aetiological investigations into different levels of childhood SNHL. The guideline for investigation into severe to profound bilateral permanent childhood hearing impairment is as follows: investigations are categorized into two tiers with level 1 investigations offered to all children and level 2 to children where there are specific indications. The indications for, and details and timing of, each investigation are discussed in the guidelines.

Level 1 investigation includes

- Thorough clinical history and examination. The details of these are provided
- Family audiograms
- ECG
- Ophthalmology assessment
- Urine examination for microscopic haematuria and proteinuria
- Cytomegalovirus testing

- Connexin 26 and 30 mutation test
- Magnetic resonance imaging of internal auditory meati and brain or, if permanent conductive component to hearing loss, CT of petrous temporal bone, both are indicated in cases of bacterial meningitis.

Level 2 investigation will be indicated by history and clinical findings and include

- Serology for congenital infection (e.g. syphilis, HIV, rubella, toxoplasma)
- Haematology and biochemistry where clinically indicated
- Investigation into autoimmune diseases
- Chromosomal studies or further genetic testing, referral to clinical genetics
- Vestibular investigation

## Critique

For the most part the algorithm proposed by Morzaria et al. (2005) has stood the test of time. Advances in technology and knowledge has contributed to additional details in the BAAP guidelines. However, much of the evidence behind the investigations for SNHL is of low grade and based on case reports, case series, or cohort studies. Despite this, the aim of the investigations is to diagnose causes that are serious, e.g. tumours, Jervell Lange Neilsen, or Alport syndromes, those that are preventable, e.g. use of ototoxic medication and m1555A>G mutation or those that can be potentially limited, e.g. impact of cytomegalovirus (Kimberlin et al. 2015). The guidelines address this aim. The investigations also provide information to inform the clinician of likely prognosis of the hearing loss and co-existing medical problems. While the evidence base is limited, the importance of a good clinical history and examination cannot be overemphasized as the first step in the investigation process.

## Additional references

Kimberlin DW, Jester PM, Sánchez PJ, Ahmed A, Arav-Boger R, Michaels MG, et al., National Institute of Allergy and Infectious Diseases Collaborative Antiviral Study Group. Valganciclovir for symptomatic congenital cytomegalovirus disease. *N Engl J Med* 2015;372:933.

Zakzouk SM, Al-Anazy F. Sensorineural hearing impaired children with unknown causes: a comprehensive etiological study. *Int J Pediatr Otorhinolaryngol* 2002;64:17–21.

# Chapter 75

# Congenital malformations of the inner ear

Veronica Kennedy

## Details of studies

An accepted classification of inner ear malformations can allow comparison of presentations and outcomes of specific malformations and guide clinicians in management planning. Children with more marked cochleovestibular abnormalities could have poorer outcomes and therefore be poorer candidates for cochlear implant surgery. Jackler et al. (1987) proposed a hypothesis that distinct morphologic patterns would result from an arrest in development during inner ear embryogenesis and developed a classification that was based on the likely time of arrested development of the cochlea. It included malformations of the osseous and membranous labyrinths. This classification became widely adopted. In 2002, Sennaroglu and Saatchi proposed a modification to expand the classification further.

## Study references

### Main studies

Jackler RK, Luxford WM, House WF. Congenital malformations of the inner ear: a classification based on embryogenesis. *Laryngoscope* 1987;**97**:2–14

### Related references

Jeong SW, Kim LS. A new classification of cochleovestibular malformations and implications for predicting speech perception ability after cochlear implantation. *Audiol Neurootol* 2015;**20**:90–101.

Sennaroglu L, Saatci I. A new classification for cochleovestibular malformations. *Laryngoscope* 2002;**112**:2230–41.

## Study details

+ Retrospective case note study (1965–85) of patients with sensorineural hearing loss and abnormal radiographs

## Outcome measures

+ Hearing thresholds
+ Speech discrimination

- ◆ Impedance
- ◆ Radiological changes on polytomes or computed tomography (CT)

## Results

- ◆ 63 patients identified
- ◆ 98 abnormal ears
  - • Cochlear abnormality in 49 patients (74 ears)
  - • Semicircular canal, vestibule or vestibular aqueduct abnormality
- ◆ Bilateral abnormalities in 65%, unilateral in 35%
- ◆ Average hearing loss for all patients was 75 dB
- ◆ Long time follow up (n = 26 ears) showed average loss of 27 dB between first and last visit

| Incidence of malformation | Mean dB score |
|---|---|
| Cochlear involvement | 120 |
| Complete labyrinthine aplasia 1 ear (1%) | 94 |
| Common cavity 19 (26%) | 117 |
| Cochlear aplasia 2 (3%) | 53 |
| Cochlear hypoplasia 11 (15%) | 75 |
| Incomplete partition 41 ears (55%) | 35 |
| Cochlea not involved | 60 |
| Enlarged vestibular aqueduct and lateral semicircular canal 7 ears | |
| Enlarged vestibular aqueduct 17 ears | |

## Classification

Based on the stages of arrested development almost weekly from the third week of embryonic development, Jackler et al. (1987) put forward the following classification:

| |
|---|
| A. With absent or malformed cochlea (vestibule and semicircular canals may be normal or malformed) |
| 1. Complete labyrinthine aplasia |
| 2. Cochlear aplasia |
| 3. Cochlear hypoplasia |
| 4. Incomplete partition |
| 5. Common cavity |
| B. With normal cochlea |
| 1. Vestibule-lateral semicircular dysplasia |
| 2. Enlarged vestibular aqueduct |

Reproduced from Jackler RK, Luxford WM, House WF. Congenital malformations of the inner ear: a classification based on embryogenesis. *Laryngoscope* 1987;97:2–14 with permission from Wiley.

## Conclusions

This classification of malformations based on radiographic appearance and stage of arrested development provides a useful means of diagnosing and managing congenital malformations of the inner ear. Generally the more severe the malformation, the more severe the hearing loss. Considerable variation in hearing was noted within some categories, particularly the incomplete partition category with some categories associated with a progressive hearing loss.

## Critique

Cochlear malformations have been reported to occur in approximately 20% of children with congenital sensorineural hearing loss. Recognition of the different types of congenital abnormalities of the inner ear can guide the clinician's management of the condition.

One of the aims of the study was to clarify the classification of the myriad dissimilar anatomic patterns that had been lumped together under the term 'Mondini dysplasia'. The study noted that the most prevalent abnormality was an incomplete partition. While the resulting classification was successful in developing a logical and clinically relevant framework for the diagnosis of inner ear malformations, Sennaroglu and Saatci (2002), with the benefit of high-resolution CT scanning, felt that further classification was needed. They proposed that the term of incomplete partition (IP) was further defined and considered as two types: IP type I to cover cystic cochleovestibular malformations in the absence of an enlarged vestibular aqueduct and IP type II for the classic Mondini malformation with the triad of cystic cochlear apex, dilated vestibule, and enlarged vestibular aqueduct. This was to allow further accuracy in defining cochlear malformations in terms of severity and in comparing outcomes of surgery, e.g. cochlear implantation. Jeong and Kim (2015) favoured a more cochlear implant related classification, classifying the cochleovestibular malformation into four subtypes based on the structure of the cochlea and modiolus.

There are some issues with this classification system. Not all abnormalities can be explained by a premature arrest in development alone, e.g. the co-existence of outer or middle ear abnormalities with those of the inner ear. Jackler et al. (1987) acknowledged that there was a surprising frequency of this co-existence despite their separate embryogenesis.

With improvements of imaging, we are aware of wider variations of malformations, not all of which fit neatly into this classification. Magnetic resonance imaging scans allow more in depth soft tissue detail as well as improved identification of intracranial pathology than can CT imaging. The complementary use of both scans can provide optimal radiological information prior to considering cochlear implant surgery (DeMarcantonio and Choo 2015). For example radiological information about the presence and size of the auditory nerve in a narrowed internal auditory meatus can be one of the factors in considering possible outcomes of surgery (Papsin 2005). The improved level of imaging is further complemented by improvements in surgical technology with different cochlear implant arrays to suit different cochlear configurations.

Although today's level of knowledge and technology has moved on since this paper was written, it is still a significant and logical paper; its findings of the correlation of arrested stage of embryogenesis and cochleovestibular findings remain relevant. It provides a good start to the consideration of the process underlying a child's sensorineural hearing loss.

## Additional references

DeMarcantonio M, Choo DI. Radiographic evaluation of children with hearing loss *Otolaryngol Clin* 2015;48:913–32.

Papsin BC. Cochlear implantation in children with anomalous cochleovestibular anatomy. *Laryngoscope* 2005;115(Pt 2 Suppl. 106):1–26.

# Chapter 76

# Cochlear implantation in children

David Selvadurai and Georgios Oikonomou

## Details of studies

Paediatric cochlear implantation has been one of the great success stories of modern medicine. We now take for granted the prospect of returning adequate hearing to those born congenitally profoundly deaf and that they will be able to develop oral communication. This prospective cohort study investigates some of the factors that were considered to be potentially important in successful outcomes. It draws important findings by following a cohort of 40 implanted children through 5 years of post-implantation development.

## Study reference

O'Donoghue GM, Nikolopoulos TP, Archbold SM. Determinants of speech perception in children after cochlear implantation. *Lancet* 2000;356:466–8.

## Study design

Prospective inception cohort study starting at time of cochlear implantation.

| Level of evidence | 1c |
|---|---|
| Number of patients | 40 |

## Inclusion criteria

Clearly defined

- Audiologically: aided hearing thresholds greater than 60 dB from 500 Hz to 4 kHz and failure to derive benefit from hearing aids. The definition of failure to derive hearing benefit was not further specified
- Onset of deafness: only those who were born deaf or lost hearing before 3 years of age
- Age at implantation: under 7 years

## Exclusion criteria

No children meeting the inclusion criteria were excluded.

## Treatment

- All patients received the same brand of implant system, Cochlear Nucleus

+ Postoperative rehabilitation was consistent within the medical sphere, but local differences in school and parental input are possible

## Follow-up

Five years.

## Outcome measures

The main outcome measure used was performance in a speech test—'connecting discourse tracking', which measures speech understanding in conversational speech without the aid of lipreading. It therefore relies on purely auditory performance. Age-appropriate words were chosen.

Assessment was made at 3, 4, and 5 years post implantation.

These results were then compared statistically using repeated measures of ANOVA against the independent variables: age at implantation, number of inserted electrodes, aetiology (congenital or meningitic), mode of communication, and social class (as defined by the UK statistical service).

## Results

The results are presented in Box 76.1 and Table 76.1

Interestingly, combining both the most influential variables (age at implantation and social class) only accounts for up to 68% of the performance variation seen.

## Conclusions

The authors reach a variety of important conclusions. Their discussion is nuanced and self critical. It appears that they have carefully considered many of the potential sources of error in the study and mitigated them. Chiefly tight control of the age of implantation and the absence of 'excluded' cases strengthens the findings.

---

### Box 76.1 CDT results at each test interval after cochlear implantation

| CDT mean words per min (SD) |
| --- |
| Preimplantation 0 |
| 3 years 26·6 (21.5) |
| 4 years 35·4 (23.0) |
| 5 years 44·8 (24.3) |

Data sourced from O'Donoghue GM, Nikolopoulos TP, Archbold SM. Determinants of speech perception in children after cochlear implantation. *Lancet* 2000;356(9228):466–8.

**Table 76.1** Correlation analysis of CDT with variables at the 5-year interval

| | Age | Number of electrodes | Origin of deafness | Communication mode | Social class |
|---|---|---|---|---|---|
| Correlation coefficient | −0.55 | −0.10 | −0.17 | 0.62 | −0.10 |
| Regression coefficient | −0.88 (−1.32 to −0.44) | −1.10 (−4.42 to 2.21) | −9.01 (−26.71 to 8.69) | 29.56 (16.63 to 42.48) | 2.15 (9.40 to 5.08) |
| p | 0.0002 | 0.50 | 0.30 | 0.00005 | 0.54 |
| Percentage of variance | 30% | 1% | 3% | 38% | 1% |

Data sourced from O'Donoghue GM, Nikolopoulos TP, Archbold SM. Determinants of speech perception in children after cochlear implantation. *Lancet* 2000;356(9228):466–8.

The chief recommendation was that early implantation is clearly and significantly associated with better implant outcome, which supports the development of neonatal screening programmes. There is only brief discussion of the importance of communication mode between individuals, but it is suggested that this is borne in mind during consideration of candidacy.

## Critique

The performance of patients following paediatric cochlear implantation has been and remains a common concern for patients and professionals alike. The authors considered the existing literature and its flaws when designing this study. This led to a more successful study and more reliable conclusions. A strong point of the study is the careful discussion around these factors.

In an area where so many factors could potentially affect long-term outcome there are some shortcomings, which the authors recognize. For instance, the postoperative involvement of parents was assessed only by the surrogate marker of social class. This may hide a variety of positive influences such as extra speech therapy, as well as masking some disadvantageous issues such as non-attendance at therapy sessions. In a multilingual society the role of bilingual or non-English-speaking environments was not commented on.

While at the time the inclusion criteria that restricted patients to under 7 years old were appropriate and novel, today the age at implantation is much lower and more robust differences might be observed by considering even tighter groups. Although number of electrodes inserted was considered, the great majority of candidates did receive full insertions. Furthermore, the group with reduced electrode insertion were largely from the post-meningitic group. Other studies have established that post-meningitic cases may perform poorly and this may not be due solely to the number of inserted electrodes. It is not clear why more detailed discussion was not centred on the mode of communication findings, which does merit further study.

In summary this is significant and well constructed study that has influenced clinical practice substantially.

# Chapter 77

# Grading subglottic stenosis

Gavin Morrison

## Details of studies

From the 1970s to the 1990s, increasing numbers of often premature neonates (typically less than 30 weeks' gestation and of low weight) with immature lungs were surviving infant respiratory distress syndrome as a result of mechanical ventilation on paediatric intensive care units. However, these babies developed chronic lung disease (bronchopulmonary dysplasia) and required long-term ventilation. Approximately 2% of infants intubated for over 48 hours then developed subglottic or laryngotracheal stenosis. Paediatric airway surgery was evolving but there was no standardized or agreed method of classifying the stenoses. This made comparisons of therapeutic procedures or treatments difficult. Under Robin Cotton's lead in Cincinnati, USA, Myer et al. (1994) proposed a grading system in 1994 which was a modification of Cotton's earlier suggestion and has become the internationally adopted gold standard classification. Its merits are reliability and ease of use, based on standard endotracheal tube sizes. It has allowed meaningful reporting of therapies and comparisons of outcomes to be made.

## Study references

### Main study

Myer CM, O'Connor DM, Cotton RT. Proposed grading system for subglottic stenosis based on endotracheal tube sizes. *Ann Otol Rhinol Laryngol* 1994;**103**:319–23

### Related references

Cotton RT. Pediatric laryngotracheal stenosis. *J Pediatr Surg* 1984;**19**:699–704.

Cotton RT, Gray SD, Miller RP. Update of the Cincinnati experience in pediatric laryngotracheal reconstruction. *Laryngoscope* 1989;**99**:1111–6.

Hollinger PH, Kutnick SL, Schild JA, Holinger LD. Subglottic stenosis in infants and children. *Ann Otol Rhinol Laryngol* 1976;**85**:591–9

## Study design

♦ Descriptive paper detailing use of a grading system to assess and record severity of subglottic stenosis

♦ Level of evidence 4

The paper 'Endotracheal tube sizing of subglottic stenosis' simply comprises a review of the prior means of assessing severity of subglottic stenosis and describes a new and unique proposal. The practical use of the grading is assisted by presentation of tables from which the percentage of stenosis can be determined. Several systems to classify subglottic stenosis were described prior to the index paper by Myer et al. These had included measuring the length, diameter, and consistency of the stenosis. The Myer–Cotton classification is limited to firm mature stenoses, and not for soft oedematous or granular and possibly reversible lesions. It is a simple to use, universally reliable, and adoptable system. In 1988 the American Society of Pediatric Otolaryngologists (ASPO) had suggested a system to collect data on Function, Lumen Diameter, Extent, Consistency and Site of stenoses (FLECS) but it had not been adopted, being too cumbersome. Another system by Hebra et al. (1991), involved a stenotic segment volume measurement from filling a balloon of an angioplasty catheter. Computed tomography (CT) scanning had also been suggested and has a role in determining the length of a stenosis if it could not be estimated endoscopically (e.g. a total stenosis with no lumen). In 1984 and 1989 Cotton had first proposed a staging system with grades I to IV based on the perceived percentage reduction of the lumen in diameter compared with a normal one of a child of the same age. The diameter of the subglottis is not exactly circular. The four-grade system readily facilitated grouping of patients for analysis and discussion. Every patient should undergo a rigid laryngoscopy, confirming that the stenosis is firm and mature.

## Outcome measures

### Primary procedure

At microlaryngoscopy/endoscopy the operator selects and passes the endotracheal tube (ET), of a size considered likely to fit the subglottis. Larger or smaller tube sizes are selected if required to achieve a comfortable passage through the subglottis with an air leak, audible or visible, when ventilating with positive pressure applied between 10 and 25 cmH$_2$O. Such a tube is a good size but not too snug or tight to cause any trauma. ET tube sizes are named according to their internal diameter (ID) but the external or outside diameter (OD) is the figure which corresponds to the stenosis diameter and is used to estimate the cross sectional airway area. By comparison of the area of the cuffless ET which fits with that of a normal, age equivalent subglottis, the percentage of airway reduction is known. Tables 77.1 and 77.2 show charts which allow the operator to read off the percentage reduction.

## Results

The paper provides two charts from which the percentage of the airways obstruction can be read with the age of the patient in descending rows and the tube size that fits the patient in adjacent columns. The second chart marks the Cotton Grade of stenosis by blocks of increasingly dark background tone.

Without a chart, the percentage could be calculated from the ET which fits, using Area = $\pi r^2$ and dividing the result by the area of the age appropriate tube size, similarly calculated.

**Table 77.1** Grading based on the percentage reduction of the airway.

| | |
|---|---|
| Grade I | 0–50% obstruction |
| Grade II | 51–70% obstruction |
| Grade III | 71–99% obstruction |
| Grade IV | No detectable lumen |

Adapted from Myer CM, O'Connor DM, Cotton RT. Proposed grading system for subglottic stenosis based on endotracheal tube sizes. *Annals of Otology Rhinology & Laryngology*, 1994;103:319–23 with permission from Sage.

**Table 77.2** The inner and outside diameter of Portex Blue Line ET tubes, commonly used.

| ET tube size | Internal diameter (ID) mm | Outside diameter (OD) mm |
|---|---|---|
| 2.5 | 2.5 | 3.6 |
| 3.0 | 3.0 | 4.3 |
| 3.5 | 3.5 | 5.0 |
| 4.0 | 4.0 | 5.6 |
| 4.5 | 4.5 | 6.3 |
| 5.0 | 5.0 | 7.0 |
| 5.5 | 5.5 | 7.6 |
| 6.0 | 6.0 | 8.3 |

Adapted from Myer CM, O'Connor DM, Cotton RT. Proposed grading system for subglottic stenosis based on endotracheal tube sizes. *Annals of Otology Rhinology & Laryngology* 1994;103:319–23 with permission from Sage.

Table 77.3 summarizes the results charts. The paper also discusses the fact that Cotton's original 1989 classification had used different percentages as the cut off between the grades (grade I was 0–50% and grade II was 50–70%, and grade III 70–99%). However, this was less useful since a big proportion of cases fell into the grade I category and very few into grade III.

## Conclusions

The grade of subglottic stenosis can be readily measured, this provides a reliable means of recording and reporting mature stenoses and allows comparisons in the published literature (Cotton 1984; Cotton et al. 1989).

## Critique

At the time of writing this paper (Myer et al. 1994), and the immediate predecessors (Cotton 1984; Cotton et al. 1989), the definitive treatment of subglottic stenosis by open

**Table 77.3** Percentage airway reduction by ET size and age.

| Age of patient | Normal OD for age (mm) | Percentage obstruction by ET tube size which fits ET sizes (mm) | | | | | | | |
|---|---|---|---|---|---|---|---|---|---|
| | | 2.5 | 3.0 | 3.5 | 4.0 | 4.5 | 5.0 | 5.5 | 6.0 |
| Premature | 3.6 | 0% | | | | | | | |
| Premature | 4.3 | 30% | 0% | | | | | | |
| 0–3 months | 5.0 | 48% | 26% | 0% | | | | | |
| 3–9 months | 5.6 | 59% | 41% | 22% | 0% | | | | |
| 9 months to 2 years | 6.2 | 67% | 53% | 38% | 20% | 0% | | | |
| 2 year | 7.0 | 74% | 62% | 50% | 35% | 19% | 0% | | |
| 4 year | 7.6 | 78% | 68% | 57% | 45% | 32% | 17% | 0% | |
| 6 year | 8.2 | 81% | 73% | 64% | 54% | 43% | 30% | 16% | 0% |

Tables after R. Cotton: with thanks to the author for permission.

reconstructive airway surgery was still evolving. The grading system was an elegant and practical contribution, which has stood the test of time. Since then it has been invaluable to the speciality. It has allowed valid comparisons between outcomes from different centres using differing techniques and has indirectly therefore led to the establishment of 'gold standard' consensus in decision-making, according to the severity of the child's mature stenosis. Thus, Myer and Cotton grades I and even II might only require endosocpic procedures and many cases of grades II and III will be more likely to need open cartilage graft laryngotracheal reconstruction (LTR) operations. The more severe grade IIIs will usually be undertaken 'staged' with the presence of a tracheostomy, and some severe grade IIIs and grade IVs might be better candidates for a cricotracheal resection procedure.

Lauren Holliger's important paper 'Subglottic stenosis in infants and children' (Hollinger et al. 1976) pre-dated that era and described management and outcomes in a series of 158 cases, but was not able to do more than discuss what the normal subglottic size should be of a newborn. In that early publication the authors considered 73% of cases to be congenital subglottic stenosis. If a 3.0 ventilating bronchoscope would not pass the subglottis, it was diagnosed as stenotic. That corresponds to 4.0–4.5 mm diameter and the normal size was considered about 6 mm in a newborn. Interestingly, these (often mild) congenital stenoses corrected themselves in time with growth, so a conservative subglottic management, if necessary with a tracheostomy for up to 4 years, was employed. In the current era, we would consider a far smaller percentage of cases to be purely congenital in origin (infants without a history of significant intubation who have an abnormally small or ill-formed and thickened cricoid cartilage from birth). Tracheostomy in the true congenital stenosis does not seem to lead to any progression, but in the child with an acquired and active stenosis it can cause the development of a more severe stenosis.

Should scanning be used instead to better define or classify a laryngotracheal stenosis? It has a place as an adjunctive investigation in a small number of cases. With modern high-resolution and three-dimensional reconstructions and software ability to 'straighten out' the airway, valuable information about the length of stenotic regions can be seen on CT or magnetic resonance imaging scanning. The drawbacks, however, are the frequent need for intubation (obscuring the details of the stenosis) and for a general anaesthetic to provide a still child. CT can acquire the images very quickly nowadays and if a laryngeal mask airway is safe it has a role. It will not replace the need for endoscopic staging.

The advent of better endoscopic therapeutic procedures and especially the success of serial radial balloon dilatations has changed the nature of paediatric airway surgery. The Myer–Cotton grading is valid for mature fixed stenoses. Currently the paediatric ENT surgeon is managing varying degrees of acute soft tissue narrowing and airway trauma. Assessment and characterization of oedema, hyperaemia, ulceration, granulation tissue, granulomatous polyps, and acquired cysts are all important factors, and to address this shortfall, Benjamin (1993) Lindholm (1970), and Colice et al. (1989) have all proposed systems. They do not replace the established grading but add to it in the management of failed extubation of infants. However, the Myer–Cotton grading has almost become a victim of its own success; it is almost universally used by authors for all types of stenosis, even soft reversible ones treated endoscopically, thus making procedure outcome comparisons misleading.

The Myer–Cotton grading is purely applied to the subglottic size. In practice, laryngotracheal stenosis frequently presents as a combined glottic and subglottic stenosis. This can influence the decision making, so even a mild subglottic stenosis, for example with acquired bilateral crico-arytenoid joint fixation, or a posterior glottic stenosis might require a posterior cricoid LTR grafting technique. Other authors such as Bogdasarsian and Olsen (1980) have proposed glottic stenosis classifications. These too have an important adjunctive role.

Cotton's grading system relates the airway size to be expected for a child of the same given age. A minor criticism is that this age is not a corrected gestational age, although two rows for premature babies do exist on the original table. In fact age might not be the best measure to assess the expected subglottic cross sectional area and a height or weight related chart could be more reliable.

Finally, while the Cotton grading defines the percentage reduction of the airway at each age, the effect of the narrowing of any given percentage will also be dependent upon the size of that child. Airflow is proportional to the forth power of the radius (Poiseuille's law), and fast air speed through a small tube causes turbulent flow. Therefore, a small reduction in radius in a neonate's airway can become quickly critical, but the same percentage of reduction in a larger airway only leads to a small compromise. The older or larger child with a 35% mature fixed airway stenosis (grade I) will manage quite well, yet the small infant with a 35% stenosis (grade I) might struggle and require single stage open LTR reconstruction. Ideally for identification of which airway is likely to be 'critical' and require open intervention, the Cotton grade or percentage reduction needs to be related to the size or weight of the child as well.

## Additional references

Benjamin, B. Laryngeal Trauma from intubation; endosopic evaluation and classification. In CW Cummings, JM Fredrickson, LA Harker, CJ Krause, DE Schuler (eds), Otolaryngology head and neck surgery, 2nd edn. St Louis, MO: Mosbey-Yearbook, 1993;1875–96.

Bogdasarian RS, Olsen NR. Posterior glottic laryngeal stenosis. *Otolaryngol Head Neck Surg* 1980;**88**:765–72.

Colice GL, Stukel TA. Dain B. Laryngeal complications of prolonged intubation. *Chest* 1989;**96**:877–84.

Hebra A, Powell DD, Smith CD, Othersen HB Jr. Balloon tracheoplasty in children: results of a 15-year experience. *J Pediatr Surge* 1991;**26**:957–61.

Lindholm CE. Prolonged endotracheal intubation (a clinical investigation with special references to its consequences for the larynx and trachea and its place as an alternative to tracheostomy). *Acta Anaesthesiol Scand* 1970;**33**(Suppl.): 1–131.

# Chapter 78

# The cricoid split

Gavin Morrison

## Details of studies

In the 1970s and 1980s increasing numbers of pre-term babies were surviving as a result of prolonged ventilatory support on intensive care units. When their lung function had matured significant numbers of these babies failed attempts of extubation and about 2.5% of these neonates were developing acquired subglottic stenosis (from factors associated with their intubation). If the extubation failure was due to upper airway obstruction, commonly in the laryngeal and subglottic region, tracheostomy had to be considered, which had been associated with progression of the subglottic pathology to severe stenosis. Cotton and Seid (1980) realized that mild, reversible, and non-fibrous narrowing might be treated by direct surgery at the cricoid level (the anterior cricoid split), as a means of avoiding the complications and morbidity of tracheostomy.

## Study references

### Main study

Cotton RT, Seid AB. Management of the extubation problem in the premature child, anterior cricoid split as an alternative to Tracheotomy. *Ann Otol Rhinol Laryngol* 1980;**89**:508–11.

### Related references

Cotton RT, Myer CM, Bratcher GO, Fitton CM. Anterior cricoid split, 1977-1987, evolution of a technique. *Arch Otlaryngol Head Neck Surg* 1988;**114**:1300–302.

Silver FM, Myer CM, Cotton RT. Anterior cricoid split, update 1991. *Am J Otolaryngol* 1991;**12**:343–6.

## Study design

- A retrospective case series study over 3 years
- Implied comparison with similar patients who would all have required tracheostomy.
- Level of evidence: 3
- Number of patients: 12
- Inclusion criteria: premature neonates requiring prolonged ventilation and failing two or more attempts at extubation, subglottic pathology: oedema ulceration, granulation tissue. Alternative management: mandatory tracheostomy

+ Exclusion criteria: those with non-airway causes of failed extubation, such as cardiac failure, sepsis
+ Follow-up: 0–3 years
+ All patients were subject to endoscopic airway assessment under general anaesthetic to confirm the laryngeal/subglottic pathology. Through an open anterior neck approach, a single vertical incision was made through the anterior cartilaginous ring of the cricoid and the first two tracheal rings, and through mucosa to expose the ET tube. The patient was then left intubated for 2–3 weeks.

## Outcome measures

+ Success in subsequent extubation from 2 weeks after cricoid split surgery
+ Need for tracheostomy

## Results

+ Nine of 12 patients were successfully extubated (75%)
+ Three who failed received a tracheostomy

The weight of the patients ranged from 1.0 kg to 2.1 kg. Two of the three failures were undertaken on infants who had glottic and subglottic pathology. Because of this, the authors advised restricting the indication for cricoid split to infants with isolated subglottic pathology. There were two subsequent deaths from non-airway or surgical causes.

## Conclusion

Pre-term infants who require ventilatory support in the neonatal period and develop subglottic oedema, ulceration, and granulations leading to failed extubation can be treated by anterior cricoid split as opposed to tracheostomy. This gives a 75% success rate in extubation without subsequent airway deterioration.

## Critique

This paper remains very important as the first description of a new and innovative surgical procedure which is successful in treating incipient or soft subglottic stenosis. Prior to its conception, the only alternative managements were continued re-intubation or tracheostomy. The pathological sequence in the baby with trauma from prolonged intubation is initially reversible airway oedema, granulations, and ulceration within the fixed lumen of the complete cricoid ring. This is followed by healing with collagen formation and even active peri-chondritis resulting in cicatrical mature, fibrous scarring, sometimes with cartilage thickening within the fixed lumen. Cotton realized that by breaking the complete cartilage ring, the pressure in the subglottic lumen from intubation was reduced and oedema fluid could escape improving local blood flow. This improves tissue viability and allowing for reversal of the pathology before mature circumferential scarring had developed.

With hindsight it is a pity the authors did not more formally report a case–control series (the controls being similar infants who underwent tracheostomy) which would have strengthened the statistical impact of the novel surgical treatment.

Cotton did however follow up on the procedure with two subsequent publications (Cotton et al. 1988; Silver et al. 1991) In 1988, he reviewed a 10-year experience retrospectively describing the evolution of his technique and extending as well as clarifying the selection criteria. Sixty-seven patients were studied of whom 60 survived. The success rate for extubation was 78% and 22% required tracheostomy. Complications of the cricoid split were uncommon but reported as accidental extubations, pneumothorax, haemorrhage, wound infection, tube occlusion, and tracheal granulation tissue. These early reports say little about the role of acid reflux in laryngeal and subglottic pathology. While its influence still remains to some extent uncertain, most units would now recommend full antireflux medications in these patients.

The (Cincinnati group's) third publication (Silver et al. 1991) reported the cricoid split series as 91 patients, and the success rate of survivors was 76%. In the whole series no death was related to the surgical procedure, but to other comorbid factors, and there was only one death between 1988 and 1991. Cricoid split failures were found to be due, in a small number of cases, to a more mature stenosis or to such things as unrecognized vocal cord palsy, severe wound infection, tracheomalacia, and neuromuscular disease.

The proposed alternative to cricoid split or tracheostomy is therapeutic reintubation (Hoeve et al. 1995). Hoeve reported a series of 23 infants showing that reintubation for a mean period of 17 days allowed 95% to be extubated. Resting the larynx to allow healing can be achieved in theory with an ET tube in situ, provided it is not snug and compromising mucosal blood flow and it does not move with shearing forces. Other sources of tissue damage such as infection or acid reflux would require control. It is difficult to reconcile Hoeve's dramatic success rate with other unit's anecdotal experiences. Possibly the Dutch team's patients were a somewhat different severity—those who had indeed confirmed tube trauma but of a milder nature and had not already received many failed attempts at extubation.

During the same period that anterior cricoid split was evolving, cartilage grafts inserted into the opened airway in LTRs were developed for more severe and mature subglottic stenosis. The published success rates for single-stage LTRs are in the region of 89% (Agrawal et al. 2007), significantly better than for cricoid split alone. This fact probably led to some authors comparing anterior cricoid split with anterior graft LTR. In 1991 Richardson and Inglis in Washington alternately assigned failed extubation patients to these two operations, reporting improved success with the LTR over cricoid split. Blake Papsin's group in Toronto (Forte et al. 2001) reported cricoid split with insertion of a small thyroid ala cartilage anterior graft as a means of reducing complications such as difficulty after accidental extubation.

So was anterior cricoid split to be superseded by the single stage LTR? It might have done so but for the subsequent evolution of endoscopic surgical therapeutic techniques; principally the advent of radial balloon dilatation and of endoscopic cricoid split. In 2010 the Florentine and Parisian group (Mirabile et al. 2010) showed that the anterior cricoid could be divided entirely endoscopically and they used adjunctive dilatation with endovascular angioplasty balloons, achieving an 83% success rate with a far less invasive procedure and with few complications for patients with grade II–IV subglottic stenoses. Three-quarters of the series required from four to seven repeat dilatations.

Comparisons between different case series always carries the risk of being misleading. With reference to cricoid split and LTR the confusing factor is frequently the lack of clarity about the nature of the subglottic stenosis. Cricoid split was originally conceived only for soft early stenosis and the Cotton grading was to be used only for mature stenosis. However authors have mixed these and regularly report the Cotton grading of III and IV for very new immature but narrow stenosis (which will be amenable to endoscopic and limited cricoid split type procedures), and have also tended to report cricoid split series as if they were established stenoses.

In my opinion, anterior cricoid split was a groundbreaking advance in the management of failed extubation and soft non-mature subglottic narrowing and trauma. However, fixed fibrous and mature subglottic stenosis is the primary indication for laryngeal framework expansion surgery with anterior, or anterior and posterior LTR. The results of the latter operations are generally very good, but fall off in tiny infants of low weight at the time of surgery. These are often the very infants presenting with failed extubation. The technical aspects of securing a stable and not too heavy or prolapsing cartilage graft in to a very small neonatal subglottis are considerable. It is in this younger neonatal population from weight 1.5–4 kg that the author considers the less invasive anterior cricoid split (endoscopically or as an open procedure, with balloon dilatation) still holds an important place.

Finally, for completeness, it is worth mentioning that the posterior cricoid split operation with cartilage grafting (posterior graft), which can also be undertaken endoscopically (Gerber et al. 2013), is a completely different procedure and is primarily employed for patients who have bilateral vocal fold immobility or posterior glottic stenosis or severe subglottic stenosis. Its objective is to open the posterior glottic and subglottic lumen, not to deal with the soft stenosis seen in failed extubation.

## Additional references

Agrawal N, Black M, Morrison G. Ten-year review of laryngtracheal reconstruction for paediatric airway stenosis. *Int J Pediatr Otorhinolaryngol* 2007;70:699–703.

Forte V, Chang M, Papsin B. Thyroid ala cartilage reconstruction in neonatal subglottic stenosis as a replacement for the anterior cricoid split. *Int J Pediatr Otorhinolaryngol* 2001;59:181–6.

Gerber ME, Modi VK, Ward RF, Gower VM, Thomsen J. Endoscopic posterior cricoid split and costal cartilage graft placement in children. *Otolaryngol Head Neck Surg* 2013;148:494–502.

**Hoeve LJ, Eskici O, Verwoerd CD.** Therapeutic re-intubation for post-intubation laryngeal injury in preterm infants. *Int J Pediatr Otorhinolaryngol* 1995;31:7–13.

**Mirabile L, Serio PP, Baggi RR, Couloigner VV.** Endoscopic anterior cricoid split and balloon dilation in pediatric subglottic stenosis. *Int J Pediatr Otorhinolaryngol* 2010;74:1409–14.

**Richardson MA, Inglis AF.** A comparison of anterior cricoid split with and without costal cartilage graft for acquired subglottic stenosis. *Int J Pediatr Otorhinolaryngol* 1991;22:187–93.

# Chapter 79

# Laryngeal papillomatosis

## Mike Saunders

## Details of studies

Recurrent respiratory papillomatosis (RRP) is a condition affecting the upper airway (mainly the larynx) which remains difficult to manage. It is characterized by papillomata occurring in the larynx and with a strong tendency to recur after treatment. It is now known to be caused by the human papilloma virus (HPV) (types 6 and 11) and this is acquired during pregnancy or delivery from a maternal source. HPV 6 and 11 also cause cervical warts.

Untreated disease will usually cause dysphonia although when the papillomata become larger, airway obstruction becomes a problem. Potentially, untreated disease can lead to fatal airway obstruction.

However aggressive the resection, the disease cannot be eradicated surgically, and most cases undergo spontaneous resolution in adolescence. Numerous variations of non-surgical treatment of the disease have been tried over the last decades, including indole-3-carbinol, topical podophyllin, and mumps vaccine with little lasting benefit. Two agents, interferon-α and topical cidofovir are effective adjuncts to control; however, the side effects of interferon limited its use to all but the most serious cases (Gerein 2005) and there are concerns about the potential side effects and long-term safety of cidofovir, particularly the possible risk of malignant transformation (Derkay 2013). The mainstay of treatment in the control of the disease is, therefore, interval surgical debridement. The aim of surgery is to improve voice and maintain the airway while causing the least possible injury to the underlying larynx.

Until the 1970s, surgical debridement was undertaken using microlaryngeal instruments to excise the disease whenever required, other techniques used were suction diathermy and cryotherapy. The main complication of surgery was damage to the underlying vocal cord and larynx leading to lasting scarring and loss of voice, even after remission of the disease.

The $CO_2$ laser was invented in 1964 (Patel 1964) and found its way into medical use in the early 1970s. Using the laser in conjunction with microlaryngoscopy offered an excellent way of ablating tissue with little blood loss and relatively modest damage to the underlying tissue compared with previously available techniques, and for many years $CO_2$ laser ablation was the 'gold standard' technique for the control of RRP (Derkay 1995). However, there remained some concerns: the laser is expensive and time-consuming to set up, there is a risk of airway fire, and some concerns about the possibility of transmission of RRP via the laser plume (Kashima 1991). In addition, laser surgery itself is not without a considerable risk of long-term scarring partly because of the depth of the thermal injury on adjacent tissue (Durkin 1986), anterior glottis webbing being a significant risk in patients undergoing repeat procedures (Crockett 1987).

In the last two decades the microdebrider has become available as an alternative tool in endolaryngeal surgery. The principal advantages it offers over the laser for the treatment of RRP are reduced cost, less theatre time lost in setting up, and, in theory, the potential for injury to underlying tissue is reduced. In surveys in the USA in 2004 (Schraff 2004) and the UK in 2013 (Manickavasagam 2013), the microdebrider has replaced the $CO_2$ laser as the surgical technique of choice in RRP.

With the introduction of the quadrivalent RRP vaccine (Gardasil™) in the UK in 2012, it is anticipated that RRP will become increasingly uncommon.

## Study references

### Main study

Strong MS, Vaughan CW, Cooperband SR, Healy GB, Clemente MA. Recurrent respiratory papillomatosis: management with the CO2 laser. *Ann Otol Rhinol Laryngol* 1976;**85**(Pt 1):508–16.

### Related references

Incze JS, Lui PS, Strong MS, Vaughan CW, Clemente MP. The morphology of human papillomas of the upper respiratory tract. *Cancer* 1977;**39**:1634–46.

## Study design

This is a retrospective review of a series of 110 patients with RRP, operated on using the $CO_2$ laser at the University Hospital, Boston, and the Boston Veterans Administration Hospital between the years 1972 and 1975.

## Outcome measures

+ Patient details: age, gender, age at presentation, details of type, and numbers of RRP procedures prior to $CO_2$ laser, history of skin warts, geographical origin, socioeconomic status
+ Operative findings: site and extent of papillomata, histology of all removed lesions
+ Antigen responses: studied in 24 patients with subcutaneous inoculation of tuberculin and other antigens
+ Complications of treatment and disease: tracheostomy, laryngeal web, pulmonary spread, and malignant degeneration

## Results

Sixty-four patients were male and 46 female. While 66% of cases were diagnosed below the age of 5 (peak between 2 and 5) years, 34% were diagnosed between 16 and 50 years of age with a second peak incidence between 21 and 30 years of age. Of 36 patients under the age of 5 years, 50% were born to mothers with vaginal warts at the time of delivery.

Previous treatment modalities included surgical excision, cryosurgery, ultrasound, autogenous vaccination, and radiotherapy.

The majority of patients had more than six previous procedures, and 12 had had over 50.

No effect of socioeconomic status was noted; the disease was found to be worldwide although differing incidences were noted in certain parts of the USA.

The commonest site affected was the larynx (103) with tracheobronchial spread in 22 and 13 on the palate. Other sites included lips, gingiva, nasal vestibule, and lungs.

All lesions were benign squamous papillomata, some exhibiting degrees of atypia. Eleven out of 24 of those tested did not react to antigen challenges.

Three patients required tracheostomy, 20% had anterior commissure webbing due to previous surgery, and seven of 110 developed webs after laser treatment. Two patients developed laryngoceles after surgery, one patient had previously developed laryngeal malignancy and presented post laryngectomy with persistent papillomatosis. Three patients had pulmonary spread at presentation.

## Conclusions

The authors make many conclusions, both in the text and in the discussion. One important point was that in the widely used description of the time 'juvenile laryngeal papillomatosis', the terms 'juvenile' and 'laryngeal' were no longer appropriate.

No variation of surgical treatment was felt to offer a long-term cure in a single treatment although the authors were certain that laser ablation offered the optimal method of papilloma removal. The authors comment that the origin of the recurrence of disease remained a mystery and that disease probably extended beyond the macroscopic limits of the visible disease at the time of surgery. Referencing a parallel histopathological study (Incze 1977) the authors suggest that the disease is probably of papovavirus origin (papovavirus being a former term for the virus family which includes HPV).

## Critique

While it would be easy to criticize the methodology of this paper using the strict scientific publication dogma of today, it is important to remember that this paper was written over 40 year ago. At the time, the majority of otolaryngology journal publications were case reports, retrospective series, and opinion. Randomized controlled trials only started to appear in the ENT literature in the 1980s, and furthermore there are still relatively few RCTs investigating the treatment of RRP.

While the apparent aim of this paper was to assess the efficacy of the $CO_2$ laser use in the treatment of RRP, the paper attempts to encompass a very wide range of aspects of the disease including aetiology, immune response, and transmission. Statistical analysis is not used at any time in the article and the numbers of patients quoted in results is often unclear, being presented in graph form only.

If published today, this study would be divided into a greater number of more focused publications, each with clearer outcome measures and analysis. However, if one assesses the information presented in its true historical context, the paper is undoubtedly a significant contributor to our knowledge of RRP.

## Related references

Crockett DM, McCabe BF, Shive CJ. Complications of laser surgery for recurrent respiratory papillomatosis. *Ann Otol Rhinol Laryngol* 1987;**96**:639–44.

Derkay CS. Task force on recurrent respiratory papillomas: a preliminary report. *Arch Otolaryngol Head Neck Surg* 1995;**121**:1386–91.

Derkay CS, Volsky PG, Rosen CA, Pransky SM, McMurray JS, Chadha NK, et al. Current use of intralesional cidofovir for recurrent respiratory papillomatosis. *Laryngoscope* 2013;**123**:705–12.

Durkin GE, Duncavage JA, Toohill RJ, Tieu TM, Caya JG. Wound healing of true vocal cord squamous epithelium after $CO_2$ laser ablation and cup forceps stripping. *Otolaryngol Neck Surg* 1986;**95**:273–7.

Gerein V, Rastorguev E, Gerein J, Pfister H. Use of Interferon-alpha in recurrent respiratory papillomatosis: 20-year follow-up. *Ann Otol Rhinol Laryngol* 2005;**114**:463–71.

Kashima HK, Kessis T, Mounts P, Shah K. polymerase chain reaction identification of human papillomavirus DNA in $CO_2$ laser plume from recurrent respiratory papillomatosis. *Otolaryngol Neck Surg* 1991;**104**:191–5.

Manickavasagam J, Wu K, Bateman ND. Treatment of paediatric laryngeal papillomas: web survey of British Association of Paediatric Otolaryngologists. *J Laryngol Otol* 2013;**127**:917–21.

Patel CKN. Continuous-wave laser action on vibrational-rotational transitions of $CO_2$. *Phys Rev* 1964;**136**:A1187–93.

Schraff S, Derkay CS, Burke B, Lawson L. American Society of Pediatric Otolaryngology members' experience with recurrent respiratory papillomatosis and the use of adjuvant therapy. *Arch Otolaryngol Neck Surg* 2004;**130**:1039.

# Chapter 80

# Infantile capillary haemangiomas

Mike Saunders

## Details of study

It seems extraordinary that an antihypertensive drug invented in the 1960s (Black 1964) and in widespread global use since, could, some 50 years later, be accidentally discovered to have a dramatic therapeutic effect on a relatively common congenital tumour of infancy. Yet in 2008 Leaute-Labreze and others reported on an unexpected beneficial effect of propranolol in infants with capillary haemangiomas treated with propranolol for cardiovascular disease.

Since that discovery, propranolol was tested as a therapeutic agent in the treatment of subglottic haemangiomas and found to be equally effective (Jephson 2009; Denoyelle 2010). In the last decade propranolol has become accepted as the first-line treatment for obstructing subglottic haemangiomas.

Capillary haemangiomas are a common benign tumour of infancy affecting 5% of the paediatric population. Lesions in the subglottis are very much rarer, affecting around 1% of infants presenting with stridor. The natural history of these lesions is to steadily increase from about 3 months of age, reaching a peak at around 9 months and then gradually involuting thereafter, although this process may take several years. Subglottic haemangiomas may be large enough to completely obstruct the subglottic and untreated may be fatal.

The traditional treatment for the condition was to bypass the obstruction using a tracheostomy and to wait until the lesion had involuted sufficiently to allow decannulation. This approach exposed the child to the physical and developmental risks of living with a tracheostomy for up to 5 years and understandably other treatments were tried to avoid tracheostomy. Implantation of a radioactive gold grain was briefly tried but abandoned because of potential side effects (Benjamin 1978). Ablation with lasers, particularly carbon dioxide (Sie 1994) but also neodymium YAG (McCaffrey 1986) and KTP (Kacker 2001) has been extensively tried but it is not without risk of long-term scarring and stenosis (Cotton 1985; Bitar 2005).

Medical treatment for subglottic haemangiomas has been effective but generally the side effects of the agents, including interferon, vincristine (Ohlms 1994), and systemic corticosteroids are considerable. The use of intralesional steroids followed by intubation for several days (Meeuwis 1990) was popular as it avoided the systemic complications of steroid therapy; however, this approach often necessitated repeated visits to the intensive care facility. One of the patients in the subject paper from Bordeaux was coincidentally being treated with propranolol for side effects of systemic steroid treatment.

Open surgical excision of the haemangioma (Wiatrak 1996; Vijayasekaran 2006) had become more widely accepted until 2008. This avoids the need for a tracheostomy and a long-term cure in one surgical procedure without long-term medical treatment; however, the surgery is similar in magnitude and risk to a single stage laryngotracheal reconstruction and requires intubation for several days postoperatively. A small number of haemangiomas do not respond to propranolol treatment and surgical excision may still have a role in these cases (Siegel 2015).

## Study reference

### Main study

Léauté-Labrèze C, Dumas de la Roque E, Hubiche T, Boralevi F, Thambo JB, Taïeb A. Propranolol for severe hemangiomas of infancy. *N Engl J Med* 2008;358:2649–51.

## Study design

The report, published in the form of a letter to the editor in the *New England Journal of Medicine*, describes two infants with capillary haemangiomas of the head and neck that had failed to respond to systemic steroid treatment and who incidentally required systemic propranolol, one for hypertrophic obstructive cardiomyopathy, the other for high output cardiac failure.

After the dramatic changes noted in the first two patients, the authors used propranolol to treat a further nine children with disfiguring infantile capillary haemangiomas. Apart from in the first case (3 mg/kg /day) propranolol was used at a dose of 2 mg per kg per day.

## Outcome measures

Age, gender of patient, previous treatment with prednisolone, age at initiation of propranolol, regression of lesion by visual assessment, ultrasound findings, other effects, age at discontinuation of propranolol, age, and lesion status at last follow-up.

## Results

Four patients were male, and seven female. Ages ranged from 2 to 6 months at the start of propranolol treatment; four had previously been treated with prednisolone.

Two were initially treated for cardiac problems, in the following nine cases treatment was aimed at the haemangioma alone.

Visual assessment confirmed regression in all cases, ultrasound scanning in four cases demonstrated reduced lesion thickness. Two cases involving the eye were able to open the eye after treatment and one case with subglottic haemangioma improved symptomatically and on appearance at microlaryngoscopy.

Age at stopping propranolol ranged from 6 months to 14 with one ongoing at the time of reporting. Haemangioma status at discontinuation was reported as stable in three cases, mild recoloration in two, mild regrowth in three, no relapse in two, and ongoing treatment in one. Age at last follow up ranged from 7 to 18 months.

## Critique

It is interesting that the authors make no specific conclusion or treatment recommendations in the published letter. The report is simply an objective statement of fact. The authors offer potential explanations for the mode of action of propranolol on capillary haemangiomas including down regulation of expression of vascular endothelial growth factor and basic fibroblast growth factor leading to endothelial apoptosis in capillary cells. By 2016 little further progress had been made in the understanding of the mechanism of action (Hardison 2016).

Since 2008 it has become apparent that compared to the other available treatments for infantile haemangioma, particularly in the subglottis, propranolol offers by far the most benefit and a relatively low incidence of side effects (bradycardia, hypotension, hypoglycaemia). Most centres have settled on a daily dose around 2 mg/kg/day (Bejaj 2013) although there remains little very good evidence to support differences in dosing regimes and a recent meta-analysis suggest that 3 mg/kg/day may be more appropriate (Hardison 2016).

It seems fatuous to criticize the methodology of a practice-changing publication of this importance (e.g. the outcome measures are variably reported and are potentially subject to observer variation). One assumes that because of the relative importance of their discovery, the authors felt that it was more important to publish the findings straight away in a major journal rather than waiting to undertaking a more scientific analysis.

## Additional references

Bajaj Y, Kapoor K, Ifeacho S, Jephson CG, Albert DM, Harper JI, et al. Great Ormond Street Hospital treatment guidelines for use of propranolol in infantile isolated subglottic haemangioma. *J Laryngol Otol* 2013;**127**:295–8.

Benjamin B. Treatment of infantile subglottic hemangioma with radioactive gold grain. *Ann Otol Rhinol Laryngol* 1978;**87**:18–21.

Bitar M, Moukarbel R, Zalzal G. Management of congenital subglottic hemangioma: Trends and success over the past 17 years. *Otolaryngol Head Neck Surg* 2005;**132**:226–31.

Black JW, Crowther AF, Shanks RG, Smith LH, Dornhorst AC. A new adrenergic betareceptor antagonist. *Lancet* 1964;**1**:1080–1.

Cotton RT, Tewfik TL. Laryngeal stenosis following carbon dioxide laser in subglottic hemangioma; report of three cases. *Ann Otol Rhinol Laryngol* 1985;**94**:494–7.

Denoyelle F, Garabédian E-N. Propranolol may become first-line treatment in obstructive subglottic infantile hemangiomas. *Otolaryngol Head Neck Surg* 2010;**142**:463–4.

Hardison S, Wan W, Dodson KM. The use of propranolol in the treatment of subglottic hemangiomas: a literature review and meta-analysis. *Int J Pediatr Otorhinolaryngol* 2016;**90**:175–80.

Jephson CG, Manunza F, Syed S, Mills NA, Harper J, Hartley BEJ. Successful treatment of isolated subglottic haemangioma with propranolol alone. *Int J Pediatr Otorhinolaryngol* 2009;73:1821–3.

Kacker A, April M, Ward RF. Use of potassium titanyl phosphate (KTP) laser in management of subglottic hemangiomas. *Int J Pediatr Otorhinolaryngol* 2001;59:15–21.

McCaffrey TV, Cortese DA. Neodymium: YAG laser treatment of subglottic hemangioma. *Otolaryngol Neck Surg* 198;94:382–4.

Meeuwis J, Bos CE, Hoeve LJ, van der Voort E. Subglottic hemangiomas in infants: treatment with intralesional corticosteroid injection and intubation. *Int J Pediatr Otorhinolaryngol* 1990;19:145–50.

Ohlms LA, McGill TJI, Jones DT, Healy GB. Interferon alfa-2a therapy for airway hemangiomas. *Ann Otol Rhinol Laryngol* 1994;103:1–8.

Sie KCY, McGill T, Healy GB. Subglottic hemangioma: ten years' experience with the carbon dioxide laser. *Ann Otol Rhinol Laryngol* 1994;103:167–72.

Siegel B, Mehta D. Open airway surgery for subglottic hemangioma in the era of propranolol: Is it still indicated? *Int J Pediatr Otorhinolaryngol* 2015;79:1124–7.

Vijayasekaran S, White DR, Hartley BEJ, Rutter MJ, Elluru RG, Cotton RT. Open excision of subglottic hemangiomas to avoid tracheostomy. *Arch Otolaryngol Neck Surg* 2006;132:159.

Wiatrak BJ, Reilly JS, Seid AB, Pransky SM, Castillo J V. Open surgical excision of subglottic hemangioma in children. *Int J Pediatr Otorhinolaryngol* 1996;34(:191–206.

# Chapter 81

# Cervical lymphadenitis in children

Andy Bath

## Details of study

Mycobacterial cervical lymphadenitis in children is caused by *Mycobacterium tuberculosis* (MTB) and complex and non-tuberculosis mycobacteria (NTM)—also known as atypical tuberculosis. They have similar presentations making them difficult to differentiate, especially as the microbiological diagnosis can take up to 8 weeks. This is important as their treatment is different: MTB is treated with prolonged antituberculous medication compared with wide surgical excision alone in NTM. Epidemiological, clinical, and laboratory data were collected prospectively to determine whether more rapid diagnosis would be possible.

## Study reference

### Main study

Spyridis P, Maltezou HC, Hantzakos A, Scondras C, Kafetzis DA. Mycobacterial cervical lymphadenitis in children: clinical, and laboratory factors of importance for differential diagnosis. *Scand J Infect Dis* 2001;**33**: 362–6.

## Study design

A prospective single-centre cohort study.

| Level of evidence | 2b: observational study |
|---|---|
| Randomization | None |
| Number of patients | 50 |
| Inclusion criteria | Children (0–14 years of age) |
| | Diagnosed with mycobacterial cervical lymphadenitis at the tuberculosis clinic of P and A Kyriakou Children's Hospital from 1982 to 1997 |
| Exclusion criteria | Serological evidence or recent infection with Epstein–Barr virus, cytomegalovirus, *Bartonella henselae* or *Toxoplasma gondii* |
| | Previous vaccination with bacillus Calmette–Guerin |

Epidemiological data including details of socioeconomic variables and parental country of origin were collected. The diagnosis of MTB complex or NTM cervical lymphadenitis was determined with a lymph node specimen (and/or gastric fluid aspirate in the case of

MTB) by culture in Lowenstein–Jensen medium or through the automatic radiometric method BACTEC.

In the absence of positive cultures, diagnosis was established by attaining two of three criteria below.

| | MTB | NTM |
|---|---|---|
| Tuberculin skin test | Positive reaction | X |
| Chest X-ray | Compatible with pulmonary tuberculosis | Normal |
| Contact with a person with infectious tuberculosis | Contact | No contact |
| Histology | X | Lymph node features compatible with mycobacterial infection |

## Outcome measures

Statistical analyses were performed on epidemiological, clinical and laboratory data.

## Results

| MTB | 24 | 18 diagnosed from 1982 to 1989 |
|---|---|---|
| NTM | 26 | 6 diagnosed from 1982 to 1989 |

Epidemiological and lymph-node features and anatomical areas were not helpful in the differential diagnosis between the two groups.

All patients with MTB were given antituberculous treatment for 6 or 9 months, surgical intervention was required in 67% due to threatened or actual node rupture. All NTM cases were managed by surgery alone.

Diagnosis of MTB by two out of three was criteria associated with 92% sensitivity.

No patients with NTM had an abnormal chest X-ray.

Microbiological confirmation from lymph node cultures:

| MTB | 55% |
|---|---|
| NTM | 88% |

Culture from specimens collected from spontaneous drainage usually inconclusive.

## Conclusions

Correct diagnosis of tuberculous lymphadenitis in children is challenging. Fulfilment of two of three of the standard criteria were highly sensitive for MTB lymphadenitis. Microbiological confirmation is also very important. Early diagnosis and treatment of mycobacterial cervical lymphadenitis in children, including total lymph node excision (not incision and drainage), will improve the chance of diagnosis and response to treatment. Early excision of all infected lymph nodes prevented spontaneous drainage and the formation of fistulae and keloids. Excellent aesthetic results were achieved in patients who presented within 1 month following the onset of lymphadenitis.

## Critique

This was a single-centre prospective observational study conducted over 15 years. It was noted that there was a change in the relative diagnosis over this time period which could have had an impact on the statistical analysis. This could have been improved by conducting a multicentre study which would have amassed more significant numbers in a shorter time. The antituberculous medication which was prescribed was not made clear.

This study highlighted the fact that in a child who presents with a cervical lymphadenitis who has not exhibited any signs or symptoms of common bacterial infections, a diagnosis of mycobacterium should be considered. The optimum treatment strategy is to perform early complete excision of the mass rather than incision and drainage. This led to good aesthetic outcomes and the authors suggest surgeons are not deterred from excision by the possibility of facial nerve problems; these all resolved over time. If the patient has a normal chest X-ray, it is more likely that they will have a diagnosis of NTM. Antituberculosis medication is necessary in patients with MTB dependent on the results of the cultures. This paper provides an excellent review of diagnostic and management strategies for mycobacterial cervical lymphadenitis

# Plastic and maxillofacial surgery

# Part VII

# Plastic and maxillofacial surgery

# Chapter 82

# Classification of fasciocutaneous flaps

Richard Haywood

## Details of study

A flap is a block of tissue that is transferred from one part of the body (a donor site) to another part (a recipient site), incorporating its own blood supply for its own nutrition. The vascular properties of a flap allow large composite blocks of tissue to be transferred to reconstruct complex three-dimensional defects and can enhance the vascularity of the recipient site. This is ideal for reconstruction after oncological resection and post-radiotherapy sites. This is in contrast to a graft that is a block of tissue transferred from one part of the body to another but it is reliant upon the recipient bed for its blood supply and nutrition. This means grafts have to have a large contact area with the recipient bed in relation to their volume and therefore have to be relatively small volume such as composite cartilage cutaneous grafts for alar reconstruction or cover a large surface area such as split thickness skin grafts. The first recognizable descriptions of flap surgery date back to 600 BCE. Sushrata described nasal reconstruction using a block of tissue transferred from the cheek to the nose. A piece of skin was cut to the shape of the nose leaving a pedicle attached to the cheek. The piece of tissue was transferred to the tip of the nose. The technique was modified to use a forehead flap and later became known as the Indian flap.

The technique of tissue transfer using pedicled flaps became the mainstay for reconstruction in modern medicine. This paper describes a classification of flaps.

## Study references

### Main study

Cormack GC, Lamberty BG. A classification of fascio-cutaneous flaps according to their patterns of vascularisation. *Br J Plast Surg* 1984;37:80–7.

## Study design

Expert opinion: level 5 evidence.

## Conclusion

Cormack and Lamberty's classification of fasciocutaneous flaps allows the reconstructive surgeon to plan how to elevate the flap but also acts as an aide-memoire to the vascular anatomy.

## Critique

To overcome the bulkiness of the musculocutaneous flaps fasciocutaneous flaps were developed after reviewing and further investigating the blood supply of the skin and fascia. These flaps allow transfer of thinner more refined blocks of tissue but do not get away from the disadvantage of needing the flap donor site to be near the recipient site. The vascular pedicle of the flap often forming the crucial pivot point for the arc of rotation of the flap.

These pioneering techniques developed a much greater knowledge of the blood supply of flaps but it was not until the advent of the binocular operating microscope in the 1960s that the limitations of having to use adjacent donor and recipient sites could be overcome. The ability to divide and anastomose small arteries and veins down to 0.5 mm in diameter coupled with the detailed knowledge of the blood supply of blocks of tissue allowed the vascular supply of the flap to be isolated, divided, and reattached by microsurgical anastomosis to blood vessels in or adjacent to the donor site. A new era of reconstruction was born, allowing harvest of blocks of specific tissue from distant donor sites to be transferred to recipient sites in one stage, negating the morbidity and time for multiple stages. This allowed the modern reconstructive microsurgeon to adhere to one of Gillies' principles of 'replace like with like' utilizing distant donor sites without the need of the multiple-staged tube pedicle. Revisiting the anatomical knowledge of previous pioneers such as Manchot and Salmon allowed separate tissue components to be harvested in isolation or as separated components on a single vascular pedicle. An example of this is the thoracodorsal artery perforator flap that can be elevated as a purely cutaneous flap composed of subcutaneous fat and skin based on the thoracodorsal vascular axis or can be elevated in combination with muscle such as seratus anterior and bone from the scapula to form a chimeric flap of skin, muscle, and bone only connected by the blood supply of each individual component and the thoracodorsal vascular axis. These chimeric flaps allow more flexibility of placement of each individual component in the recipient defect.

Numerous different classifications have been written in an attempt to classify the bewildering array of types of flap. However, not one classification can suit all and different classifications are required to help select the correct flap to use, plan the flap, help elevate the flap, and transfer the flap. To aid flap selection the flap can be classified according to its composition, i.e. bone, muscle, nerve, fat, fascia, skin. For example, a pectoralis major flap with a skin paddle would be classified as a musculocutaneous flap with its component parts of muscle, fat, and skin; a radial forearm flap would be classified as a fasciocutaneous flap with its component parts of fascia, fat, and skin. Cutaneous skin flaps are frequently described according to shape and geometry—transposition flap, rotational flap, rhomboid flap, bilobed flap. Understanding the geometry and pivot point is vital to plan the flap so it transfers into the recipient site correctly.

Chapter 83

# Vascular territories

Richard Haywood

## Details of studies

Early works by Manchot in the late nineteenth century and later works by Salmon in the early twentieth century gave accurate descriptions of not only the entire skin but also every muscle in the body. Comparison with modern imaging techniques has shown the accuracy of these early descriptions. Neither Manchot nor Salmon described the connections between the blood supply of the deep tissues and the skin, Salmon hinted at a relationship between the two. The pioneering works of Gillies and colleagues (1949) with the tube pedicle overlooked the French texts of Manchot and Salmon, and to overcome the 'battle between blood supply and beauty' strict length to breath ratios were formulated for the tube pedicle design to avoid the constant threat of necrosis of the distal and most crucial part of these flaps. Taylor and Palmer's seminal paper on vascular territories recognizes the importance of these works by Manchot and Salmon.

## Study reference

### Main study

Taylor GI, Palmer JH. The vascular territories (angiosomes) of the body: experimental study and clinical applications. *Br J Plast Surg* 1987;40:113–41.

### Relate studies

Gillies H. Team surgery in cancer. *Proc R Soc Med* 1949; **42**: 176–83.

## Study design

Level of evidence 4: cadaveric studies.

## Results

Based on over 2,000 cadaveric dye studies, radiological studies, and dissections by the Melbourne team, Taylor and Palmer undertook 50 further cadaveric studies to formulate their angiosome model. They modestly state the aim of their paper was to 'provide the reader with a basic understanding of the vascular anatomy which will help clarify nomenclature, aid in the planning of flaps and incisions and provide the basis for explaining certain pathological processes'.

## Conclusion

Four important anatomical concepts recognized from their own work and that of others are highlighted.

1  The blood supply of the body courses within or adjacent to the connective tissue framework whether it is bone, septa, or fascia

2  Vessels course from fixed foci to mobile areas

3  The vascular outflow is a continuous system of arteries linked predominantly by reduced calibre vessels—the choke arteries and arterioles

4  The body is a three dimensional jigsaw made up of composite blocks of tissue supplied by named source arteries. The arteries supplying these blocks of tissue are responsible for the supply of the skin and the underlying structures. These composite units were named angiosomes

## Critique

Taylor and Palmer expand on these concepts in their discussion and are essential reading for the reconstructive surgeon to aid flap dissection, design, and ensure safe reliable outcomes for our patients. Knowing the anatomy of the blood supply of tissue courses within or adjacent to the connective tissue framework allows the reconstructive surgeon to identify the vascular anatomy of a flap with greater ease and dissect the vascular pedicle safely and efficiently. The connective tissue framework and vascular system co exist as interconnecting systems. As the specialized tissues of the mesoderm (i.e. muscles, nerves, fat, and bone) develop within these interconnecting systems the vascular system is captured within and between these specialized tissues. We see the vascular pedicles following their course along intramuscular and intermuscular septae, for example if we split the septum between rectus femoris and vastus lateralis we can easily identify the descending branch of the lateral circumflex femoral artery forming the pedicle for the anterolateral thigh flap.

More distal dissection of the pedicle within the muscle can usually be achieved by splitting the muscle along the intramuscular septae rather than dividing the muscle hence preserving more muscle function at the donor site. The loose connective tissue with an associated cuff of fat may be the first indication of the position of the main pedicle during the dissection of a perforator flap.

Identification of the perforator its self can be made easier knowing it is likely to be found in the septae attaching the skin to the deeper tissue. This is particularly noticeable where there are denser firmer attachments such as the buttock and the inferior gluteal artery perforator flap (IGAP flap).

Perforators are not encountered where there is great mobility and shearing of the superficial tissue over deep tissue but emerge from more stable points with the blood supply of the skin often radiating from fixed concave areas such as the groin into mobile convex areas such as the upper thigh. The perforators can often be identified near the origins of muscles, at the edges of muscles and at intermuscular septae.

The three dimensional concept of the angiosome allows the reconstructive surgeon to develop composite flaps of multiple tissue elements such as bone, muscle, fat and skin. Essential when returning to one of Gillies's core principles of 'replacing like with like' tissue.

# Chapter 84

# Microvascular free flaps in head and neck surgery

Richard Haywood

## Details of study

The vast majority of head and neck flap reconstructions are undertaken after oncological resection within the upper aerodigestive tract. This poses several problems for the reconstructive surgeon. Aggressive oncological resection frequently removes a composite block of specialized tissues such as the tongue, mandible, or palate that has specific high-index quality-of-life functions such as eating, drinking, and talking. An old adage to indicate the success of a head neck reconstruction is that a patient should be able to walk into a pub, order a pint, and be able to drink it. Ensuring they have the confidence in their appearance to be seen in public, have good function for their speech to be intelligible, and appropriate control and swallow to drink without drooling and coughing. The patient group are often elderly with several comorbidities and may be malnourished. However we are seeing a younger age group with human papilloma virus-associated cancers who present a further challenge with them surviving longer and developing second primary tumours requiring higher function and less donor site morbidity from multiple donor sites. The treatment of their cancer frequently involves radiotherapy either as primary treatment or as a adjuvant treatment to surgery. This can mean salvage cases after recurrence can be within a field of irradiated tissue or the reconstruction has to be robust enough to tolerate post operative radiotherapy. The recipient bed is frequently contaminated with nasal and oral secretions making infection, sinus, and fistula formation constant threats to the success of any reconstruction. The dirty oral and nasal cavities may be made in continuity with the sterile intracranial cavity posing a specific life-threatening threat of intracranial sepsis if the intracranial cavity is beached as in complex skull base resection. These factors mean these patients are high risk patients with significant risks of flap failure and system complications. To combat these factors the reconstructive surgeon needs a broad armamentarium of flaps at their disposal.

## Study reference

### Main study

Urken ML, Weinberg H, Buchbinder D, Moscoso JF, Lawson W, Catalano PJ, Biller HF. Microvascular free flaps in head and neck reconstruction. Report of 200 cases and review of complications. *Arch Otolaryngol Head Neck Surg* 1994;**120**:633–40.

## Study design

Level 4: case studies—200 cases

## Conclusion

An overall success rate of 93.5% for free tissue transfers was reported.

## Critique

Small lining defects can be reconstructed with local flaps; however, there is always the concern the defect has been reconstructed with tissue that has been exposed to the same precipitating cancer factors and within the same field change. Regional pedicled and islanded flaps from the head and neck offer good reconstructive options for smaller less complex defects, particularly lining. Examples of these are the forehead flap, temporal flap, nasolabial flap, platysma flap, and submental flaps. For larger defects tissue can be brought in from the trunk with flaps such as the deltopectoral flap, pectoralis major flap, latissimus dorsi flap, and trapezius flap. These have the limitations of their arc of rotation around the pivot point of their vascular pedicle along with their limited composition and bulk. The development of microsurgical free flaps has given a new era to the recon-structive head and neck surgeon enabling complex composite flaps of different tissue to be transferred as single-stage procedures with complex composite tissue defects being reconstructed with similar tissue. The free anterolateral thigh flap has taken over from the free radial forearm flap as the workhorse flap for lining but can be large enough to easily tube for pharyngeal defects. The free fibula bone flap in combination with a skin paddle based on a perforator from the peroneal artery offers boney reconstruction of the mandible with lining. A chimeric flap of bone from the scapula, serratus anterior muscle, latissimus dorsi muscle, and thoracodorsal artery perforator skin flap based on the subscapular artery can provide composite tissue for very large complex defects. There was early scepticism in the use of free flaps in head an neck reconstruction due to its complexity, learning curve, and limited units undertaking free tissue transfer. In 1994 when the clear benefits of free tissue transfer were understood and the learning curve for large units had levelled, Urken et al. (1994) looked at their series of 200 microvascular free flaps to review the morbidity and mortality. They present an early postoperative mortality rate of 1.6% reflecting the high-risk patient group and high-risk surgery. They recognized the specific problems with infection when operating within a dirty field and saw an increased infection rate if multiple cavities were opened. If infection involved the vascular pedicle this lead to complete flap failure. Overall they had a success rate of 93.5% only loosing 13 free flaps. They recognized their learning curve with 13 is-chaemia-related flap complications occurring in the first 75 cases of the series compared to 5 in the last 125 cases of the series. In selected cases they used pedicled flaps to sal-vage cases but also to cover the vascular pedicle and microsurgical anastomosis. We are coming to the end of the fifth decade of microvascular free flap surgery and the early pioneers have allowed us to view microvascular free flap surgery as a standard technique with surgeons being trained to avoid the steep learning curve of those brave patients of the early pioneers. The rehabilitation benefits of single stage complex composite tissue reconstruction far outweigh the risks.

# Chapter 85

# The free thigh flap

Richard Haywood

## Details of studies

In head and neck oncological reconstruction a thin pliable flap is frequently required; in the new microsurgical era the radial forearm flap became the workhorse flap in head and neck reconstruction. It is thin, pliable, can be contoured easily to reconstruct intra-oral defects, has a long vascular pedicle, large calibre artery, large calibre vein, is easy to harvest, and can be harvested synchronously during head and neck tumour resection. However, its harvest can cause significant donor site morbidity; its harvest sacrifices one of the main axial arteries to the hand (the radial artery). Larger flaps require the donor site to be skin grafted. A larger flap with less donor site morbidity was required. Song et al.'s paper on the free thigh flap brought this ideal flap and set the scene for a new era of perforator flap reconstruction.

## Study references

Song YG, Chen GZ, Song YL. The free thigh flap: a new free flap concept based on the septocutaneous artery. *Br J Plast Surg* 1984;37:149–59.

## Study design

Descriptive study: level 5—expert opinion

## Conclusion

Song et al. (1984) described the anterolateral thigh flap. The vascular pedicle of this flap is the descending branch of the lateral circumflex femoral artery and its venae commitantes which give off branches that perforate the deep fascia to supply the skin; hence the name perforator flap. The flap is thin and pliable, has a long vascular pedicle of greater than 8–12 cm in length, and a large calibre artery and vein, greater than 2 mm in diameter. The donor site can usually be closed directly with flaps up to 6 cm wide and 20 cm long. Very large flaps of up to 800 cm$^2$ can be harvested if the donor site is skin grafted to gain closure. If the flap is thick due to the patient's body habitus it can be thinned by carefully dissecting excess fat while preserving the vascular pedicle and its branches. Cutaneous nerves can be included in the flap to anastomose to nerves in the recipient site giving a degree of sensation of the flap. The flap can be elevated synchronously during head and neck tumour resection, and being further away from the head and neck the flap elevation team will be less intrusive into the tumour resection teams space.

## Critique

In the modern era of perforator flap reconstruction flap elevation is relatively simple once the basic technique of individual perforator identification, protection, and dissection is mastered. If two perforators are used the flap can be divided into two to reconstruct full thickness defects of the cheek. The long potential length of the flap means it is easily tubed to reconstruct pharyngeal defects. These qualities mean it has taken over from the radial forearm flap as the work horse flap in head and neck reconstruction.

In their seminal paper, Song et al. (1984) also describe the medial thigh flap and posterior thigh, also based on perforators from other deeper vessels in the thigh. This illustrates the versatility of perforator flap technique and numerous further perforator flaps have since been described mirroring the original anatomical descriptions described by Manchot over 100 years before. Since Song et al.'s paper the reconstructive microsurgeon has even more choice to harvest ideal tissue from numerous body areas and reduce donor site morbidity and preserve the function of underlying muscles. For example, the supraclavicular artery perforator flap can offer a local pedicled flap to cover defects of the neck without the need for microsurgical anastomosis and utilizing the skin over the lateral leg supplied by a perforator of the peroneal artery allows the use of a reliable skin paddle in combination with the fibula bone yet separated enough to allow convenient insetting. We are now entering an era where microsurgeons are selecting a block of tissue which is suitable, identifying the perforator, and dissecting this back to a vessel that is large enough and long enough to anastomose to vessels at the recipient site—the free-style free flap.

Chapter 86

# Skull base flaps

Rajiv Bhalla

## Details of study

In the paper by Hadad et al. (2006), work by Hirsch from the early 1950s examining random pattern rotation flaps in the nose was further refined by designing a much more robust, neurovascular pedicled flap of the nasal septum mucoperiosteum and mucoperichondrium. Rather than being a random pattern flap, the Hadad–Bassagasteguy flap (HBF) is based on the posterior nasoseptal arteries, which are branches of the posterior nasal artery, which is one of the terminal branches of the internal maxillary artery. The objective was to reduce postoperative cerebrospinal fluid (CSF) leak after expanded endonasal approaches (EEAs) of the ventral skull base.

## Study references

### Main study

Hadad G, Bassagasteguy L, Carrau RL, Mataza JC, Kassam A, Snyderman CH, et al. A novel reconstructive technique after endoscopic expanded endonasal approaches: vascular pedicle nasoseptal flap. *Laryngoscope* 2006;**116**:1882–6.

### Related reference

Hegazy HM, Carrau RL, Snyderman CH, Kassam A, Zweig J. Transnasal endoscopic repair of cerebrospinal fluid rhinorrhea: a meta-analysis. *Laryngoscope* 2000;**110**:1166–72.

## Study design

A retrospective review of patients undergoing endonasal skull base surgery at two university medical centres: University of Rosario, Argentina, and University of Pittsburgh Medical Center, USA.

| | |
|---|---|
| Level of evidence | 4 |
| Randomization | None |
| Number of patients | 43 |
| Inclusion criteria | Patients undergoing expanded endonasal approaches for CSF leaks (traumatic and spontaneous), meningoencephalocoeles, clival chordomas, aesthesioneuroblastoma, craniopharyngioma, meningiomas, and extrasellar extension of pituitary tumours |

| Exclusion criteria | None |
| --- | --- |
| Follow-up | Minimum of 2 months postoperative endoscopic examinations and imaging |

## Outcome measures

### Primary endpoint

Completion of an EEA, with a resulting large dural defect, requiring repair with a HBF.

### Secondary endpoints

None.

## Results

+ Forty-three patients, 31 men and 12 women, age range from 22 to 74 years
+ No CSF leak in 41 patients
+ Transient leak in two patients, successfully repaired with focal fat graft
+ No other infectious or wound complication such as partial or total loss of the flap
+ One posterior epistaxis arising from the posterior nasal artery controlled with electrocautery
+ Minor asymptomatic synechiae requiring no treatment

## Conclusions

Use of the pedicled vascularized HBF has greatly reduced the incidence of postoperative CSF leak after expanded endonasal approaches to the ventral skull base compared with traditional multilayer repair techniques.

## Critique

Postoperative CSF leak in patients with large dural defects after anterior and ventral skull base surgery can be problematic. Small defects of the ventral skull base may be reconstructed using a variety of techniques with a success rate of greater than 95%, as described in the meta-analysis from Hegazy et al. Extrapolating these subdural inlay and onlay techniques in larger defects proved not to be an efficient means of reducing postoperative CSF leak, with failures generally occurring due to graft migration and poor adherence. The HBF and the series of cases presented in this paper have transformed the management of large anterior skull base dural defects by greatly reducing postoperative CSF leak rates. It is one of the extremely important reasons why, along with better anatomic understanding, improved training and enhanced instrumentation, that the sub-specialty area of extended endoscopic approaches to the ventral skull base has gained acceptance in the past 10–15 years.

## Additional references

Chin D, Harvey RJ. Endoscopic reconstruction of frontal, cribriform and ethmoid skull base defects. *Adv Otorhinolaryngol* 2013;74:104–18.

Hirsch O. Successful closure of cerebrospinal fluid rhinorrhea by endonasal surgery. *Arch Otolaryngol* 1952;**56**:1–12.

Zuniga MG, Turner JH, Chandra RK. Updates in anterior skull base reconstruction. *Current Opin Otolaryngol Head Neck Surg* 2016;**24**:75–82.

Additional references

Chapter 87

# Classification of facial fractures

Andrew Sidebottom

## Details of studies

Professor Le Fort aimed to determine the lines of least resistance in fractures of the face. His original studies defined how we describe fractures of the midfacial skeleton. They are based on a series of experiments on cadaveric bodies and decapitated heads using blunt impact such as clubs, sides of tables, or even a vice! Clearly cadaveric ethics were limited at the turn of the twentieth century.

## Study reference

### Main study

Le Fort R. Experimental study of fractures of the upper jaw parts 1, 2 and 3. *Rev Chir de Paris* 1901;23:208–27, 360–79, 479–507. The review of this article is from a translation by Paul Tessier *Plastic Reconstruc Surg* 1972;**50**:497–506, 600–605.

## Study design

Caderveric study of humans with a range of traumas inflicted to determine the pattern of facial fractures in response to different types of blunt trauma.

## Outcome measures

Observation and description of fractures and injuries sustained.

## Results

Anteroposterior blows to the region of the upper lip produce the first type of fracture originally described by, and named after, Guerin. This is a separation of the upper teeth and dentoalveolar bone from the remainder of the upper jaw and is presently known as the Le Fort type 1 fracture. A transverse fracture which runs from below the nostrils (below or above the anterior nasal spine), 1 cm below the zygoma and extends into the lower part of the pterygoid plates. This fracture may be unilateral and associated with a midline palatal split.

Lateral blows on the lower part of the upper jaw produced a different fracture pattern. While these produced Le Fort type 1 fractures; in addition, contracoup mandibular fractures and ipsilateral malar fractures were also seen. If the force were from somewhat below, then the fracture would extend upwards to give higher level fractures particularly on the contralateral side.

A force directed from below against the upper anterior alveolus leads to the second type of fracture pattern—Le Fort 2. This is a pyramidal fracture extending from the nasal bones above into the orbital floor behind the nasolacrimal ducts, through the orbital rim and below the zygomatic buttress and into the mid portion of the pterygomaxillary fissure through the pterygoid plates. This type of fracture should be considered when a significant blow occurs rather than just nasal bone fracture.

Blows backward on the midface produced similar or localized fractures patterns including Le Fort 2 type injuries with a midline palatal split.

Blows to the mandible exerting force then onto the midface leads to a pattern which depends on whether the mouth is open or closed at the time of force application. When open the injuries are the same as when the force is directly applied to the alveolus, Le Fort 2 type pattern, because of the mandible generating the same impact on the upper jaw. When closed there is a compression between the mandible and skull base.

Direct blows to the lateral face over the malar lead to the classic zygomaticomaxillary fracture with fracture lines described at the zygomaticofrontal area, infraorbital rim, zygomatic arch, and between the malar buttress and the maxilla. Currently, this remains the most common injury seen in UK practice and is due to interpersonal violence.

Swinging blows to the zygomatic region resemble what may be seen following a fall from height. These similarly produce a zygomatic complex fracture, but with increasing force this may extend to include separation at the Le Fort 1 level unilaterally with a midline palatal split and include one side of the nose—naso-orbito-zygomatic fracture.

Blows to the anterolateral malar with the head supported again produce a similar zygomatic injury with an associated bilateral Le Fort 1 type injury with involvement of the ipsilateral nasal bone. In contrast, when the head was supported over the opposite malar the fracture pattern was more symmetrical; however, when compressed in a vice both zygomas fractured followed by the temporal bones.

An anteroposterior force onto the whole of the face produced separation of the whole of the midface from the skull—Le Fort 3. The remainder of the midfacial bones were separately fractured in differing positions. Le Fort goes on to describe the third fracture pattern in detail, advising that higher level fractures around the nasal bone involve the cribriform plate of the ethmoid, extend back through the frontal process of the maxillary bone and posteriorly through the lacrimal bones and ethmoid air cells. It extends back towards the optic canal and drops below this extending to the lateral wall of the orbit separating the sphenoid process and frontal bone from the zygomatic bone through the pterygomaxillary fissure to the base of the pterygoid process, the zygomatic arch often breaking in several places.

## Conclusion

Le Fort describes the trauma necessary to produce a fracture of the face. The fragile parts of the facial skeleton are not very easily accessible to direct trauma since they are so covered with soft tissue which means the energy of a blow to the face is dissipated. Fractures occur, but in a different manner from long bones. The study eloquently describes the exact patterns which occur due to various traumatic injuries. This was particularly helpful in times preceding the ready availability of imaging and the classification is still in widespread use today.

## Critique

This study remains key to our understanding of the principles of stability and reconstruction required for trauma management. Gruss (1985, 1986, 1990) understood this in his series of articles which investigated repositioning of the facial pillars to facilitate accurate repositioning of the facial structures. This principle, from Le Forts work, relies on placing the horizontal and vertical buttresses back into anatomical alignment by surgical exposure and direct internal fixation, with the intervening minor fragments being largely ignored. If necessary bone grafts should be harvested to use to support the pillars. Paul Manson (1980) subsequently expanded on these principles particularly in relation to the management of subunits and soft tissues. The reader is referred to these articles as a basis which is still relevant today in the management of traumatic injuries to the midface but is beyond the scope of this text.

### Additional references

Gruss JS. Naso-ethmoid-orbital fractures. Classification and role of primary bone grafting. *Plast Reconstr Surg* 1985;**75**:303–15.

Gruss JS, Mackinnon SE. Complex maxillary fractures: role of buttress reconstruction and immediate bone grafts. *Plast Reconstr Surg* 1986;**78**:9–22.

Gruss JS, Pollock RA, Phillips JH, Antonyshyn O. Combined injuries of the cranium and face. *Br J Plast Surg* 1989;**42**:385–98.

Gruss JS, Van Wyck L, Phillips JH, Antonyshyn O. The importance of the zygomatic arch in complex midfacial fracture repair and correction of post-traumatic orbitozygomatic deformities. *Plast Reconstr Surg* 1990;**85**:878–90.

Lee RH, Gamble B, Robertson B, Manson PN. The MCFONTZL classification system for soft-tissue injuries to the face. *Plast Reconstr Surg* 1999;**103**:1150–7.

Manson PN, Clark N, Robertson B, Slezak S, Wheatly M, Van der Kolk C, Iliff N. Subunit principles in midface fractures: the importance of sagittal buttresses, soft tissue reductions and sequencing treatment of segmental fractures. *Plast Reconstr Surg* 1999;**103**:1287–306.

Manson PN, Hoopes JE, Su CT. Structural pillars of the facial skeleton: an approach to the management of Le Fort fractures. *Plast Reconstr Surg* 1980;**66**:54–61.

# Chapter 88

# The temporomandibular joint

Andrew Sidebottom

## Details of studies

Temporomandibular joint (TMJ) disorders are common, affecting an estimated 8–15% of women and 3–10% of men. Most involve either muscular or skeletal structures or both and lead to pain and dysfunction. The term 'internal derangements' refers to conditions when the articular disc is displaced from its original position on the condyle of the mandible. The TMJ is a complex joint, with a range of movements including hinge-like, sliding, lateral, protrusive, and retrusive movements.

Classification and explanation of both normal and pathological movements is important to facilitate correct diagnosis and optimal management.

## Study reference

### Main study

Wilkes CH. Internal derangements of the temporomandibular joint: pathological variations. *Arch Otolaryngol Head Neck* 1989;115:469–77.

## Study design

A retrospective single surgeon comparison of clinical, radiologic, and operative data Analysis of 540 operations and 740 joints.

## Outcome measures

Correlation between clinical signs, radiologic findings either with tomography, arthrography or magnetic resonance imaging (MRI) and clinical findings at open joint surgery.

## Results

The data presented are based on 740 joints. Female predominance in a 7:1 ratio. This is common in TMJ practice. The mean age was 31 years with a peak in the third decade. A pre-existing correlation was stated based on previous studies and tabulated in the paper. Wilkes classifies five stages of TMJ disease: stage 1 'Early', stage 2 'Early/Intermediate', stage 3 'Intermediate', stage 4 'Intermediate/Late', and stage 5 'Late'. For each stage, Wilkes details the typical clinical and radiological features that are usually identified.

The majority (97%) of treated patients were in stages 3–5. Periods of increased activity and quiescence were noted. Indeed, there were periods when the bite of the teeth was affected (malocclusion). Patients with late stage disease tended to be older with longer standing problems.

The hypothesis then followed that the predisposing factor was disc displacement and that over time this progressed through the various stages of severity with periods of quiescence. Inflammatory changes were noted in the posterior attachment and these were correlated with forwards displacement of the condyle and associated malocclusion. As the disease progressed it is proposed that the posterior disc becomes thickened with catching and therefore locking occurring. Ultimately the disc becomes permanently stuck anterior to the condyle and does not move as the normal disc–condyle complex would in unison.

Causality was hypothesized to be due to macro-trauma potentially in around 50% of cases and repetitive micro-trauma in the remainder. While bruxism may be a predisposing factor it is stated that those with stress largely had normal radiologic imaging and that this was not a predisposing factor.

## Critique

This is a large retrospective case series and therefore dependent on accurate note keeping. It categorizes several stages of disease which merge with each other, but seem to be correlated to outcome. With many such studies the correlations made may be related to the authors interpretation of the findings in relation to their understanding of the disease process.

It is clear from subsequent literature that progression through the Wilkes categories does not necessarily occur and that disease progress can be arrested with remodelling occurring leaving the patient with a functional and manageable joint without the need for surgical intervention. Similarly, there is evidence that even without treatment the long-term outcome for patients with a clicking joint is generally benign.

Limitation of movement may be related to disc position but increasingly lubrication is felt to play a major factor and may be one of the reasons why arthroscopy and arthrocentesis is so successful in improving symptomatology. Muscle spasm may also contribute to limited motion as a response to pain from the intra-articular inflammatory changes or independently due to muscle hyperactivity. Reducing intra-articular inflammatory mediators by the dilutional process of arthrocentesis may contribute to the success of this procedure.

This remains a landmark paper in the assessment and management of TMJ disorders as it is a large series with pertinent findings.

## Discussion

While this is considered the definitive paper (Wilkes 1989), Wilkes described the pathological variants much earlier than this using double contrast arthrography (Wilkes 1978). Subsequent studies used other methods of radiologic analysis (Wilkes 1978a,b, 1990, 1991; Schell 1987). Double contrast arthrography is a technique where radio-opaque dye is injected into the upper then a different dye into the lower joint space to determine the disc position and integrity. It is noteworthy that while this has largely been superseded by MRI as a diagnostic tool for assessment of TMJ dysfunction (TMD), arthrography is considerably more accurate in diagnosing disc tear, with MRI being accurate in around 50% of cases in the best hands (Shen 2014; Tura 2015). The current gold standard for diagnosis in TMD is arthroscopy (Ahmed 2012; Weedon 2013; Tzanidakis 2013). Despite now being more able to assess the stage of TMD the outcomes of management are not statistically related to Wilkes stage although most studies show a trend towards worse outcome in lower Wilkes stage (Tzanidakis 2013).

Despite the Wilkes staging being now nearly 40 years old, it remains the mainstay of assessment of severity of TMD. It is, however, like many staging protocols, a guide rather than an absolute indicator for further treatment. It has not been superseded by a better system and until either arthroscopy or MRI can be shown to directly correlate outcome with currently unknown findings it will remain the only choice in outcome studies on TMD.

## References

Ahmed N, Sidebottom A, O'Connor M, Kerr H-L. Prospective outcome assessment of the therapeutic benefits of arthroscopy and arthrocentesis of the temporomandibular joint. *Br J Oral Maxillofac Surg* 2012;**50**;745–8.

Schellhas KP, Wilkes CH, Omlie MR, Block JC, Larsen JW, Idelkope BI. Temporomandibular joint imaging. Practical application of available technology. *Arch Otolaryngol Head Neck Surg* 1987;**113**:744–8.

Shen P, Huo L, Zhang SY, Yang C, Cai XY, Liu XM. Magnetic resonance imaging applied to the diagnosis of perforation of the temporomandibular joint. *J Craniomaxillofac Surg* 2014;**42**:874–8.

Tzanidakis K, Sidebottom AJ. How accurate is arthroscopy of the temporomandibular joint? A comparison of findings in patients who had open operations after arthroscopic management failed. *Br J Oral Maxillofac Surg* 2013;**51**:968–70.

Tzanidakis K, Sidebottom AJ. Outcomes of open TMJ surgery following failure to improve after arthroscopy: Is there an algorithm for success? *Br J Oral Maxillofac Surg* 2013;**51**:818–21.

Weedon S, Ahmed N, Sidebottom AJ. Prospective assessment of outcomes following disposable arthroscopy of the TMJ. *Br J Oral Maxillofac Surg* 2013;**51**:625–9.

Wilkes CH. Arthrography of the temporomandibular joint in patients with the TMJ pain-dysfunction syndrome. *Miss Med* 1978a;**61**:645–52.

Wilkes CH. Structural and functional alterations of the temporomandibular joint. *Northwest Dent* 1978b;**57**:287–94.

Wilkes CH. Internal derangements of the temporomandibular joint: pathological variations. *Arch Otolaryngol Head Neck* 1989;**115**;469–77.

Wilkes CH. Internal derangements of the temporomandibular joint. Pathological variations. *Northwest Dent* 1990;**69**:25–32.

Wilkes CH. Surgical treatment of internal derangements of the temporomandibular joint. A long-term study. *Arch Otolaryngol Head Neck Surg* 1991;**117**:64–72.

Yura S, Harada S, Kobayashi K. Diagnostic accuracy on magnetic resonance imaging for the diagnosis of osteoarthritis of the temporomandibular joint. *J Clin Diagn Res* 2015;**9**:95–7.

# Chapter 89

# Drooling

## Andrew Sidebottom

## Details of studies

Drooling or sialorrhoea affects up to 58% of children with neurological impairment with around 33% being severely affected. The management of this condition has largely been symptomatic with use of anticholinergic drugs (mainly scopolamine), although these had significant systemic side-effects. More recently transdermal hyoscine patches have been used with fewer side-effects and medical management should remain the first-line therapy for these individuals.

Wilkie et al. (1967) attempted to suggest a surgical management strategy based on a physiological understanding that a reduction in production of saliva could be achieved. This was by eliminating the glands which produce the majority of the saliva (submandibular glands have a constant flow and deliver around 75% of saliva). Similarly redirecting the flow of the other major glands (parotids) should reduce the salivary amount by around 85%.

## Study references

### Main study

Wilkie TF. The problem of drooling in cerebral palsy: a surgical approach. *Can J Surg* 1967;**10**:160–72.

### Related references

Wilkie TF. The surgical treatment of drooling. A follow-up report of five years' experience. *Plast Reconstr Surg* 1970;**45**:549–54.

Wilkie TF, Brody GS. The surgical treatment of drooling. A ten-year review. *Plast Reconstr Surg* 1977;**59**:791–7.

## Study design

Retrospective review of outcome data of a new surgical technique—bilateral submandibular gland excision and rerouting of Stensen's duct (Wilkie procedure). The further two studies show outcomes up to 10 years with minimum duration of follow-up of 18 months.

## Outcome measures

### Primary endpoint

Reduction in drooling.

### Secondary endpoint

Complications.

## Results

Successful in reducing drooling in 86% of patients. No significant morbidity reported.

## Conclusion

Bilateral submandibular gland removal with redirection of the parotid ducts provides a successful method of management of children with drooling secondary to cerebral palsy.

## Critique

The reported morbidity for this procedure was said to be low but is not recorded. Subsequent surgical approaches have addressed the issue of reducing salivary flow in a number of ways, such as transtympanic division of the chorda tympani and the tympanic nerve and plexus which control the salivary flow for the submandibular gland. These procedures have been shown to be effective in 83% of cases when combined but only 62% of cases when just the chorda tympani was sectioned. A variant of the 'Wilkie procedure' with ligation of the parotid ducts produced similar results with 86% success. Unfortunately, while the authors report less morbidity, in common with many older studies actual figures are difficult to find. Redirection of just the submandibular duct was the next suggestion. This is again a 'simpler procedure with less morbidity' than gland excision. Unfortunately, most studies report rates of submandibular swelling, ranula formation, and sialadentis occurring in 10–20% of cases. The reported satisfaction from carers remained high.

A meta-analysis of the data from surgical management strategies still suggests that the most successful outcomes are achieved using the original 'Wilkie procedure' (86%), with the least successful outcomes using four-duct ligation (61%). The use of botulinum injections into the gland parenchyma has been suggested as a long-term management strategy. While this gives good short-term results, the injections require repeats every 6 months. In the patient population studied, cooperation is difficult and hence general anaesthesia, albeit for a short period of time, has to be utilized and hence the associated risks of this with respiratory complications have to be considered. Ultrasound guidance, while it provides an accurate positioning of the needle, does not seem to add benefit. The use of botulinum has however shown a benefit in reducing the incidence of respiratory complications in this group of patients by reducing aspiration.

Owing to the need for repeated general anaesthesia the author would suggest a trial of botulinum injected into the submandibular gland, and if successful bilateral submandibular gland removal, as this proved effective in every case of our series. The physiologic principle behind this is also sound as there is no excess saliva directed into the compromised pharyngeal space. Also, the submandibular glands deliver 75% of saliva and are constantly active, but from a dental perspective there remains the 'on demand' flow of the parotids allowing cleansing of the teeth after oral intake. This should help to maintain oral hygiene and reduce the risk of dental caries and periodontal disease. There is minimal scarring and the procedure in an otherwise healthy gland has proven to be safe as well as effective, and is routinely performed as a day case procedure as drainage is not needed.

## Additional references

Brundage SR, Moore WD. Submandibular gland resection and bilateral parotid duct ligation as a management for chronic drooling in cerebral palsy. *Plast Reconstr Surg* 1989;**83**:443–6.

Grewal DS, Hiranandani NL, Rangwalla ZA, Sheode JH. Transtympanic neurectomies for control of drooling. *Auris Nasus Larynx* 1984;**11**:109–14.

Reed J, Mans C, Brietzke SE. Surgical management of drooling: a meta-analysis. *Arch Otolaryngol Head Neck Surg* 2009;**135**:924–31.

Rosen A, Komisar A, Pphir D, Marshak G. Experience with the Wilkie procedure for sialorrhea. *Ann Otol Rhinol Laryngol* 1990;**99**(Pt 1);730–2.

Sidebottom AJ, May JE, Madahar AK. Role of botulinum toxin A injection into the submandibular salivary glands as an assessment for the subsequent removal of the submandibular glands in the management of children with sialorrhoea. *Br J Oral Maxillofac Surg* 2013;**51**:113–6.

Tabmassebi JF, Curzon ME. Prevalence of drooling in children with cerebral palsy attending special schools. *Dev Med Child Neurol* 2003;**45**:613–7.

Part VIII

# Miscellaneous

Chapter 90

# Steroids for children undergoing tonsillectomy

Phil Hodgson

## Details of studies

After tonsillectomy pain, nausea, vomiting, and delays returning to eating are common, particularly in children. Dexamethasone is sometimes given in a single intravenous dose at the time of surgery to try to prevent vomiting in the early postoperative period. A Cochrane Review about the efficacy of this practice was first published in 2003. The objective was to quantify whether a single dose of dexamethasone reduced postoperative morbidity in paediatric tonsillectomy and adenotonsillectomy.

## Study references

### Main study

Steward DL, Grisel J, Meinzen-Derr J. Steroids for improving recovery following tonsillectomy in children (Review). *Cochrane Database Syst Rev* 2011;**10**:CD003997.

### Related reference

Steward DL, Welge JA, Myer CM. Steroids for improving recovery following tonsillectomy in children. *Cochrane Database Syst Rev* 2003;**1**:CD003997.

## Study design

| Type | Meta-analysis |
|---|---|
| Level of evidence | 1a |
| The intervention | A single dose of intraoperative dexamethasone at a dose ranging from 0.15 mg/kg to 1 mg/kg |
| Inclusion criteria | Randomized, double-blind, placebo-controlled trials containing patients under 18 years of age undergoing tonsillectomy or adenotonsillectomy |
| Number of included trials | 19 (10 new studies combined with nine studies identified in the earlier 2003 review)<br>Studies sought in all language formats as of 29 October 2010 |

| Three primary endpoints | The number of children experiencing emesis in the first 24 hours following tonsillectomy or adenotonsillectomy (15 studies, 1,273 participants) |
| | The number of children returning to a soft or solid diet by postoperative day one (five studies, 452 participants) |
| | Pain in the first 24 hours as measured by a visual analogue scale (VAS) using a 0–10 scale range, where 0 is no pain and 10 the most pain imaginable (eight studies, 652 participants) |

## Results

The overall incidence of emesis was compared. The incidence of emesis and return to diet were also reported using the 'risk ratio' (RR) of the group receiving dexamethasone relative to the placebo group, hence also known as 'relative risk'. This is the ratio of the risk of the event occurring in the two groups. Ninety-five per cent confidence intervals (CI) were also given. The number needed to treated (NNT) was also determined.

Pain scores were reported as the mean difference in the VAS pain scores between the two groups.

Sensitivity analyses were also conducted to exclude potential reporting bias. The authors further analysed the data with the assumption that those studies with missing data had missing data that matched the pooled average result of all the studies. When the process was applied to pain scores, the missing data was assumed to have a null result and the mean difference recalculated. In each case, the statistical significance remained, effectively excluding significant reporting bias.

| | Steroid vs. placebo | p |
|---|---|---|
| Emesis rate % (SD) | 21% vs. 48% | <0.00001 |
| Emesis RR value (95% CI) | 0.49 (0.41 to 0.58) | <0.00001 |
| NNT value | 4.17 | |
| Diet RR value (95% CI) | 1.45 (1.15 to 1.83) | <0.001 |
| NNT value | 4.76 | |
| Mean difference in pain score value (95% CI) | −1.07 (−1.73 to −0.41) | 0.001 |

## Conclusion

In children, a single dose of perioperative dexamethasone is associated with reduced vomiting rates and earlier return to food intake on the first postoperative day. It also appears to exert a modest analgesic effect. From the data presented, the broad headlines are that if children are given perioperative dexamethasone, their chances of vomiting are halved and they are 50% more likely to eat on the first day. They are also likely to report being more comfortable.

## Critique

Despite well-debated limitations, meta-analyses such as this study undoubtedly provide more persuasive, quantitative outcome data than smaller individual trials or a review article. The authors highlight the difficulties in pooling different surgical and anaesthetic techniques, dexamethasone dose, and patient demographics.

The almost 10-fold range of dexamethasone dosage across the included studies is noteworthy. The lower dose in the range included in the analysis (0.15 mg/kg) is more representative of that used in anaesthetic clinical guidelines both in the USA and UK. Therefore, although suboptimal dosing in the included studies in unlikely, the effects observed may be a function of higher doses of dexamethasone not routinely given.

Although beyond the scope of this discussion, the surgical technique of tonsil removal is reported to have an influence on early pain scores. Likewise, anaesthetic agents and techniques vary in their analgesic and emetogenic profiles. The reduction in pain score, although statistically significant, is modest (1 point on a 10-point scale) and may not be clinically visible. Furthermore, studies using facial and behavioural pain assessment tools such as used in younger age groups are not included.

The inter-relationship between nausea, appetite, food intake, and postoperative pain in children is undoubtedly complex. The antiemetic mechanism of action of dexamethasone is still not understood. Although early feeding may be a reflection of nausea reduction, the drug also appears to directly stimulate appetite and well-being in adults. The beneficial effects quantified in this review are mirrored in adult studies where dexamethasone has been shown to reduce postoperative emesis as well as reducing inflammation, tissue oedema, and pain. The stimulation of appetite, maintenance of glucose levels, and feeling of well-being appear to contribute to earlier discharge of adult patients after routine daycare surgery.

Given other physiological effects of corticosteroids, there is an understandable reluctance to use higher, or repeated, dosing of dexamethasone to gain further benefit. It is worth noting that a more recent meta-analysis and systematic review (referenced below) found that the risk of postoperative haemorrhage in children is not increased by dexamethasone use with or without non-steroidal anti-inflammatory drugs. The reader is directed to two linked editorials also referenced below stating the case for and the case against routine use of dexamethasone in adult surgical patients. Both give an excellent overview of the other considerations when using the drug.

The use of intravenous dexamethasone perioperatively is now widespread in paediatric anaesthesia. This well-constructed paper reassures surgeons and anaesthetists that there is much to be gained from its use.

## Additional references

**Association of Paediatric Anaesthetists of Great Britain & Ireland.** Guidelines on the prevention of post-operative vomiting in children. London: APAGBI, 2016.

**Bartlett R, Hartle AJ** Routine use of dexamethasone for postoperative nausea and vomiting: the case for. *Anaesthesia* 2013;**68**:892–6.

**Bellis JR, Pirmohamed RM, Nunn AJ, Loke YK, De S, Golder S, Kirkham JJ** Dexamethasone and haemorrhage risk in paediatric tonsillectomy: a systematic review and meta-analysis *Br J Anaesthes* 2014;**113**: 23–42.

**De Oliveira GJ, Almeida M, Benzon H, McCarthy R.** Perioperative single dose systemic dexamethasone for postoperative pain: a meta-analysis of randomized controlled trials. *Anesthesiology* 2011;**115**:575–88.

**Gan TJ, Meyer T, Apfel CC, Chung F, Davis PJ, Eubanks S,** et al. Consensus guidelines for managing postoperative nausea and vomiting. *Anesthes Analges* 2003;**97**:62–71.

**Kakodkar PS.** Routine use of dexamethasone for postoperative nausea and vomiting: the case for. *Anaesthesia* 2013;**68**:889–91.

**Steward DL, Grisel J, Meinzen-Derr J.** Steroids for improving recovery following tonsillectomy in children (Review). *Cochrane Database Syst Rev* 2011;**10**:CD003997.

# Chapter 91

# Implications of codeine administration after tonsillectomy

Phil Hodgson

## Details of studies

Historically, codeine was thought to be a weak opioid analgesic and was widely used after adenotonsillectomy. It was considered synergistic with paracetamol, less likely than non-steroidal anti-inflammatory drugs to affect platelet function and less likely to cause postoperative respiratory depression in patients presenting with obstructive sleep apnoea (OSA) than other opioids. However, with the mapping of the human genome and the advances in the study of pharmacogenetics, the metabolism of codeine has been shown to show genetic variation within the population that questions the assumption that it is a safe and effective opioid analgesic in all patients.

The analgesic activity of codeine depends on its conversion to morphine by the hepatic cytochrome P-450 isoenzyme 2D6 (CYP2D6). Unfortunately, the gene encoding this isoenzyme shows variation within the patient population. Around 90% of the population are 'extensive metabolizers' and so respond in a predictable way by bioactivating 10% of codeine to morphine and gaining clinical benefit. However, 5–10% of the population have no functional alleles for CYP2D6 and are 'poor metabolizers' and so gain little to no benefit from the drug. Of most concern is a final population of 'ultrametabolizers' who have two or more functional alleles for the isoenzyme and show a gene–dose effect in converting codeine into 50–75% more morphine than usual and may be at risk of opioid overdose. Ultrametabolizers are over-represented in certain demographic groups, most notably those of North African and Middle Eastern heritage where an incidence of up to 15% has been reported.

Opioid sensitivity is also affected by other factors. Of note, patients of all ages with OSA are known to show particular sensitivity to opioid-induced respiratory depression. Although 70–80% of children lose their OSA in the long term following adenotonsillectomy, many see their symptoms paradoxically worsen immediately after surgery. Having previously presented a fatal case report in 2009 of a toddler with OSA who had received codeine, the same authors present a further three cases.

## Study references

### Main study

**Kelly LE, Rieder M, Van den Anker J, Malkin B, Ross C, Neely MN**, et al. More codeine fatalities after tonsillectomy in North American children. *Pediatrics* 2012;**129**:1343–7.

### Related references

**Racoosin JA, Roberson DW, Pacanowski MA, Nielsen DR.** New evidence about an old drug—risk with codeine after adenotonsillectomy. *N Engl J Med* 2013;**268**:2155–7.

## Study design

| Type | Case study series of three patients<br>Paediatric adenotonsillectomy<br>Age and weight standard dosing with codeine |
| --- | --- |
| Patient group | Elective |
| Level of evidence | 4 |
| Case 1 | 4-year-old, 27.6-kg boy. First Nations Canadian descent<br>Prescribed 8 mg oral codeine five times per day<br>After four doses given at home had fatal cardiorespiratory arrest<br>Plasma codeine level in the expected therapeutic range<br>Plasma morphine level 17.6 ng/mL (therapeutic morphine range 2.4–6.6 ng/mL) |
| Case 2 | 3-year-old, 14.4-kg girl. Middle Eastern descent<br>15 mg 4–6 hourly. Two doses in hospital and two at home<br>Respiratory depression and unresponsive. Successfully resuscitated<br>Plasma morphine level 17 ng/mL (therapeutic morphine range 2.4-6.6 ng/mL) |
| Case 3 | 5-year-old, 29 kg boy. Snoring history<br>Prescribed 12 mg oral codeine every 4 hours<br>24 hours post surgery found dead at home<br>Plasma codeine level in the expected therapeutic range<br>Plasma morphine level 30 ng/mL (therapeutic morphine range 2.4–6.6 ng/mL) |

## Conclusion

These cases demonstrate that codeine after adenotonsillectomy may not be safe in young children with OSA syndrome

## Critique

In response to the paper, the FDA used their Adverse Event Reporting System (FAERS) to evaluate the safety record of codeine in children. Their search identified 10 deaths and three near fatal respiratory events in the USA between 1969 and 2012. Eight had been in children undergoing adenotonsillectomy. However, a search for morphine, hydrocodone, and oxycodone revealed no such unexplained cases. Therefore in late 2012, the FDA made codeine contraindicated in paediatric patients undergoing adenotonsillectomy and manufacturers of codeine distributed in the USA are required to highlight this risk.

The American Academy of Otolaryngology, Head and Neck Surgery (AAO-HNS) also reported two additional fatalities in OSA children having adenotonsillectomy having received codeine. They subsequently released a consensus view following a survey of its membership stating that the risks of codeine outweighed its value. This was based on the risk of catastrophic events in ultrametabolizers, its ineffectiveness in poor metabolizers and the availability of other analgesics.

In early 2013, the European Medicines Agency sent out an alert bulletin stating that 'the use of codeine for cough and cold is now contraindicated in children below 12 years. This means it must not be used in this patient group. Use of codeine for cough and cold is not recommended in children and adolescents between 12 and 18 years who have breathing problems'.[1]

In July 2013 in the UK, the Medicines and Healthcare products Regulatory Agency (MHRA) released the following statement:

> Codeine should only be used to relieve acute moderate pain in children older than 12 years and only if it cannot be relieved by other painkillers such as paracetamol or ibuprofen alone. Furthermore, a significant risk of serious and life-threatening adverse reactions has been identified in children with OSA who received codeine after tonsillectomy or adenoidectomy (or both). Codeine is now contraindicated in all children younger than 18 years who undergo these procedures for obstructive sleep apnoea.[2]

This message was further reinforced by the Association of Paediatric Anaesthetists of Great Britain and Ireland (APAGBI) and the Royal College of Paediatrics and Child Health (RCPCH) in a joint statement. They use the statement to helpfully suggest potential, alternative, opioid analgesic strategies.

This paper highlights how a case report series, while not in themselves considered high level evidence by the scientific community, can be a landmark paper in being the initial catalyst for a subsequent reaction and action within both the medical community and medicines regulatory authorities.

This landmark paper was undoubtedly instrumental in preventing further paediatric fatalities with codeine. It is clear that it should be avoided in paediatric practice. Other safer, more efficacious opioid strategies are increasingly available if required. Given what we now know of the pharmacogenetics of its metabolism, codeine may also be an unreliable analgesic choice in other age groups.

---

1 Reproduced from European Medicines Agency: Press release: codeine not to be used in children below 12 years for cough and cold 2014. http://www.ema.europa.eu/ema/index.jsp?curl=pages/news_and_events/news/2015/04/news_detail_002316.jsp&mid=WC0b01ac058004d5c1, December 2017.

2 Reprinted from MHRA 'Codeine for analgesia: restricted use in children because of reports of morphine toxicity' (2013) under the Open Government License v.30.

## Additional references

Patino M, Sadhasivam S, Mahmoud M. Obstructive sleep apnoea in children: perioperative considerations. *Br J Anaesth* 2013;111:83–95.

Association of Paediatric Anaesthetists of Great Britain and Ireland. Guidance for the administration of codeine and alternative opioid analgesics in children. London: APAGBI, 2013.

# Chapter 92

# Effects of general anaesthesia in children

Phil Hodgson

## Details of study

This 'General anaesthesia compared to spinal anaesthesia ('GAS') study' is one of a series of ongoing prospective clinical trials whose objective is to provide high-level evidence whether exposure to general anaesthesia in early life can adversely affect a child's neurodevelopmental outcome.

## Background

Most general anaesthetic agents in common use exert their effect by stimulating $GABA_A$ receptors in the central nervous system. These agents include propofol and inhalational agents such as sevoflurane and isoflurane. Other agents such as ketamine and nitrous oxide have an alternative mechanism action that inhibits NMDA receptors. Unfortunately, in vitro studies have repeatedly implicated all these receptor interactions as precipitating irreversible structural damage, cellular dysfunction, and even apoptosis in developing neurones. Subsequent observational animal and human studies have produced conflicting, but occasionally concerning, results whether exposure to these agents in infancy precipitates long-term cognitive and behavioural changes. This has left the medical profession and parents unable to quantify the risks (if any) of general anaesthesia in infancy. An international, multi-agency collaboration 'SmartTots' (Strategies for Mitigating Anesthesia-Related Neuro-Toxicity in Tots) has been established to coordinate and fund large-scale research in this field and disseminate any high level evidence generated. Their webstite smarttots.org is an invaluable resource for both the medical profession and members of the public.

## Study references

### Main study

Davidson AJ, Disma N, de Graaff JC, Withington DE, Dorris L, Bell G, et al; GAS consortium. Neurodevelopmental outcome at 2 years of age after general anaesthesia and awake-regional anaesthesia in infancy (GAS): an international multicentre, randomised controlled trial. *Lancet* 2016;387:239–50.

## Related reference

Sun LS. Early childhood general anaesthesia exposure and neurocognitive development. *Br J Anaesth* 2010;**105**(Suppl. 1):61–8.

# Study design

Infants were randomized to receive sevoflurane (GA group) or awake regional anaesthesia (RA group) for inguinal hernia repair. The GA group received sevoflurane in air and oxygen. No nitrous oxide was used. The RA group had their surgery while awake after a local anaesthetic solution was injected by either spinal or caudal epidural route. In both groups, further local anaesthetic blockade for per- and postoperative analgesia were allowed at the discretion of the anaesthetist. Paracetamol could be used in both groups but opioids were avoided.

Each child's neurodevelopmental outcome was then assessed when they reached their second birthday. Assessments by both psychologists and paediatricians and structured parental questionnaires were used to obtain a numerical score for key neurodevelopmental outcomes. The study will also report when the children reach their fifth birthday. This paper presents the interim findings at 2 years of age.

| | |
|---|---|
| Type | International, multicentre, observer blind, prospective, randomized controlled trial. |
| Level of evidence | 1a |
| Number of patients | 722 |
| Institutions | 28 (in UK, USA, Canada, Australia, Italy, and Netherlands) |
| Inclusion criteria | Infants up to 60 weeks' post-menstrual age<br>Born at greater than 26 weeks' gestation<br>Unilateral or bilateral herniotomy |
| Exclusion criteria | Contraindication to either anaesthetic technique<br>Mechanical ventilation immediately before surgery<br>Congenital heart disease requiring treatment<br>Known neuronal injury<br>Chromosome or congenital abnormalities<br>Prior exposure to anaesthetic agent or benzodiazepine |
| Randomization | Web based<br>Stratified by institution and gestational age |
| Follow-up | Formal assessment within 2 months either side of the child's second birthday (corrected for prematurity). |
| Primary endpoint | Cognitive score by psychologists using the Bayley III Scale |
| Secondary endpoints | Language, motor, adaptive behaviour and social-emotional scores using the Bayley III Scale and parents' structured questionnaire<br>Formal diagnosis of cerebral palsy or autism.<br>Visual or hearing defects |

# Results

Of the 722 recruited, two misrandomizations and one withdrawal of consent left 361 in the RA group and 358 in the GA group. There were subsequently 74 protocol violations in the RA group (mostly due to needing rescue general anaesthesia) and two in the GA group (surgery cancelled). Fifty-two were then lost to follow-up in the RA group and 47 in the GA group.

# Key findings

| | RA group Assessed (n = 287) | GA group Assessed (n = 356) |
|---|---|---|
| Cognitive composite score, mean (SD) | 98.6 (14.2) | 98.2 (14.7) |
| Language composite score, Mean (SD) | 94.6 (15.4) | 94.0 (15.6) |
| Motor composite score, Mean (SD) | 98.3 (13.2) | 97.9 (13.4) |
| Social-emotional score, Mean (SD) | 97.4 (19) | 95.4 (18.3) |
| Adaptive behaviour score, Mean (SD) | 93.1 (15.6) | 94.3 (14.7) |
| Cerebral palsy diagnosis, n (%) | 1 (<1%) | 4 (1%) |
| Autism diagnosis, n (%) | 2 (1%) | 0 |
| Hearing defect, n (%) | 9 (3%) | 9 (3%) |

Data sourced from Davidson et al. GAS consortium. Neurodevelopmental outcome at 2 years of age after general anaesthesia and awake-regional anaesthesia in infancy (GAS): an international multicentre, randomised controlled trial. *Lancet* 2016;387:239–50.

Note: Composite scores are all standardized to have a mean (SD) of 100 (15) within the reference population. The addition of the patients who violated protocols did not significantly alter any of the composite scores or incidence data, confirming that no bias was introduced by treatment failure.

# Conclusion

The outcome data support strong equivalence between the two groups in all measures of neurodevelopmental outcome at the age of 2. The 95% confidence intervals fell within one-third of a SD, which is well inside the investigator boundaries of clinical equivalence.

# Critique

This is a landmark paper, as it is the first published, randomized, prospective trial that is both methodologically robust and adequately powered to assess whether receiving a general anaesthetic in early life predisposes to adverse neurodevelopmental outcomes later in childhood. The study method corrected potential cofounding variables that could introduce bias at the time of original surgery (hypoxaemia, hypotension, or hypoglycaemia). Furthermore, the incidence of other confounding variables that could introduce subsequent bias are quantified and found to be similar in the two groups (examples are significant head injury, history of seizures, chronic illness, and a general anaesthetic).

The cognitive composite score was chosen as the primary outcome. Unlike the other outcome scores generated, cognition is said to rely on several brain regions and is theoretically more sensitive to the diffuse neuronal damage by general anaesthetic agents documented in previous preclinical studies.

The authors acknowledge that it is difficult at 2 years of age to accurately diagnose some hearing and visual disorders and some cerebral palsy and autistic spectrum disorders. The incidence is documented, but low and the study is not adequately powered to detect differences between the groups.

Although previous studies have implicated prolonged and repeated general anaesthesia agents as causing most concern, the duration and concentrations of sevoflurane administered in this study are similar to those reported in some previous studies reporting adverse outcomes. The authors also highlight that the median duration of general anaesthesia of 54 minutes in this study is a similar value to around 50% of anaesthetics administered in their practice and so well represents a real life scenario. However, they are careful to point out that the study does not exclude adverse outcomes after more prolonged exposure.

Another SmartTots' coordinated prospective trial has also recently been published and is referenced at the end of this critique. The Pediatric Anesthesia NeuroDevelopment Assessment (PANDA) Trial found no statistically significant differences in IQ scores in later childhood among healthy children after a single anesthesia exposure before age 36 months when compared with unexposed healthy siblings.

Many have been keenly awaiting the results of this and other high profile prospective trials for some time. The GAS study group will report again when the children are 5 years of age. In the meantime, the outcome of this (and the PANDA) study is provisionally reassuring.

## Additional references

Sun LS, Li G, Miller TL, Salorio C, Byrne MW, Bellinger DC, et al. Association between a single general anesthesia exposure before age 36 months and neurocognitive outcomes in later childhood. *JAMA* 2016;**315**:2312–20.

Rappaport R, Mellon DR, Simone A, Woodcock J. Defining safe use of anesthesia in children. *N Engl J Med* 2011;**364**:1387–90.

SmartTots. Current thinking regarding potential neurotoxicity of general anesthesia in infants. 2016 http://smarttots.org/resources/faq (accessed March 2013).

# Chapter 93

# Managing perioperative anticoagulation

Hamish Lyall

## Details of studies

Increasingly, patients scheduled for elective surgery are noted to have an anticoagulant listed as one of their regular medications. The most frequent indication for anticoagulation is prevention of arterial thromboembolism in persons with atrial fibrillation (AF). Currently, one of the most widely used anticoagulants for this indication is the vitamin K antagonist, warfarin. Surgeons have a dilemma: what is the best way to interrupt anticoagulation to permit surgery to be performed, while minimizing the risk of thromboembolic stroke? What is the risk of stroke if warfarin is stopped and what is the risk of bleeding with anticoagulation after surgery? There is general agreement that for procedures with a risk of bleeding, warfarin needs to be stopped preoperatively until the anticoagulant effect has ceased, followed by restarting postoperatively. Debate surrounds whether the pre- and postoperative days when warfarin is subtherapeutic should be covered by heparin, a rapid onset, short half-life parenteral anticoagulant. This practice is known as bridging therapy. In this landmark paper researchers performed a randomized control trial of bridging versus no bridging therapy across a wide range of surgical procedures.

## Study references

### Main study

Douketis JD, Spyropoulos AC, Kaatz D, Becker RC, Caprini JA, Dunn AS, et al; BRIDGE investigators. Perioperative bridging anticoagulation in patients with atrial fibrillation. *N Engl J Med* 2015;37:823–33.

### Related reference

Keeling D, Tait RC, Watson H. and the British Committee of Standards for Haematology. Perioperative management of anticoagulation and antiplatelet therapy. *Br J Haematol* 2016;175:602–13.

## Study design

Randomized double blind, placebo-controlled trial.

Warfarin was stopped 5 days prior to surgery. Trial participants were randomized to receive bridging treatment with subcutaneous injections of low molecular weight heparin (dalteparin 100 units/kg twice daily) or placebo. The study drug was commenced 3 days before surgery, stopped 24 hours before surgery, and restarted postoperatively. The timing of restarting the study drug postoperatively was 12–24 hours post procedure for low bleeding risk surgery and 48–72 hours for high bleeding risk surgery. Warfarin was restarted on the evening after surgery or the first postoperative day. The study drug was discontinued postoperatively after 5–10 days when the international normalized ratio (INR) was >2.

| Level of evidence | 1b |
|---|---|
| Number of participants | 1,884 patients. 950 randomized to placebo, 934 assigned bridging therapy Results available for 1,813 participants |
| Inclusion criteria | Age over 18 years |
| | Chronic atrial fibrillation receiving warfarin for >3 months INR target 2.0–3.0 |
| | ≥1 CHADS$_2$ stroke risk factor (congestive heart failure/left ventricular dysfunction, hypertension, age >75 years, diabetes, previous stroke/transient ischaemic attack (TIA)/systemic embolism) |
| Exclusion criteria | Mechanical heart valve |
| | Stroke/systemic embolism/TIA within previous 12 weeks |
| | Major bleeding within preceding 6 weeks |
| | Creatinine clearance <30 mL/min |
| | Platelets <100 × 10$^9$/L |
| | Planned intracranial, intraspinal or cardiac surgery |
| Outcomes | Primary outcomes: arterial thromboembolism (stroke, TIA, systemic embolism), major bleeding Secondary outcomes: death, myocardial infarction, venous thromboembolism, minor bleeding |
| Duration of follow-up | 30 days |

## Results

| | Stroke/TIA/systemic embolism | Major bleeding |
|---|---|---|
| No bridging, N = 918 | 0.4% | 1.3% |
| Bridging, N = 895 | 0.3% | 3.2% |
| Statistical significance | p = 0.01 (non-inferiority—no bridging is not inferior to bridging) | p = 0.005 (superiority—no bridging has less major bleeding than bridging) RR 0.41 (95% CI 0.2–0.78) |

Secondary outcomes for death, myocardial infarction, and venous thromboembolism showed no significant difference. Minor bleeding was significantly higher with bridging therapy.

## Conclusion

In persons with atrial fibrillation stopping warfarin prior to surgery, perioperative bridging therapy resulted in similar rates of arterial thromboembolism to no bridging therapy. Bridging therapy was associated with an increased risk of bleeding.

## Critique

This is an important study, implying that for many patients taking warfarin for AF undergoing surgery, bridging anticoagulation is not beneficial. An important caveat to this study is that the number of patients undergoing high bleeding risk procedures was small (10.6%), not all types of surgery were represented, and the proportion of highest thrombotic risk AF patients (CHADS$_2$ score 5–6) included was also low. Increasingly, alternatives to warfarin, e.g. direct oral anticoagulants are used for long-term anticoagulation; these patients were not included in this study. Clinical guidelines published since this paper continue to advocate an individualized approach to perioperative anticoagulation, considering both the patients risk factors for thromboembolism and the bleeding risks of the procedure.

Chapter 94

# Postoperative venous thromboembolism

Hamish Lyall

## Details of studies

Venous thromboembolism (VTE) is a recognized and feared complication of surgery, causing significant morbidity or mortality. Surgeons need to understand VTE risk when discussing consent with patients for a surgical procedure. Knowledge of VTE risk is also required when considering thromboprophylaxis measures and deciding duration of thromboprophylaxis.

## Study references

### Main study

Sweetland, S, Green J, Liu B, Berrington de Gonzalez A, Canonico M, Reeves G, Beral V; Million women study collaborators. Duration and magnitude of the risk of venous thromboembolism in middle aged women: prospective cohort study *BMJ* 2009;**339**:b45483.

### Related references

Guyatt GH, Akl EA, Crowther M, Gutterman DD, Schuünemann HJ; American College of Chest Physicians Antithrombotic Therapy and Prevention of Thrombosis Panel. Antithrombotic therapy and prevention of thrombosis, 9th ed: American College of Chest Physicians evidence based clinical practice guidelines. *Chest* 2012;**141**(2_suppl):7S–47S.

National Institute for Health and Clinical Excellence (NICE). Clinical guideline 92: Reducing the risk of venous thromboembolism (deep vein thrombosis and pulmonary embolism) in patients admitted to hospital. London: NICE, 2010.

## Study design

Prospective cohort study

Information from 1.3 million participants enrolled in a UK National Health Service (NHS) breast screening programme was linked to centralized NHS records for hospital admissions, deaths, cancer registrations, and emigrations. Data on participants who had a surgical procedure or were admitted for VTE or died from VTE during the study period were collected. From this, incidence and relative risk of postoperative VTE was determined by comparing study participants who had a surgical procedure with those that had not.

| Level of evidence | 1b |
|---|---|
| Number of participants | 947,454 study participants, 239,614 surgical procedures, 5,689 VTE events |
| Inclusion criteria | Females, registered with NHS breast screening programme between 1996 and 2001, aged 50–64 years as part of the million women study |
| | Completed recruitment questionnaire |
| | Informed consent |
| Exclusion criteria | Prior history of VTE |
| | History of treatment for clotting problems |
| | >1 surgical procedure during follow-up or surgery in the year prior to recruitment |
| Follow up data | Data from centralized NHS records |
| | Follow up questionnaires |
| Duration of follow-up | 5.84 million person years (~6.2 years per woman) |

## Main outcome measures

Relative risks and incidence rates for hospital admission or death from VTE, by time since surgery and type of surgery

## Results

### Incidence of VTE

| No surgery | 0.058/1,000 person months |
|---|---|
| 0–12 weeks post inpatient surgery | 2.6/1,000 person months |
| 4–12 months post inpatient surgery | 0.4/1,000 person months |
| 0–12 weeks post day case surgery | 0.4/1,000 person months |
| 4–12 months post day case surgery | 0.2/1,000 person months |

Over a 12-week period without surgery the incidence of hospital admission and death for VTE was 1:6200, compared to 1:140 after inpatient surgery and 1:815 after day case surgery.

### Relative risk of VTE after inpatient surgery compared with no surgery

| Type of surgery | 0–6 weeks post surgery | 7–12 weeks post surgery | 4–12 months post surgery | ≥1 year post surgery |
|---|---|---|---|---|
| Cancer | 91.6 | 53.4 | 34.4 | 6.1 |
| Hip or knee replacement | 220.6 | 39.7 | 4.6 | 2.7 |

| Fracture | 89.0 | 39.8 | 2.9 | 0.6* |
|---|---|---|---|---|
| Other orthopaedic | 57.3 | 5.6 | 1.4* | 1.6* |
| Vascular | 87.0 | 15.8 | 3.9 | 2.2 |
| Gynaecological | 22.7 | 1.1 | 1.4* | 1.7 |
| Gastrointestinal | 56.3 | 18.5 | 5.1 | 1.3* |
| All other surgery | 36.0 | 8.4 | 3.7 | 1.7* |

*95% confidence intervals include 1.0.

The highest relative risk for VTE occurred 3 weeks post surgery.

## Relative risk of VTE after day case surgery compared with no surgery

| Type of surgery | 0–6 weeks post surgery | 7–12 weeks post surgery | 4–13 months post surgery | ≥1 year post surgery |
|---|---|---|---|---|
| Cancer | 80.4 | 47.7 | 12.1 | 1.7* |
| Other orthopaedic | 22.9 | 5.4 | 3.1 | 1.6 |
| Vascular | 26.4 | 5.1 | 5.2 | 1.6 |
| Gynaecological | 2.5* | 4.5 | 2.3 | 1.5 |
| Gastrointestinal | 5.3 | 4.5 | 2.9 | 1.6 |
| All other surgery | 6.2 | 4.0 | 2.3 | 1.7 |

*95% confidence intervals include 1.0.

## Conclusion

The risk of VTE after surgery is increased in the first 12 postoperative weeks, with a peak incidence after in patient surgery at 3 weeks. The risk varies substantially by type of surgery. Day surgery has a lower incidence of postoperative VTE than inpatient surgery but is significantly higher than no surgery.

## Critique

The strength of this study is the large number of participants, followed prospectively and exposed to a wide range of surgical procedures with a long duration of follow-up. Limitations of the study are that it included only female participants, within an age range which does not reflect the full range of patients receiving surgery in everyday practice. In addition, the incidence of VTE will have been modified by existing thromboprophylaxis measures employed. Therefore, the incidence rates have to be interpreted in light of thromboprophylaxis measures that were likely to have been used within the UK at the time of the study.

This is an epidemiological study and care must be taken when translating the conclusions to everyday practice. The likelihood of a patient developing postoperative VTE depends not only on the type of surgery, but also on any pre-existing patient-specific risk factors for VTE, for example active malignancy, previous history of VTE, advanced age. This is reflected in international clinical practice guidelines such as those from the National Institute of Health and Social Care Excellence and American College of Chest Physicians, which advocate a patient-specific risk assessment to consider both the thrombotic risks of the procedure and the patient specific risk factors as well as contraindications to thromboprophlyaxis when making thromboprophylaxis decisions.

# Chapter 95

# Tranexamic acid

Hamish Lyall

## Details of studies

Tranexamic acid is an antifibrinolytic drug used to treat or prevent bleeding. Clinical trials in surgery have demonstrated that tranexamic acid reduces the probability of needing a blood transfusion by approximately one-third. CRASH-2 is the first randomized controlled trial of tranexamic acid in major trauma, adding to the large volume of evidence already accumulated in the surgical setting.

## Study references

### Main study

CRASH-2 trial collaborators. Effect of tranexamic acid on death, vascular occlusive events, and blood transfusion in trauma patients with significant haemorrhage (CRASH-2): a randomised, placebo controlled trial. *Lancet* 2010;376:23–32.

CRASH-2 Collaborators. The importance of early treatment with tranexamic acid in bleeding trauma patients: an exploratory analysis of the CRASH-2 randomised control trial. *Lancet* 2011;377:1096–101.

## Study design

CRASH-2 was an international study performed in 274 hospitals in 40 countries. Adult trauma patients within 8 hours of injury were randomized to receive tranexamic acid (1 g intravenously infused over 10 minutes followed by 1 g of intravenous infusion over 8 hours) or placebo.

| | |
|---|---|
| Level of evidence | 1b |
| Number of participants | 20,211 |
| Inclusion criteria | Adult patients |
| | Significant haemorrhage (blood pressure <90 mmHg, heart rate >110 beats per minute) or at risk of significant haemorrhage |
| | Within 8 hours of injury |
| Exclusion criteria | Cases considered as having a clear indication for tranexamic acid or if tranexamic acid was considered a clear contraindication |
| Duration of follow-up | 28 days after injury |

## Main outcome measures

### Primary outcome

Death in hospital within 4 weeks of injury.

### Secondary outcomes

Vascular occlusive events, surgical intervention, receipt of blood transfusion, and units of blood products transfused.

## Results

### Primary outcome

| | Tranexamic acid | Placebo | RR (95% CI) |
|---|---|---|---|
| Death (all causes) | 1,463 (14.5%) | 1,613 (16.0%) | 0.91 (0.85–0.97) |

Sub-analysis of causes of death.

All causes of mortality (bleeding, vascular occlusion, multi-organ failure, head injury, and other causes) had a lower relative risk of death in the tranexamic acid arm, although only a reduction in death due to bleeding reached statistical significance.

### Secondary outcomes

Vascular occlusive events, transfusion requirements and surgery demonstrated a trend towards fewer events in the tranexamic arm but these did not reach statistical significance.

### Dependency on discharge

Discharge with no symptoms was higher in the tranexamic acid arm with a relative risk of 1.11 (CI 1.04–1.19). Other categories of dependency (minor symptoms, some restriction, dependant, fully dependant) showed a trend towards a benefit from tranexamic acid but did not reach statistical significance.

## Conclusion

Tranexamic acid reduces death in bleeding trauma patients.

## Critique

The CRASH-2 trial provides high-quality evidence for the benefit of tranexamic acid in the setting of major trauma. Importantly, adverse events due to thromboembolism (both arterial and venous were lower (not significantly) in the tranexamic arm, providing further reassurance regarding the safety of this drug. A subsequent publication from the trial investigators concluded that the benefit was restricted to patients receiving treatment within 3 hours of injury.

For the otolaryngologist, this trial was of trauma patients and therefore would not have included spontaneous epistaxis, a common emergency presentation. A review by

Kamhieh and Fox (2016) identified five randomized controlled trials of tranexamic acid in epistaxis. A trend towards more favourable outcomes with tranexamic acid was observed, concluding further studies of intravenous or topical tranexamic acid are required.

## Additional references

Kamhieh Y, Fox H. Tranexamic acid in epistaxis: a systematic review. *Clin Otolaryngol* 2016;41:771–6.

Ker K, Edwards P, Perel P, Shakur H, Roberts I. Effect of tranexamic acid on surgical bleeding: systematic review and cumulative meta-analysis. *BMJ* 2012;**344**:e3054.

# Chapter 96

# Bolam v. Friern Hospital Management Committee

Peter Webber

## Details of studies

The cost of clinical negligence claims in any healthcare system almost always constitutes a limitless drain on a finite amount of money allocated to the health service in question. The figures, which are available for the UK National Health Service (NHS), amply illustrate this point.

In 1990/1991, the cost of clinical negligence claims to the NHS was estimated at around £52 million. Although in 2015/2016, the number of new clinical claims reported, 10,965, was lower than in 2013/2014 (11,945), the damages payments to patients had risen to £950.4 million, and with the addition of Claimant and Defence legal costs, the total for 2015/2016 was £1,488.5 million. This represented a significant increase over the previous financial year.[1]

It is against this background, that the role of key judgements in medico-legal matters will be discussed. This will be very much in the context of UK practice and particularly in terms of the law as applied in England and Wales, but the principles are similar elsewhere in the world.

## Study reference

### Main study

*Bolam v. Friern Hospital Management Committee* [1957] 1 WLR 582

This is in English law the landmark case in establishing liability and causation for medical practitioners, and incorporates many, if not all, aspects involved in medical litigation, i.e. consent, duty of care (liability), differences in reasonable practice, and causation. Liability is defined as a breach of the doctor's duty of care to his or her patient, and causation is the demonstrable harm, which flows from the liable act. Both need to be present for clinical negligence to be proven.

At the time of the Bolam case, it can be safely stated that the medical profession was both paternalistic and largely unregulated. Doctors tended to enjoy unquestioning compliance from patients, and were treated with great deference by society in general.

---

1 NHS Litigation Authority, Annual report and accounts 2015/16 © NHS Litigation Authority 2016.

## Circumstances of the case

In 1954, John Hector Bolam, a patient suffering from depression, was voluntarily admitted to the Friern Hospital to undergo electroconvulsive therapy (ECT). ECT was delivered 'unmodified', that is to say no muscle relaxant drugs were administered. He was not restrained, apart from the presence of nursing staff to prevent him from falling. During the administration of the ECT, Mr Bolam suffered violent muscle spasms, which caused pelvic fractures by way of acetabular fractures. He thus pursued a claim for negligence on the grounds that had he been warned of the risk of pelvic fracture, he would not have undergone the treatment, and had he received a muscle relaxant drug, his injuries would not have occurred, or in the alternative that the lack of restraints directly contributed to the fractures.

At the trial, which in those days, unlike such cases in English law now, was heard before a jury, expert evidence confirmed that there was a range of professional opinion whether or not the ECT should have been undertaken unmodified. The treating doctor, Dr De Bastarrechea, stated that he (the doctor) was aware of the risk of fractures arising as a result of unmodified ECT, but he did not so inform Mr Bolam of the risk, because as the latter's treating clinician, he considered that the risk was very small, and that Mr Bolam was clearly in need of the treatment. Concerning the use of 'unmodified' ECT, expert opinion differed as to whether or not a muscle relaxant should have been used. The judge, McNair J, considered that the opinions of the competing testimony of the experts, was something that he could respect equally. McNair J thus contended that a doctor is 'not guilty of negligence if he has acted in accordance with practice accepted as proper by a responsible body of medical men, skilled in that particular art ... putting it the other way round, a man is not negligent if he is acting in accordance with such a practice, merely because there is a body of opinion who would take a contrary view.'

McNair J also made it clear to the Jury that a doctor could not go on 'obstinately and pigheadedly carry on with some old technique if it has been proved to be contrary to really what is substantially the whole of informed medical opinion.' In all the issues, i.e. that of consent, duty of care, and causation, the Jury found for the Defendant, i.e. against Mr Bolam. In so doing, McNair J's statement regarding test of negligence for a doctor, emerged as a legal benchmark, stating that the burden of proof lay with the patient bringing the action, to demonstrate that no responsible body of professional opinion would have endorsed the particular course of action, be it the disclosure or risk or the method of treatment. This became known as the Bolam Test.

A similar case had occurred before Bolam, in Scotland, namely *Hunter* v. *Hanley*, where the presiding judge, Lord President Clyde, stated that 'the true test for establishing negligence in diagnosis or treatment on the part of a doctor is whether he has been proven to be guilty of such failure as no doctor of ordinary skill would be guilty of if acting with ordinary care.' This was quoted by McNair J in the Bolam case.

It can be stated that the principle of the Bolam Test is that doctors are allowed to make mistakes, so long as they are mistakes that might be made by a responsible or reasonable body of doctors with equivalent skills and experience, exercising a reasonable standard of care.

In the subsequent case of *Maynard* v. *West Midlands Health Authority*, it was established that the judge could not determine negligence by simply preferring one expert's opinion over another. The presiding judge, Lord Scarman, again stated that it was a failure to exercise the ordinary skill of a doctor in order for that doctor to be found guilty of negligence.

## Critique

Although undoubtedly a landmark judgement, there are a number of difficulties with the Bolam Test, one of which is that it can be stated that it is easy to invoke Bolam on the basis of a single expert's opinion, conversely too difficult for the Claimant, i.e. the patient making the claim against the doctor or hospital, to show that no other doctor would have acted similarly. In terms of a doctor's duty of care or liability, Bolam determines what medical practice is (or what contemporary practice was), rather than what practice should be. Thus, instead of considering a standard of care that is good, Bolam defaults to a standard of care that can be supported, i.e. just adequate.

In terms of Bolam as applied to consent, and the disclosure of risks of treatment, matters have moved forward over the years since the judgement, to a position more in alignment with that of North American jurisdiction.

## Additional references

### Cases

*Bolam* v. *Friern Hospital Management Committee* [1957] **1** WLR 582
*Hunter* v. *Hanley* [1955] S.C. 200
*Maynard* v. *West Midlands Regional Health Authority* [1984] **1** WLR 634
*Bolitho (Deceased)* v. *City and Hackney Health Authority* [1997] **3** WLR 1151
*Reynolds* v. *North Tyneside Health Authority* [2002] All ER (D) 523
*Chapel* v. *Hart* [1998] **156** ALR 517
*Chester* v. *Afshar* [2004] UKHL 41
*Montgomery* v. *Lanarkshire Health Board* [2015] UKSC 11

### Article

**Lord Woolf.** Are the Courts Excessively Deferential to the Medical Profession? [2001] **9** Med Law Rev 1

# Chapter 97

# *Bolitho* v. *City & Hackney Health Authority*

Peter Webber

## Details of studies

This case indicated a sense of judicial dissatisfaction with the Bolam Test, and a shift towards redressing of the balance in favour of the patient (Claimant).

## Study reference

### Main study

*Bolitho* v. *City & Hackney Health Authority* [1996] 4 All ER 771

## Circumstances of the case

Patrick Nigel Bolitho, a 2 year old, suffered catastrophic brain damage as a result of cardiac arrest induced by respiratory failure, following his admission with croup to St Bartholomew's Hospital in 1984. He had been initially admitted with croup and discharged home after 24 hours. The following day, he was re-admitted, as his parents had become concerned about his condition. The day following his admission, he suffered an episode of respiratory distress, about which the nursing sister was sufficiently concerned that she bleeped the Senior Paediatric Registrar, rather than go through the usual medical chain of command by first contacting the Senior House Officer (SHO). The Senior Registrar, Dr Horn, responded to the bleep by telephone, and stated that she would attend as soon as possible. In the event, she did not attend to see the child. However, Patrick appeared to recover very rapidly, and again appeared very well.

About 2 hours later, a second episode of respiratory distress occurred. Dr Horn was contacted again, and stated that she could not attend and had asked the SHO to see Patrick. During the course of this conversation, the nurse attending Patrick noted that he was now well again, and not in distress.

About 30 minutes later, Patrick's condition deteriorated again and the nurse who was attending him left to inform the nursing sister to bleep the doctors again. This time, Patrick went into respiratory arrest, followed by a cardiac arrest. He was revived, but as there was a delay of some 9–10 minutes before restoration of respiratory and cardiac functions, Patrick suffered severe brain damage, and later died.

At the initial trial, it was accepted that Dr Horn was in breach of her duty of care not to have attended Patrick, after receiving the telephone calls, or not to have arranged a suitable deputy to do so. Dr Horn averred that had she come to see Patrick at the second episode of respiratory difficulty, she would not have arranged for him to be intubated. Expert evidence from medical experts called on behalf of Patrick were of the view that at least after the second episode, any competent doctor would have intubated. On the side of the Defendant, three experts stated that intubation at this stage would not have been appropriate.

The case hung on the premise that Patrick was experiencing a progressive state of respiratory distress, which led to the cardiorespiratory arrest. The Defendant's experts, on the other hand, considered that the facts appeared to indicate that Patrick was quite well, apart from the two quite sudden episodes preceding the final respiratory arrest. The judge held the view that, although the opinion of the experts for the Defence and Plaintiff were diametrically opposed, both represented a responsible body of professional opinion. Thus, according to the Bolam Test, if Dr Horn had attended but not intubated, she would have come up to the proper level of skill and competence, i.e. the standard represented by the Defendant's expert. The case was thus dismissed.

An appeal was made to the Court of Appeal. This too found for the Defendant, stating that if Dr Horn had attended Patrick and failed to intubate, she would have been acting in accordance with a responsible body of medical opinion, i.e. the Bolam Test. However, one of the judges stated that 'it is not enough for a Defendant to call a number of doctors to say that what he had done or not done was in accord with accepted clinical practice. It is necessary for the Judge to consider that evidence and decide whether that clinical practice puts the patient unnecessarily at risk.'

Following the dismissal of that appeal, a further appeal was made to the House of Lords, and was dismissed on similar grounds. However, in his summing up, Lord Browne-Wilkinson, made caveats to the Bolam Test, in particular that the reasonableness of professional opinion has to withstand logical analysis. He stated

> In the vast majority of cases, the fact is that distinguished experts in the field of a particular opinion will demonstrate the reasonableness of that opinion ... but if, in a rare case, it can be demonstrated that the professional opinion is not capable of withstanding logical analysis, the Judge is entitled to hold that the body of opinion is not reasonable or responsible

and he added:

> I emphasise that in my view it will very seldom be right for a Judge to reach the conclusion that views genuinely held by a competent medical expert are unreasonable ... it is only where a Judge can be satisfied that the body of expert opinion cannot be logically supported at all that such opinion will not provide the benchmark by reference to which the Defendant's conduct falls to be assessed.

Lord Browne-Wilkinson considered that the expert evidence for the Defendant in Patrick's case was logical and reasonable, and thus this appeal was dismissed. In other words, the Bolam Test had been upheld, but the judiciary had laid down a marker that simply giving a view that doctors actions were reasonable, could not in itself be sufficient to exonerate that doctor of any negligence; the opinion held must withstand logical analysis. This was later demonstrated, in 2002, with *Reynolds v North Tyneside Health Authority*. The judgement here held that the Defendant Midwife negligently failed to perform a vaginal examination at an appropriate time, missing an abnormal presentation of a foetus, with resulting adverse consequences. Finding for the Claimant, Gross J dismissed the argument on behalf of the Defence as follows:

> Where the sole reason relied upon in support of a practice is untenable, it follows ... that the practice itself is not defensible and lacks a logical basis. That is the case here. The suggested contrary practice (or body of opinion) is neither defensible nor logical.

Another issue where matters have moved on from the Bolam Test, is in the matter of consent. The basis of consent as shown in the Bolam Test, is the rather paternalistic one of 'doctor knows best'. This has increasingly moved on from that attitude to one of the 'prudent patient'. This is well illustrated by a case from Australia, which also gives an illuminating insight into the way evidence by an expert is presented.

## Additional references

### Cases

*Bolam* v. *Friern Hospital Management Committee* [1957] **1** WLR 582
*Hunter* v. *Hanley* [1955] S.C. 200
*Maynard* v. *West Midlands Regional Health Authority* [1984] **1** WLR 634
*Bolitho (Deceased)* v. *City and Hackney Health Authority* [1997] **3** WLR 1151
*Reynolds* v. *North Tyneside Health Authority* [2002] All ER (D) 523
*Chapel* v. *Hart* [1998] **156** ALR 517
*Chester* v. *Afshar* [2004] UKHL 41
*Montgomery* v. *Lanarkshire Health Board* [2015] UKSC 11

### Article

**Lord Woolf.** Are the Courts Excessively Deferential to the Medical Profession? [2001] **9** Med Law Rev 1

Chapter 98

# *Chappel* v. *Hart*

Peter Webber

## Study references

### Main case

*Chapel* v. *Hart* [1998] **156** ALR 517

### Related cases

*Montgomery* v. *Lanarkshire Health Board* [2015] UKSC 11

## Circumstances of the case

Mrs Hart, an Education Officer, underwent an operation for a pharyngeal pouch, carried out by Dr Chappel, in 1983. The pouch was giving rise to severe symptoms, and surgery offered the only prospect of relief.

At the preoperative discussion, the options of excision of the pouch through an external neck incision, or the endoscopic Dohlman procedure, were discussed. The Dohlman procedure utilizes a specially adapted rigid endoscope, and the use of cutting diathermy, to divide the mucosal and muscular septum between the pouch and the oesophagus—effectively an internal cricopharyngeal myotomy, thus creating a single lumen. Since the first description of this technique by Dohlman in 1935, the popularity of the endoscopic technique, particularly since the 1960s, has increased, with endoscopic stapling over recent years having become a popular method of treatment.

Mrs Hart chose the Dohlman operation. Dr Chappel warned her of the risk of perforation, giving a frequency for this complication of between 6% and 18%. Unfortunately, a few hours postoperatively, it was evident that Mrs Hart had developed a perforation. She eventually recovered in another hospital, and while there complained of hoarseness and was seen by another ENT surgeon, Professor Bruce Benjamin, and diagnosed with a right vocal cord palsy. This was assumed to be the result of injury to the right recurrent laryngeal nerve. Because of the hoarseness, Mrs Hart was unable to continue in her work as an Education Officer. She thus commenced legal proceedings against Dr Chappel, on the basis of a failure to warn of the risk of a vocal cord palsy. In the trial before the New South Wales Supreme Court in 1994, it was accepted by Mrs Hart that the operation had been carried out with due care by Dr Chappel, that the perforation was a recognized complication, and it was agreed by both Defendant and Plaintiff, that the likely cause of the vocal cord palsy was the effect on the recurrent laryngeal nerve of mediastinitis caused by the perforation.

Mrs Hart claimed in evidence, that during her preoperative discussion of the risks with Dr Chappel, she had told him that 'I don't want to wind up like Neville Wran'. Mr Wran was at that time a famously hoarse Australian politician. It was later noted that Mrs Hart's comment was not contested, thus it was stated that therefore there was a duty of care, on Dr Chappel's part, to warn of the risk to the voice, due to possible recurrent laryngeal nerve injury. Furthermore, Counsel for Mrs Hart argued that if she had been warned of the risk of cord palsy, she would have chosen to undergo the operation at a later date, and by a more experienced surgeon, and thus the risks of pharyngeal perforation, mediastinitis, and vocal cord palsy would have been less likely.

Dr Chappel was found negligent in failing to warn of the risk of vocal cord palsy; he appealed, the matter eventually went to the High Court, who in 1998 dismissed the appeal.

However, the reasonable question as to how common was the incidence of vocal cord palsy was never satisfactorily answered at trial. Professor Benjamin had said in evidence that vocal cord palsy was very uncommon, while other experts stated that it was highly unusual after the Dohlman operation. This evidence did not accord with the published literature, which showed that prior to 1983 there was no report of any vocal cord palsy in association with the Dohlman procedure. One case was reported in a publication by Professor Benjamin in 1991, but based on the details of the age, sex, and history of the patient described in that paper, this case of a vocal cord palsy following a Dohlman's procedure was likely to have been that of Mrs Hart.

Furthermore, it was unclear as to how the vocal cord palsy had occurred beyond the obvious and likely damage to the recurrent laryngeal nerve. The aetiology in Mrs Hart's case was ascribed to mediastinitis, and although mediastinitis had previously been described following perforation in the Dohlman procedure, vocal cord palsy had not.

Thus, Dr Chappel was judged to not have informed Mrs Hart of all material risks, based on a material risk which was probably negligible. However, the principle has held forth since.

The decision in this case, took the standard concerning warning about material risks to a new level. The significance of this judgement was obviously not lost in the UK, well-illustrated by the case of *Chester* v. *Afshar* (2004). This case involved a young journalist, Miss Chester, undergoing urgent back surgery, and suffering cauda equina syndrome, about which she was not warned preoperatively. The neurosurgeon's own audited series of similar back operations had shown an incidence of less than 0.9% of cauda equina syndrome. He thus used the same defence as in Bolam, that the patient was in urgent need of surgery, and probably would have consented to surgery even if informed of the risk. However, Miss Chester's evidence in Court was the same as that which was used by Mrs Hart, i.e. if she had been warned about the risk, she may well have decided not to have had the operation done at the time it was carried out, or indeed consulted another surgeon, and thus had the operation done on a different day, and therefore on probabilities, would have avoided the complications which befell her. As with the earlier Australian case, Miss Chester won her case.

## Subsequent cases

It was thus not surprising that the principle of being required as the treating doctor to warn the patient of all material risks, finally became enshrined in English law, in 2015, with the judgement of *Montgomery* v. *Lanarkshire Health Authority*.

Nadine Montgomery, of small stature and a diabetic, gave birth to a baby boy on 1 October 1999; the baby was born with severe disabilities. It was contended that she should have been advised of the risk of shoulder dystocia with vaginal delivery, being diabetic, and hence with the risk of delivering a large baby, and thus should have been informed of the alternative treatment, i.e. C-section. Her obstetrician contended that risk of dystocia was very small (9–10%) and thus it was not her routine practice to discuss the risk; the obstetrician also averred that it was more preferable for women to have a vaginal delivery rather than a C-section. Mrs Montgomery contended that had she been so advised, she would have elected for a C-section. After her case had been dismissed in the lower courts, judgement was made in her favour by the UK Supreme Court, who considered that it should now be a legal requirement that doctors explain all material risks of a procedure, to the patient. This finally brought the principle of informed consent into line with many other countries, notably the USA.

In conclusion, while the Bolam Test could well be considered an anachronistic throwback to 1950s medical paternalism, the Test, certainly in English Law (and by way of *Hunter* v. *Handley* in Scottish Law), remains a cornerstone in clinical negligence litigation. However, the cases of Bolitho, and what has followed after the judgement in *Chapel* v. *Hart*, has certainly modified the way the Bolam Test is used.

This was recognized by Lord Woolf, former Lord Chief Justice of England and Wales, in an article discussing whether Courts were excessively deferential to the medical profession, stated 'when interference is justified (the Courts) must not be deterred from doing so by any principle such as the fact that what has been done is in accord with a practice approved of by a respectable body of medical opinion.'

## Additional references

### Cases

*Bolam* v. *Friern Hospital Management Committee* [1957] **1** WLR 582
*Hunter* v. *Hanley* [1955] S.C. 200
*Maynard* v. *West Midlands Regional Health Authority* [1984] **1** WLR 634
*Bolitho (Deceased)* v. *City and Hackney Health Authority* [1997] **3** WLR 1151
*Reynolds* v. *North Tyneside Health Authority* [2002] All ER (D) 523
*Chapel* v. *Hart* [1998] **156** ALR 517
*Chester* v. *Afshar* [2004] UKHL 41
*Montgomery* v. *Lanarkshire Health Board* [2015] UKSC 11

### Article

**Lord Woolf**. Are the Courts Excessively Deferential to the Medical Profession? [2001] **9** Med Law Rev 1

# Chapter 99

# Noise-induced hearing loss

Robert Dobie

Noise-induced hearing loss (NIHL) (also known as industrial deafness or occupational deafness) is a common cause of litigation. Prior to the advent of guidelines, varation in clinical opinion led to large differences in management and settlement of such cases.

## Details of study

Coles' guidelines are widely used in British legal settings and perhaps elsewhere, probably because they offer a step-by-step approach that can be used by both experienced experts (such as the authors) and less experienced people such as junior clinicians and even attorneys in their management of NIHL. Their use has reduced both variance among expert reports and overhead costs in hearing loss litigation in the UK (Lutman, personal communication 18 January 2017). Adding the noise bulge to the better-known noise notch as criteria for NIHL was a well-justified innovation of the method.

## Study references

### Main study

Coles RR, Lutman ME, Buffin JT. Guidelines on the diagnosis of noise-induced hearing loss for medicolegal purposes. *Clin Otolaryngol Allied Sci* 2000;25:264–73.

### Related reference

Lutman ME, Coles RR, Buffin JT. Guidelines for quantification of noise-induced hearing loss in a medicolegal context. *Clin Otolaryngol* 2016;41:347–57.

## Study design

This paper offers a valuable collection of expert opinions, grounded in both research and the clinical experience of the highly respected authors. The authors propose that a diagnosis of occupational NIHL can be made on a 'more probable than not' basis when there is (1) high-frequency sensorineural hearing loss; (2) hazardous noise exposure; and (3) a notch or bulge in the 3–6 kHz region. Each of these criteria is explained in detail, with caveats and exceptions. For example, hazardous occupational exposure is defined as noise emission level (NIL) $\geq$100 dBA, or $\geq$90 dBA if the audiometric evidence for NIHL is especially strong. NIL = sound level in dBA plus 10 $\log_{10}$ (years); thus, the latter criterion can be met with as little as 3 years' exposure at 85 dBA, an exposure that few would consider likely to cause measurable threshold shift. An audiometric notch or bulge is considered genuine if its depth is ≥10 dB in the 3–6 kHz region.

Bulge detection requires estimating the age-related audiogram that the claimant might have had in the absence of occupational noise, by comparing the claimant's actual thresholds at 1 and 8 kHz to tables of expected loss for people of the same age and sex, but varying susceptibility. The bulge depth at each frequency is simply the difference between the actual threshold and the putative age-related threshold. There will often be little difference between the results of this procedure and a simpler one in which age-related thresholds are estimated by drawing a straight line between the 1 and 8 kHz anchor points.

Four modifying factors are proposed. The 'clinical picture' includes reports of temporary threshold shifts as well as hearing aid use compatible with NIHL. 'Compatibility with age and noise exposure' means that the audiogram is not worse than the 5th percentile for the claimant's age and noise exposure. Robinson's (1985) criteria would be used to identify cases that were unusual in audiometric shape and (especially) symmetry. For 'complicated cases,' the authors offer suggestions for dealing with marked asymmetry, conductive hearing loss, and the presence of other otologic disorders.

## Critique

Although these guidelines reduce the role of clinical judgment, there are multiple points in the modifying factors where judgment is essential; one wonders whether these topics are simply ignored by less experienced clinicians and attorneys. As an American otologist with interest and experience in medical-legal settings (Dobie 2015), these guidelines do not appear to have been used in the USA, perhaps because they are not well known and require a fair amount of computation.

There are two significant gaps in the Coles guidelines. First, they ignore the important information available in a series of audiograms and a parallel series of noise exposure estimates. Many claimants will have annual audiograms from pre-employment to retirement. When available, data such as these often deserve greater weight than noise exposure estimates that may be unreliable (often based on general knowledge about exposure in a particular craft rather than measurements in the claimant's workplace). These audiograms may show excellent hearing without notching or bulging until mid-career, then an accelerating growth of hearing loss, in a worker who began to use hearing protection in mid-career. In such cases, a bulge or even a frank notch cannot fairly be attributed to occupational noise, regardless of noise levels present prior to the use of hearing protection. In other cases, early notching and a decelerating trajectory can justify a diagnosis of NIHL even if later audiograms do not meet notch or bulge criteria.

The second gap is the lack of validation; these guidelines are based largely on clinical experience. Notches are common in people who deny noise exposure (Nondahl et al. 2009; Osei-Lah and Yeoh 2010; Schlauch and Carney 2011; Lie et al. 2015). If the Coles bulge criteria were applied to a large group of audiograms from such people, it may be that the prevalence of false positives would be quite high. In addition, comparing the diagnostic conclusions of multiple clinicians to the same datasets could test the reliability of the method.

A smaller issue: the 10-dB criterion for a notch or bulge is initially justified based on what is 'reliably measurable', but later claimed to identify a 'material contribution to the claimant's overall hearing impairment'. These are distinct concepts that cannot be assumed to be equivalent. A 10-dB shift in hearing at 6 kHz may create a notch that is measurable without changing a person's impairment in activities of daily living (ADLs). Internationally, thresholds above 4 kHz are almost always ignored in assessing the effects of hearing loss on ADLs.

From an American perspective, the guidelines lack appropriate emphasis on non-occupational noise exposure. Unprotected recreational firearm use is very common in the USA and probably accounts for about as much NIHL as occupational noise. Shooting accounts for much of the asymmetry seen in individual cases (for right-handed shooters, the left ear gets most of the noise).

## Amendments to the study

In Lutman et al. (2016), the same three authors note that the method of bulge estimation in their 2000 paper relied on the shaky assumption that there was no noise-induced permanent threshold shift (NIPTS) at the anchor frequencies of 1 and 8 kHz. This could lead to underestimation of the actual contribution of occupational noise to a claimant's hearing loss. They estimate that 1 kHz NIPTS is typically about 10% as large, and 8 kHz NIPTS about 30% as large, as 4 kHz NIPTS, and correct the putative age-related thresholds to account for this. If disability is based on the pure-tone average of 1, 2, and 3 kHz, as is typical in Britain, the authors show that the new method increases the estimate of noise contribution by about one third; their short-cut method simply multiplies the bulge depth, averaged across these frequencies using the 2000 method, by 1.33.

In contrast, ISO-1999 includes no estimates for 8 kHz NIPTS due to the scarcity of data, and predicts no NIPTS at 1 kHz for daily noise exposures below 92 dBA. Since most claimants will have been exposed at these lower levels, the Lutman et al. (2016) method could therefore overestimate noise contribution. On the other hand, the ISO model includes a compression factor: predicted hearing levels are less than the sum of age-related thresholds and NIPTS. This suggests that estimated NIPTS (current audiogram compared with putative age-related thresholds) could underestimate the actual NIPTS.

The 2016 method requires more computation than the 2000 method; it would be interesting to know its reliability across examiners.

Both methods rely heavily on the current audiogram. As noted previously, a series of audiograms may add important information. In addition, the trichotomization of exposure levels (NIL <90, 90–99, and ≥100) obscures important differences. As a rough rule of thumb, every 5 dB increase in exposure level will double the expected NIPTS. Based on the ISO 1999 model and the 1, 2, 3 kHz average, an exposure with an NIL of 100 (10 years at 90 dBA) should produce median NIPTS of only 3 dB, compared with 13 dB for an exposure 10 dB higher (10 years at 100 dBA). These lines of evidence (current audiogram, audiometric trajectory, and expected hearing loss based on both occupational and non-occupational noise exposure) may conflict and may differ markedly in reliability. Only solid clinical judgment can appropriately weigh them and arrive at a fair estimate of the magnitude of noise contribution.

In summary, both Coles et al. (2000) and Lutman et al. (2016) are innovative methodological papers that combine a deep understanding of the NIHL literature with impressive clinical experience both in practice and in medical-legal consulting. Their methods would be most helpful in cases where little is known about a claimant's noise exposure and there are few previous audiograms, or in legal settings that emphasize expeditious settlement to achieve inexpensive 'rough justice' (e.g. workers compensation programs in most US states). In other cases, either of these methods can provide one of several lines of evidence for a clinician to consider.

## Additional references

Dobie RA. Medical-legal evaluation of hearing loss, 3rd edn. San Diego: Plural Publishing, 2015.

ISO 1999. Acoustics: estimation of noise-induced hearing loss, 3rd edn. Geneva: International Organization for Standardization, 2013.

Lie A, Skogstad M, Johnsen TS, Engdahl B, Tambs K. The prevalence of notched audiograms in a cross-sectional study of 12,055 railway workers. *Ear Hear* 2015;36:e86–92.

Nondahl DM, Shi X, Cruickshanks KJ, et al. Notched audiograms and noise exposure history in older adults. *Ear Hear* 2009;30:696–703.

Osei-lah V, Yeoh LH. High frequency audiometric notch: an outpatient clinic survey. *Int J Audiol* 2010;49:95–8.

Robinson DW. The audiogram in hearing loss due to noise: a probability test to uncover other causation. *Ann Occup Hyg* 1985;29:477–93.

Schlauch RS, Carney E. Are false-positive rates leading to an overestimation of noise-induced hearing loss? *J Speech Lang Hear Res* 2011;54: 679–92.

# Index of Authors

# General Index